Basic Immunology

Immune Mechanisms in Health and Disease

Stewart Sell, M.D.

Professor and Chairman
Department of Pathology and Laboratory Medicine
Medical School
University of Texas Health Science Center at Houston

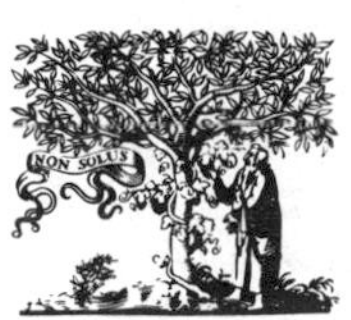

Elsevier
New York • Amsterdam • London

No responsibility is assumed by the Publisher for any injury and/or damage to persons or property as a matter of products liability, negligence or otherwise, or from any use or operation of any methods, products, instructions, or ideas contained in the material herein. Because of rapid advances in the medical sciences, the Publisher recommends that independent verification of diagnosis and drug dosages should be made.

Elsevier Science Publishing Company, Inc.
52 Vanderbilt Avenue, New York, New York 10017

Sole distributors outside the United States and Canada:
Elsevier Applied Science Publishers Ltd.
Crown House, Linton Road, Barking, Essex IG11 8JU, England

Library of Congress Cataloging-in-Publication Data

Sell, Stewart, 1935–

Basic immunology: immune mechanisms in health and disease.

Includes bibliographies and index.
1. Immunology. I. Title
QR181.S387 1987 616.07′9 86-32990
ISBN 0-444-01138-2

Current printing (last digit)
10 9 8 7 6 5 4 3 2

Manufactured in the United States of America

To the late Jose Sala-Trepat—
one of the best scientists and kindest people I have known

Contents

Preface

Since World War II understanding of immunology has grown from a description of phenomena (Arthus reaction, anaphylaxis, delayed hypersensitivity reaction, precipitin reaction, complement fixation, etc.) to a detailed knowledge of the chemistry of antibody and receptor molecules, the structure of the genes for antibodies and receptors, the development and interaction of cells responsible for expression of immunity, and the inflammatory mechanisms that not only provide protection when directed to foreign invaders, but also cause tissue damage (immunopathology). The growth in understanding and knowledge has gone hand in hand with an increased effort that must be made by students to learn the basic principles of immunology required for understanding of immune-mediated diseases.

This text is designed to provide to students of the health and biologic sciences the information needed to understand the present "state of the art" of immunology. It is intended to be an introduction to immunology that will be sufficient to undertake study of the role of immunology in human physiology and disease. *Basic Immunology: Immune Mechanisms in Health and Disease* comprises the first of three sections of a larger book entitled *Immunology, Immunopathology, and Immunity,* which addresses the role of immunology in protective and destructive reactions in humans. The present text covers the background information of "basic" immunology needed to begin study of "clinical" aspects of immunology. It is not a "preview" or "outline" that covers the subject in a superficial way, but includes sufficient information to give the reader a meaningful introduction to the biologic aspects of immunology.

I would like to thank the following individuals, who read all or parts of the manuscript and made many valuable suggestions for improvement:

Nicholas Cohen
Stanley Cohen
Joseph C. Fantone
Paul M. Knopf
D. Scott Linthicum
Scott Rodkey
Thomas G. Wegmann

A special thanks goes to Ira Birkhower, who provided detailed critiques that led to major improvements in the text, and to Ann Rose for reading, typing, and organizing the rough drafts that were provided.

Basic Immunology

Immune Mechanisms in Health and Disease

1 Introduction to Immunology

The human organism, from the time of conception, must maintain its integrity in the face of a changing and often threatening environment. Our bodies have many physiological mechanisms that permit us to adjust to basic variables such as temperature, supply of food and water, and physical injury. In addition, we must defend ourselves against invasion and colonization by foreign organisms. This defensive ability is called *immunity.*

Immunity

Immunity comes from the Latin word *immunitas* and means "protection from." In legal terms, immunity means that an immune person is not subject to certain laws (e.g., diplomatic immunity) or is exempt from certain duties (e.g., not required to serve in the armed forces). In medical terms immunity means protection from certain diseases, particularly infectious disease. For instance, the commonly used statement "She is immune to measles" implies that the person indicated has had measles once and will not get measles again. Immunology (*-ology,* study of) is the study of immunity.

The protective mechanisms of the body may be divided into two major groups: innate and adaptive (Table 1-1). Innate

Table 1-1. Comparison of Innate and Adaptive Immunity

Characteristic	Innate Resistance	Adaptive Resistance
Specificity	Nonspecific, indiscriminate	Specific, discriminating
Mechanical	Epithelium	Immune induced reactive fibrosis (granuloma)
Humoral	pH, lysozyme, serum proteins	Antibody
Cellular	White blood cells	Specifically sensitized lymphocytes
Induction	Does not require immunization; constitutive	Requires immunization

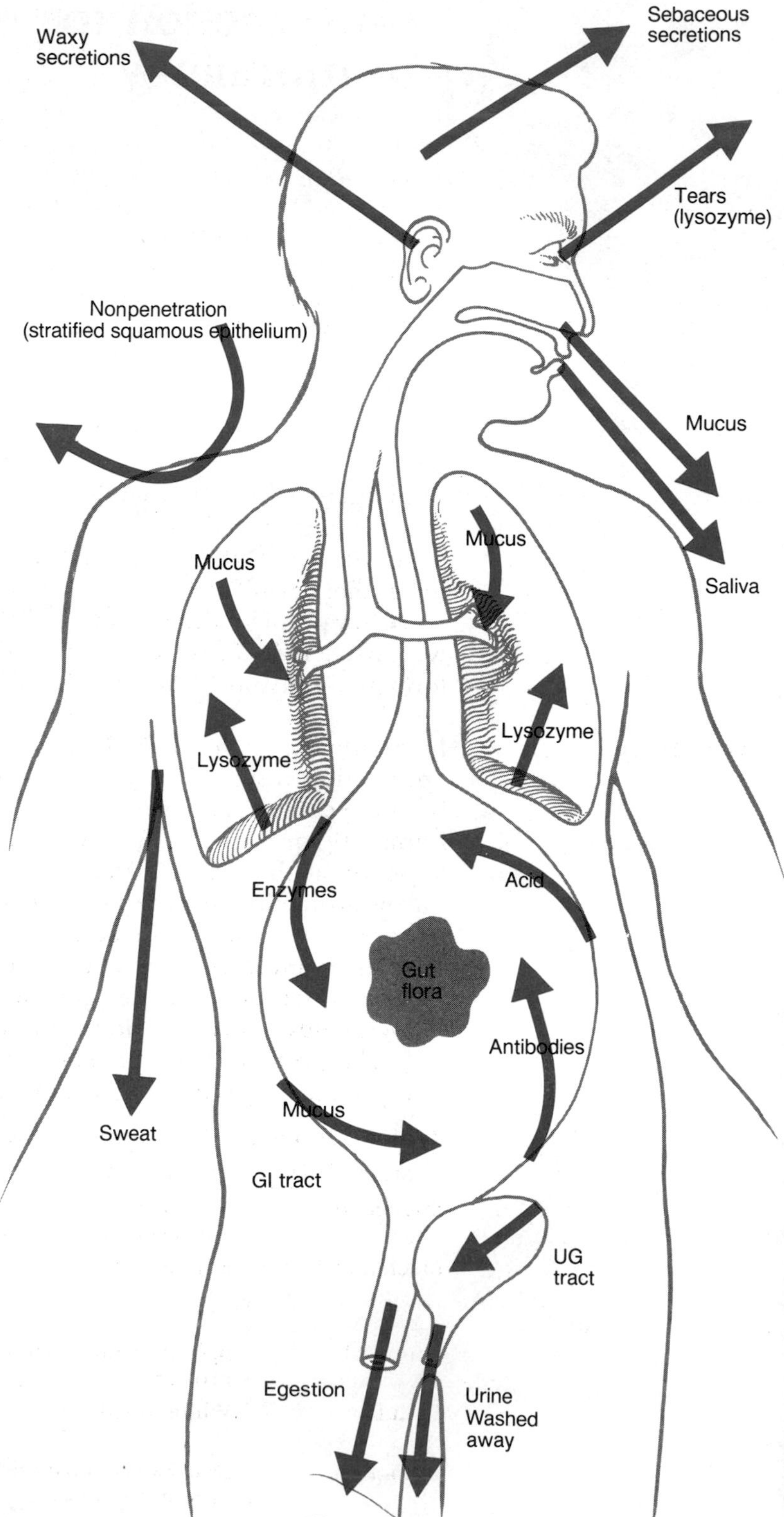

Figure 1-1. Innate immune mechanisms.

resistance is present in all normal individuals and operates on different infectious agents in the same way every time the individual is exposed to the agent. The adaptive, specific immune defense system is not actively present in all individuals. It requires stimulation or *immunization* to become activated, and is mediated by products that specifically recognize one organism and do not act on other organisms. In an infectious disease, such as measles, the adaptive immune system is activated during the first infection, so that upon subsequent contact with the same infectious agent no disease will occur. The immune system has learned to recognize the agent previously contacted and react specifically to it with an accelerated response. This is termed *immune memory*.

Innate Resistance

Innate defense mechanisms against foreign invaders include mechanical barriers, secreted products, and inflammatory cells (Fig. 1-1). Innate resistance is present at all times in normal individuals, modulated by physiological conditions (nutrition, age, hormones, etc.); does not distinguish among microorganisms of different species; and does not alter in intensity upon reexposure. One of the major nonspecific defense systems is the epithelial surface of the body. Externally the skin, and internally the mucous membrane linings of the gastrointestinal tract and the epithelium of the airways of the lung, provide mechanical barriers to invasion. Secreted products such as acid in the stomach, lysozyme in tears, sebaceous gland secretions, and certain proteins in the blood are toxic to potential invaders. White cells of the blood (macrophages and polymorphonuclear leukocytes) are attracted to sites of infection by products of infecting organisms or necrotic tissue and attack the invaders.

The protective epithelial barriers are frequently breached (as by a cut or abrasion of the skin or by penetration of invading organisms past the protective lining of the airways in the lung). Once organisms get through the innate defensive mechanisms and begin to grow in the tissues of the body, a more specific and more powerful backup defense system is needed. Since most infectious organisms can multiply rapidly and the defensive mechanisms in tissues must be directed specifically to the infection and not host tissue, this system must be activated quickly, be effective against relatively large numbers of organisms, and be able to react specifically with the infectious agent. This backup is provided by the adaptive immune system.

Adaptive Resistance

The adaptive immune system is quiescent until stimulated by a specific infection (*immunizing event*); it is capable of exquisitely distinguishing among microorganisms and significantly alters in its intensity and response time upon reexposure. Thus, in normal individuals, the adaptive immune system contains the potential to be activated. This potential is converted to actuality by one of two major arms of the immune response: specific antibodies (*humoral immunity*) or specifically sensitized white blood cells (*cellular immunity*). The cells responsible for antibody production are in the B lymphocyte series, those for cellular immunity in the T lymphocyte series (Table 1-2). Antibodies

Table 1-2. Two Major Arms of Immunity

	Humoral	Cellular
Cell line	B cells, plasma cells	T cells
Product	Antibody	Sensitized cells
Protection against	Bacteria	Viruses, mycobacteria, fungi

are protein molecules that react specifically with structures (*antigens*) on infecting organisms through specialized receptors (*binding sites*) on the antibody molecule. Specifically sensitized T cells also have an antibody-like receptor that recognizes antigens. Antibodies belong to a family of molecules found in the blood or external secretions, termed *immunoglobulins.* Antibodies and sensitized cells are made in response to specific stimulation after contact with an immunizing agent (*immunogen*). They are manufactured by specialized organs in the body (the *lymphoid system*) and released into the blood, which allows rapid delivery to other parts of the body.

Immunization (or vaccination) is the process of stimulating adaptive resistance; once induced, a discrete *state of immunity* exists. The response of the immune system to immunization has been compared to a motor neuron reflex arc, in that it has an afferent, an efferent, and a central limb (Fig. 1-2). *Afferent* refers to delivery of the immunogen to cells of the

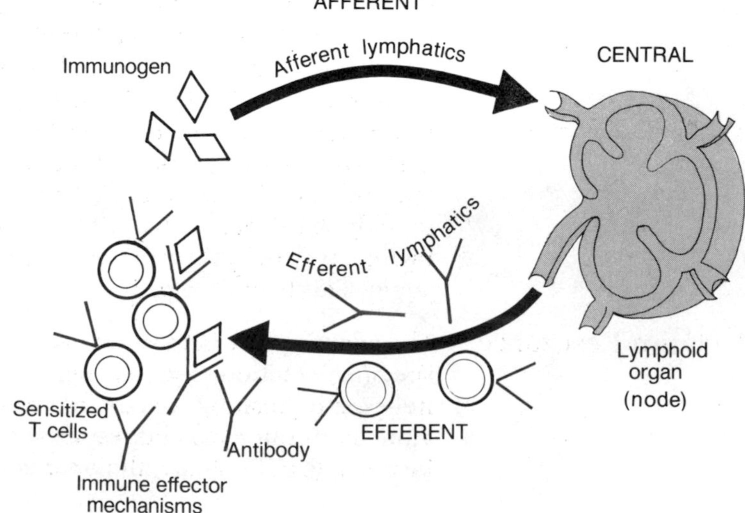

Figure 1-2. Afferent, central, and efferent limbs of the immune response. Afferent: delivery of immunogen to lymphoid organ (lymph node). Central: recognition of antigen by cells of the immune system and production of specifically sensitized cells and humoral antibody. Efferent: delivery of immune products to site of antigen localization and activation of immune effector mechanisms.

immune system; *central* to the response of the reacting organs, resulting in production of antibody and sensitized cells; *efferent* to the delivery of these products to the site of antigen deposition and activation of immune defense mechanisms. Once immunization has occurred, the immunized individual will respond with a more rapid and more intense response upon second exposure to the same immunogen.

The infectious invaders of our bodies have many ways of evading both the innate and the adaptive resistance. These include such properties as the release of *toxins,* the formation of protective coatings, the ability to localize in inaccessible sites, and the ability to exist within our own cells or even be incorporated into our DNA and thus evade recognition or destruction. Important properties for the effectiveness of the adaptive immune system are listed in Table 1-3.

Table 1-3. Functional Abilities of the Adaptive Immune System

1. *Recognition* of many different foreign invaders specifically
2. *Rapid synthesis* of immune products upon contact with invaders
3. *Delivery* of the immune products quickly to the site of infection
4. *Diversity* of effector defensive mechanisms to combat infectious agents with different properties
5. *Direction* of the defensive mechanisms specifically to foreign invaders rather than one's own tissue
6. *Deactivation* mechanisms to turn off the system when the invader has been cleared

Inflammatory Response

The response of our bodies to an infection occurs in the form of *inflammation.* The hallmark of an inflammatory response is the passage of proteins, fluid, and cells from the blood into focal areas in tissues. The result is the local delivery of agents that can effectively combat infections. During an inflammatory response, components of the innate and adaptive resistance mechanisms are shared. These include *inflammatory cells,* products of inflammatory cells, certain blood proteins *(inflammatory mediators),* and common pathways of response (see Chapter 12).

Initiation of an inflammatory response begins with increasing blood flow to infected tissues and with the opening of the cells lining the blood vessels or capillaries (Fig. 1-3). This allows fluid and/or cells to enter into the tissues. The manifestations of acute inflammation were first clearly described by Celsus about 25 BC. The cardinal signs of inflammation (Table 1-4) are manifestations of the increased blood flow and infiltration of tissues by inflammatory proteins and cells. Increased blood flow causes redness and increased temperature. The presence of fluid and red blood cells in tissues is grossly recognized by swelling (edema) and redness. White blood cell (inflammatory cell) infiltrations cause a white color. If the site of

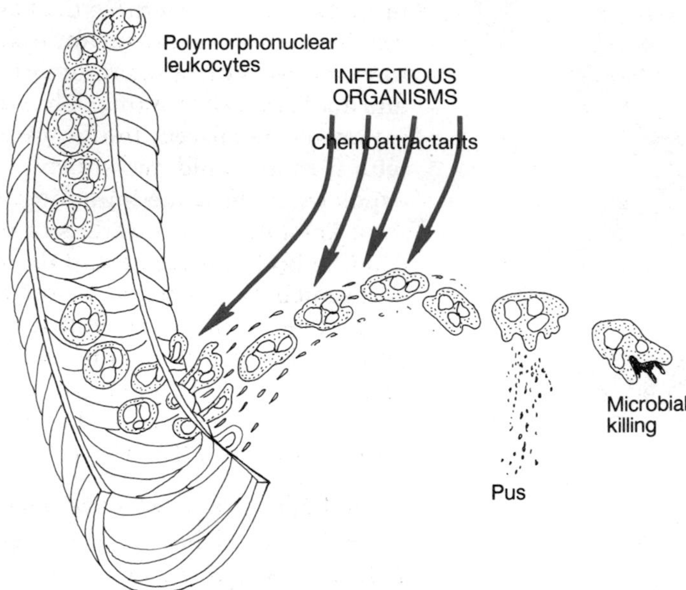

Figure 1-3. Acute inflammatory response to infection. Infectious organisms release chemicals or initiate tissue damage, which produces substances that are chemotactic toward (attract) inflammatory cells (polymorphonuclear leukocytes) and cause constriction of vascular endothelial cells. This results in release of fluid into the tissue (edema) and/or infiltration of tissue with inflammatory cells. Polymorphonuclear leukocytes may ingest and kill the infecting organisms or may release proteolytic enzymes into tissue, causing necrosis and formation of pus. Antibody serves to enhance this response and direct the inflammatory cells by reacting with the infecting organisms and activating bloodborne inflammatory mediators brought into the tissue during edema formation. These mediators react with cell surface receptors on the inflammatory cells and enhance the ability of the cells to ingest (phagocytose) the organisms.

inflammation is necrotic and filled with white cells, the inflammatory site will be seen as pus. If red blood cells are present, the pus may be yellow or bloody red depending on the proportion of red cells. The cellular evolution of an inflammatory response eventually results in the healing or scarring of the lesion. The inflammatory process is presented in detail in Chapter 12.

Table 1-4. The Four Cardinal Signs of Acute Inflammation: Celsus (25 BC)[a]

Rubor	Redness
Tumor	Swelling
Calor	Heat
Dolor	Pain

[a] The fifth classic sign of acute inflammation, *functio laesa* (loss of function), was added by Virchow (1821–1902).

Evolution of Immunity (Phylogeny)

Adaptation to the environment is the driving force in the evolution and survival of a species. Organisms must not only accommodate to changes in temperature, pH, nutrients, oxygen, and water, but also be able to defend against potentially fatal effects of other organisms. The most primitive defense system is the ability to recognize that something is foreign (nonself). This capacity may have evolved from the primitive alimentation function of phagocytosis, the ingestion of material by a cell. That is, protozoa are able to recognize other protozoa as different because of different enzymes in different species and can defend themselves by phagocytosis. In this process they are able to differentiate foreign from self (same species).

Invertebrate

A simplified phylogenetic tree as related to evolution of immune functions in invertebrates is presented in Figure 1-4. The ability to identify foreign species and strains is present in each species. Specific immunoglobulin antibody and T and B cell lymphocyte differentiation are not seen in invertebrates. The ability to recognize tissue of different species (histocompatibility differences) clearly exists in sponges. Identical pairs will fuse when mixed, whereas foreign pairs show a cytotoxic (necrotic) rejection response at their interface. The strength of rejection depends on the degree of genetic difference. A more rapid and extensive rejection occurs when two allogenic (different) species are put together a second time (secondary response or immune memory). In higher organisms this phenomenon is tested by whether or not an individual will accept a graft of tissue from another individual (graft rejection implies recognition of foreign tissue). In coral the extent of parabiotic incompatibility suggests that each clone of coral is different. This principle of the uniqueness of the individual also applies to humans (see Chapter 9).

White blood cell differentiation appears first in echinoderms and protochordates (for a description of white blood cells, see Chapter 2). In the coelomic cavity of earthworms are primitive white blood cell types that combine features of polymorphonuclear cells and lymphocytes. These cells appear to be responsible for graft rejection in these species, and some appear to respond to mitogen stimulation. Protochordates contain nodules of lymphatic cells and circulating lymphocytes that respond to stimulation. Lymphocyte-like cells also infiltrate grafts of sea urchins. Humoral factors also appear in earthworms, and hemolysins (which cause lysis of red blood cells) and hemagglutinins (which cause agglutination of red blood cells) are found in starfish and shellfish. However, these are not immunoglobulins and are not antigen specific. Tunicates express both cellular and humoral immune factors, including some differentiation of lymphocytes. Immune

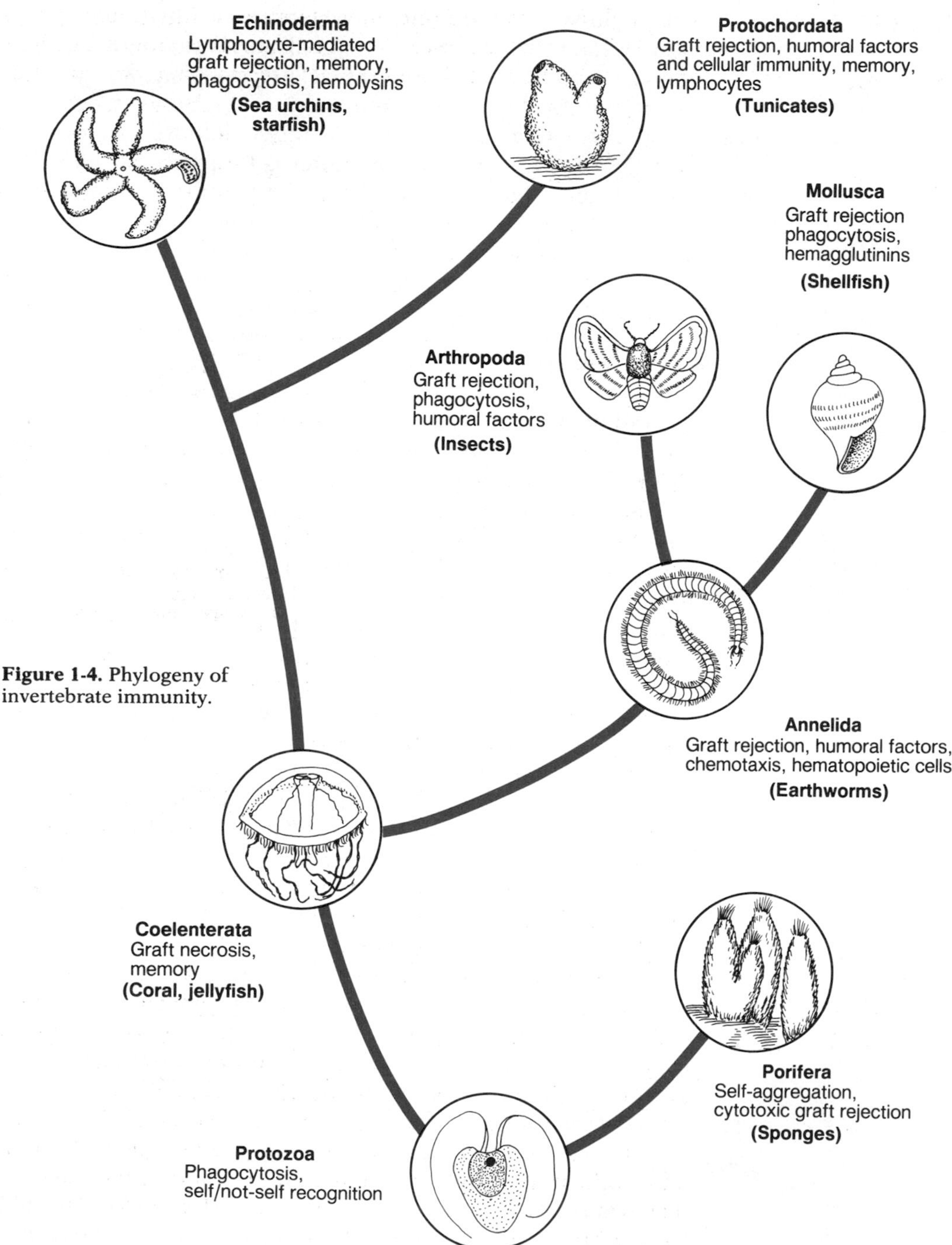

Figure 1-4. Phylogeny of invertebrate immunity.

memory, expressed as a shorter time to induce necrosis in grafts of different strains upon second exposure, is seen in coral. Cellular immune responses appear to precede the development of humoral responses during evolution.

Vertebrate

The phylogeny of immunity in vertebrates is illustrated in Figure 1-5. The immune system in vertebrates is characterized by a true two-component (T and B cell) system, specific immuno-

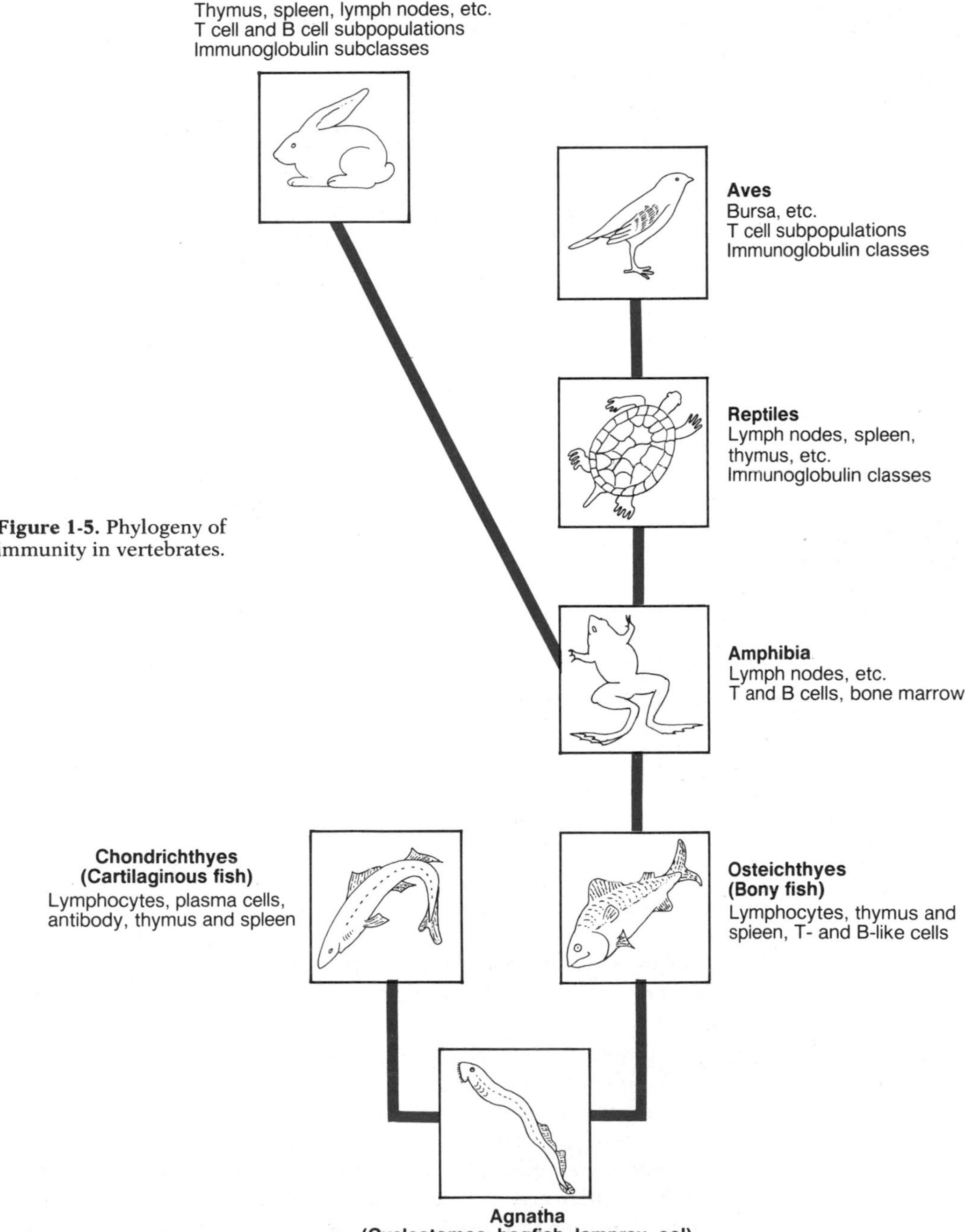

Figure 1-5. Phylogeny of immunity in vertebrates.

globulin antibody production, highly developed specific cellular immunity, and specific immune memory. T- and B-like cells exist in teleost fishes but are not clearly defined in agnatha, although a primitive T cell response can be demonstrated. Table 1-5 outlines the evolution of lymphoid organs in vertebrates (for a description of lymphoid organs see Chapter 3).

Table 1-5. Phylogeny of the Immune System from Primitive Fishes to Mammals

Class or Group	Thymus	Bone Marrow	Lymph Glands or Nodes	Blood Granulocytes and Lymphocytes	Reactions to Primary Tissue Allografts (Cell-Mediated Immunity[a])	
					Moderate	Strong
Hagfish and lampreys	0	0	0	+	+	0
Sharks and rays	+	0	0	+	+	0
Bony fishes	+	+	0	+	+	+
Amphibians	+	+	+	+	+	+
Reptiles	+	+	+	+	+	0
Birds	+	+	+	+	+	+
Mammals	+	+	+	+	+	+

+ indicates presence of corresponding types of cells or reactivity.

[a] Moderate histocompatibility barriers are found in animals representing all vertebrate classes, but strong barriers are the rule in advanced bony fishes, anuran amphibians, and most birds and mammals.

From Hildemann WH: "Immunophylogeny," in Hildemann WH (ed): *Frontiers in Immunogenetics*, Elsevier, 1981.

Agnatha demonstrate diffuse lymphoid tissue in the gut but do not have other lymphoid organs. Thymus and spleen appear in fishes, and lymph nodes in amphibians.

Clearly defined T and B cells are first seen in amphibians. Reptiles have demonstrable T regulatory cells, cells with surface immunoglobulin, and lymphoid organs that resemble those of mammals. Most amphibians do not have graft rejection, but some have graft rejection reactions that are slow and chronic compared with those of reptiles, birds, and mammals. The evolutionary trend from slow to fast graft rejection may reflect expression of histocompatibility antigens rather than a weakness in the immune reaction.

Epithelium and Lymphoid Organ Evolution

Associations of epithelial tissue and lymphoid tissue in some lymphoid organs appear to be of critical importance in the development of the mammalian immune system. In order to make survival on land possible, changes in the gill pouches and cloacal bursa of amphibians had to evolve in birds and mammals. In primitive coelenterates the coelomic cavity serves not only to absorb nutrients, but also to absorb oxygen. To perform this function, gills evolved in the neck (foregut) of fishes and the hindgut of mollusks and arthropods. During embryogenesis of higher vertebrates the five paired gill pouches cease absorbing oxygen and develop to supply epithelium for cervical organs. The five gill pouches in fish become vestigial in amphibia, but the epithelial tissue of the third pharyngeal pouch provides the stroma of the medulla of the thymus. This epithelial stroma produces thymic hormones essential for the maturation of thymocytes (see Chapter 3). The hindgut gills evolve into the cloaca in turtles and further into the cloacal bursa of Fabricius in birds. The bursa of Fabricius is essential for the development of the B cell system in birds. In mammalia, there is evidence that the gastrointestinal associated lymphoid tissue (GALT) plays an important role in the development of the B cell system.

In Summary

1. Some form of recognition of self and nonself is present in the simplest animal species.
2. Cellular immunity precedes humoral immunity in evolution.
3. A bifunctional (T and B cell) system with developed lymphoid organs is the most recent immunological development.
4. Epithelium that evolves from the gills of fishes (i.e., pharyngeal pouches) plays a major role in the development of the lymphoid organs of mammals (thymus and GALT).

Selective pressures during evolution are believed to have resulted in the development of protective immune mechanisms. Primitive immune mechanisms may have had a number of other functions in lower organisms, such as recognition of cell surface markers required for aggregation of cell types in the early stages of development of multicellular structures (recognition of self and nonself). Immune recognition mechanisms may be variants of the cell–cell interactions that occur during embryologic development. It is likely that the immune system, as we now see it, is expanding and being modified to perform even other new functions such as regulation of neuroendocrine or hormonally expressive cells.

Immunopathology, the Double-Edged Sword

The evolution of the immune system did not occur without flaws. This same system that functions so well to protect against foreign invaders may also be turned against us. The term *immunopathology* incorporates a double meaning: *immune* means protected or exempt; *pathology* is the study of disease. Thus immunopathology literally means the study of the protection from disease, but in usage it actually means the study of how immune mechanisms cause diseases. Immunity is a double-edged sword: on the one hand immune responses protect us from infections; on the other hand, immune mechanisms may cause disease. The most compelling evidence that immune reactions are protective is provided by the naturally occurring immune deficiency diseases of man. Individuals with an inability to mount an effective immune response to infectious agents invariably succumb to infections unless vigorously treated. However, immune reactions may also cause disease. The terms *allergy* and *hypersensitivity* are used to denote deleterious immune reactions. *Allergy* is frequently used for a particular type of reaction *(anaphylactic)*, and *hypersensitivity* for delayed or cell-mediated immune reactivity. The term *immunity* was once restricted to the protective effects of immune reactions but, by common usage, this is no longer the case. In some diseases immune mechanisms may actually be directed against our own tissues. This is termed *autoimmunity*.

History of Immunology and Immunopathology

A short history of immunology is given in Table 1-6. Recognition of adaptive immunity occurred in the ancient societies of China and Egypt. Application of this phenomenon by introduction of smallpox organisms into lesions scratched on the skin—"variolation"—or by their inhalation into the nasal cavity was practiced by the Chinese about AD 1000, and artificial vaccination was introduced in England in 1798. In the late 1800s and early 1900s many immune-mediated phenomena were described. The cellular immune system was emphasized by Metchnikoff and the humoral system by von Behring. Modern immunology can be said to have begun in the late 1950s with the recognition of histocompatibility antigens, identification of structure of antibodies, and study of immune mechanisms that cause disease. Today studies in immunology are revealing the nature of the different cell types involved in immune responses, how cellular receptors are made, how immune cells are activated, and the nature and expression of the genetic information required for specific immune recognition.

Summary

Higher organisms have evolved effective defense systems to protect themselves against foreign invaders. One system is constitutive and consists of mechanical barriers, pH, temperature, phagocytosis, and nonspecific inflammation (innate resistance). The other is induced and consists of specific products that recognize invaders as foreign (adaptive immunity). After induction (immunization) the adaptive system responds more rapidly and with greater intensity than after first exposure (immune memory). The two major arms of the adaptive immune response are humoral (antibody) and cellular (specifically sensitized cells). Cells of the body known as lymphocytes are responsible for the adaptive immune response (T lymphocytes for cellular immunity and B lymphocytes for humoral immunity). In response to infection both adaptive and innate inflammatory mechanisms may be activated.

During evolution the adaptive immune response has become increasingly complex. Humans have different classes of antibody and different subsets of T cells that have different functions as immune effectors.

Table 1-6. A Short History of Immunology

Fever	Mesopotamia	3000 BC
Recognition of adaptive immunity	Egypt, China	2000 BC
Anatomic identification of organs	Hippocrates	400 BC
Acquired resistance to poisons	Mithridates Eupator, King of Pontus	80 BC
Four cardinal signs of inflammation	Celsus	AD 25
"Snuff" variolation for smallpox	Sung Dynasty, China	1000
Renaissance of anatomy	Vesalius	1540
Bursa of birds described	Fabricius	1590
Peyer's patch	Peyer	1690
Cowpox vaccination	Jenner	1798
Tuberculous granulomas	Rokitansky	1855
Langhans' giant cell	Langhans	1868
Waldeyer's ring	Waldeyer	1870
Cellular pathology	Virchow	1880
Attenuated vaccines	Pasteur	1880
Phagocytosis	Metchnikoff	1882
Neutralization (antitoxin)	von Behring	1890
Delayed hypersensitivity skin test	Koch	1890
Bacteriolysis (antibody and complement)	Bordet	1894
Blood groups	Landsteiner	1900
Side-chain theory, tumor immunity, horror autotoxicus	Ehrlich	1900
Anaphylaxis	Richet and Portier	1902
Arthus' phenomenon	Arthus	1903
Serum sickness	von Pirquet and Schick	1905
Organ transplantation	Carrel and Guthrie	1905
Delayed hypersensitivity to viruses	von Pirquet	1906
Immune surveillance of cancer	Ehrlich	1909
Viral cancer immunity	Peyton Rous	1910
Passive cutaneous anaphylaxis	Prausnitz and Kustner	1921
Chemical mediators of inflammation	Lewis	1925
Quantitative precipitin reaction	Heidelberger	1935
Gamma globulin	Tiselius and Kabat	1938
Hemolytic disease of newborn (Rh)	Levine	1941
Immunofluorescence	Coons	1942
Concept of collagen disease	Klemperer	1942
Immune tolerance	Medawar and Burnet	1944
Mechanism of glomerulonephritis	Dixon	1956
Histocompatibility antigens	Snell, Dausset	1958
Structure of antibodies	Porter, Edelman	1959
Lymphocyte recirculation	Gowans	1959
Mitogenic activation of lymphocytes	Nowell	1961
Function of the thymus	Miller and Good	1961
Classification of immune mechanisms	Gell and Coombs	1962
Lymphocyte surface immunoglobulin and lymphocyte activation	Sell and Gell	1964
Immunoglobulin gene rearrangements	Dreyer and Bennet	1965
Identification of T and B cells	Claman	1966
In vitro primary immune response	Mischell and Dutton	1967
Accessory cell role in immune response	Mosier	1968
Immune response genes	Benacerraf and McDevitt	1969
Idiotype network	Jerne	1974
Hybridoma (monoclonal antibodies)	Kohler and Milstein	1975
T cell receptor	Allison, Kappler, et al	1982
T cell receptor gene	Hedrick, Davis	1984

The immune response is not always protective; in many instances the same immune effector mechanisms that defend against foreign invaders may be turned against us and produce disease (the double-edged sword of immunopathology). In the following chapters the immune response is described.

General References

Periodicals

Advances in Immunology, Academic Press, New York.

Annual Review of Immunology, Annual Reviews Inc., Palo Alto, Calif.

Comprehensive Immunology, Plenum, New York.

Progress in Allergy, Karger, Basel, Switzerland.

Immunological Reviews, Munksgard, Copenhagen.

Immunology Today, Elsevier, Amsterdam.

Basic Immunology Texts

Barrett JT: Textbook of Immunology, 4th ed. St. Louis, Mosby, 1983.

Dale MM, Foreman JC: Textbook of Immunopharmacology. London, Blackwell, 1984.

Eisen H: Immunology, 2nd ed. Hagerstown, Md., Harper & Row, 1980.

Golub ES: The Cellular Basis of the Immune Response, 2nd ed. Sunderland, Mass., Sinauer Assocs., 1981.

Hildemann WH: Fundamentals of Immunology. New York, Elsevier, 1984.

Hood L, Weissman IL, Wood WB, Wilson JH: Immunology, 2nd ed. Menlo Park, Calif., Benjamin Cummings, 1984.

Humphrey SH, White RG: Immunology for Students of Medicine, 3rd ed. Oxford, Blackwell, 1970.

McConnel I, Munro A, Waldemann H: The Immune System, 2nd ed. Oxford, Blackwell, 1981.

Roitt I: Essential Immunology, 5th ed. Oxford, Blackwell, 1984.

Stites DP, Stobo JD, Fudenberg HH, Wells JV: Basic and Clinical Immunology, 5th ed. Los Altos, Calif., Lange, 1985.

Clinical Immunology Texts

Holborow EJ, Reeves WG: Immunology in Medicine. London, Academic Press, 1977.

Lachmann PJ, Peters DK: Clinical Aspects of Immunology, 4th ed. Oxford, Blackwell, 1982.

Miescher PA, Muller-Eberhard HJ: Textbook of Immunopathology, 2nd ed. New York, Grune & Stratton, 1976.

Sampter M: Immunological Diseases, 2nd ed. Boston, Little, Brown, 1965.

Historical

Haggard HW: Mystery, Magic and Medicine. Garden City, N.Y., Doubleday, Doran and Co., 1933.

Kabat EA: Structural Concepts in Immunology and Immunochemistry. New York, Holt, Rinehart & Winston, 1968.

Landsteiner K: The Specificity of Serological Reactions. New York, Dover, 1962.

Long ER: A History of Pathology. New York, Dover, 1965.

Majno G: The Healing Hand. Cambridge, Mass., Harvard University Press, 1975.

Silverstein AM: History of immunology: a history of theories of antibody formation. Cell Immunol 91:263–283, 1985.

Phylogeny of Immunity

Cohen N: Phylogeny of lymphocyte structure and function. Am Zool 15:119–133, 1975.

Goetz D (ed): Evolution and function of the major histocompatibility system. Berlin, Springer-Verlag, 1977.

Hildemann WH (ed): Frontiers in Immunogenetics. New York, Elsevier, 1981.

Hildemann WH, Clark EA, Raison RL: Comprehensive Immunogenetics. New York, Elsevier, 1981.

2 The Immune System I: Cells and Vessels

The organs of our bodies that provide the products (proteins and cells) of immunity make up the *lymphoid system*. The lymphoid system is a complex network of lymphatic vessels, lymphoid nodules, lymph nodes, tonsils, spleen, and other organs (Fig. 2-1). The cells and vessels of the lymphoid system are described in this chapter; the lymphoid organs and their development are the subjects of Chapters 3 and 4.

Cells of the Immune System

The major constituents of the immune system are lymphocytes. However, other cells (macrophages) are also involved in induction of immune responses, and other white blood cell types such as macrophages and polymorphonuclear leukocytes take an active part in various parts of inflammatory responses associated with immune reactions (Fig. 2-1). The term *white blood cell (leukocyte)* is applied because when unclotted blood is allowed to stand, these cells sediment in a thin, white layer between the denser erythrocytes (red blood cells) and the plasma. This layer of white cells is called the *buffy coat*. The mature forms of these cells are most easily recognized in peripheral blood smears. The basic structure and function of white blood cells are now described; their role in immune responses and inflammation is presented in more detail in the following chapters.

Blood Cells

In smears of peripheral blood stained with Wright's stain, *erythrocytes* are small and light pink and have no nuclei. Because erythrocytes are by far the most numerous cells in blood smears, it is the percentage of nonerythroid cells (white blood cells) that is normally counted.

White Blood Cells (Leukocytes)

The terms used by pathologists, immunologists, and hematologists for the different white blood cells reflect different ways of looking at complex cell populations. A simple classification is presented in Figure 2-2.

Cell Type	% of White Blood Cells in Blood	Diameter (μm)	Nucleus	Cytoplasm and Granules	Drawings
Erythrocytes	—	7.5	None	Pink, homogeneous cytoplasm	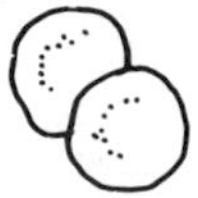
LEUKOCYTES					
Polymorphonuclear					
Neutrophils	50–70	10–12	2–5 lobules connected by thin bridges, coarse chromatin	Abundant cytoplasm/fine pinkish granules	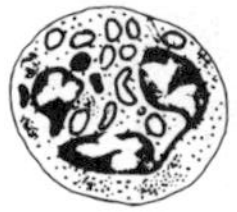
Eosinophils	1–3	10–12	Usually two oval lobes connected by bridge	Abundant cytoplasm/coarse reflective granules stained red	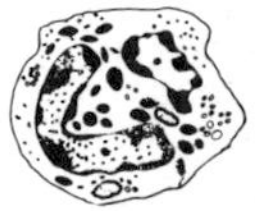
Basophils	<1	8–10	Bent in S with two or more constrictions; obscured by cytoplasmic granules	Large and irregular granules stained deep blue	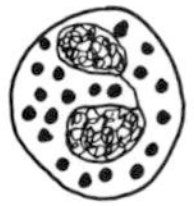
Mononuclear					
Lymphocytes	25–35	6–15	Round to oval; coarse chromatin	Bluish cytoplasm/about 10% of cells fine azurophilic granules	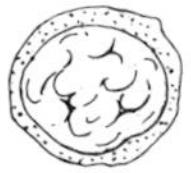
Monocytes	3–7	12–18	Kidney shaped, indented; fine chromatin	Bluish cytoplasm/fine azurophilic granules	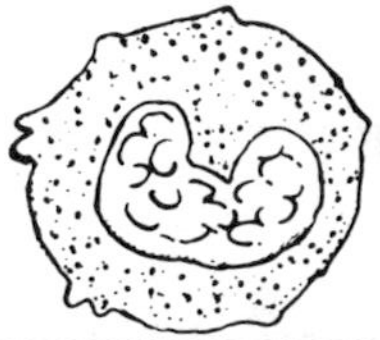

Figure 2-1. Leukocytes. Composite drawing indicating relative size (micrometers) and morphology of cells involved in immune reactions and in nonimmune inflammatory reactions. The erythrocyte is included for size reference, since it is the most easily identified cell in blood smears and in many tissue sections. The drawings illustrate the characteristic appearance of cells in a peripheral blood smear stained with Wright's stain.

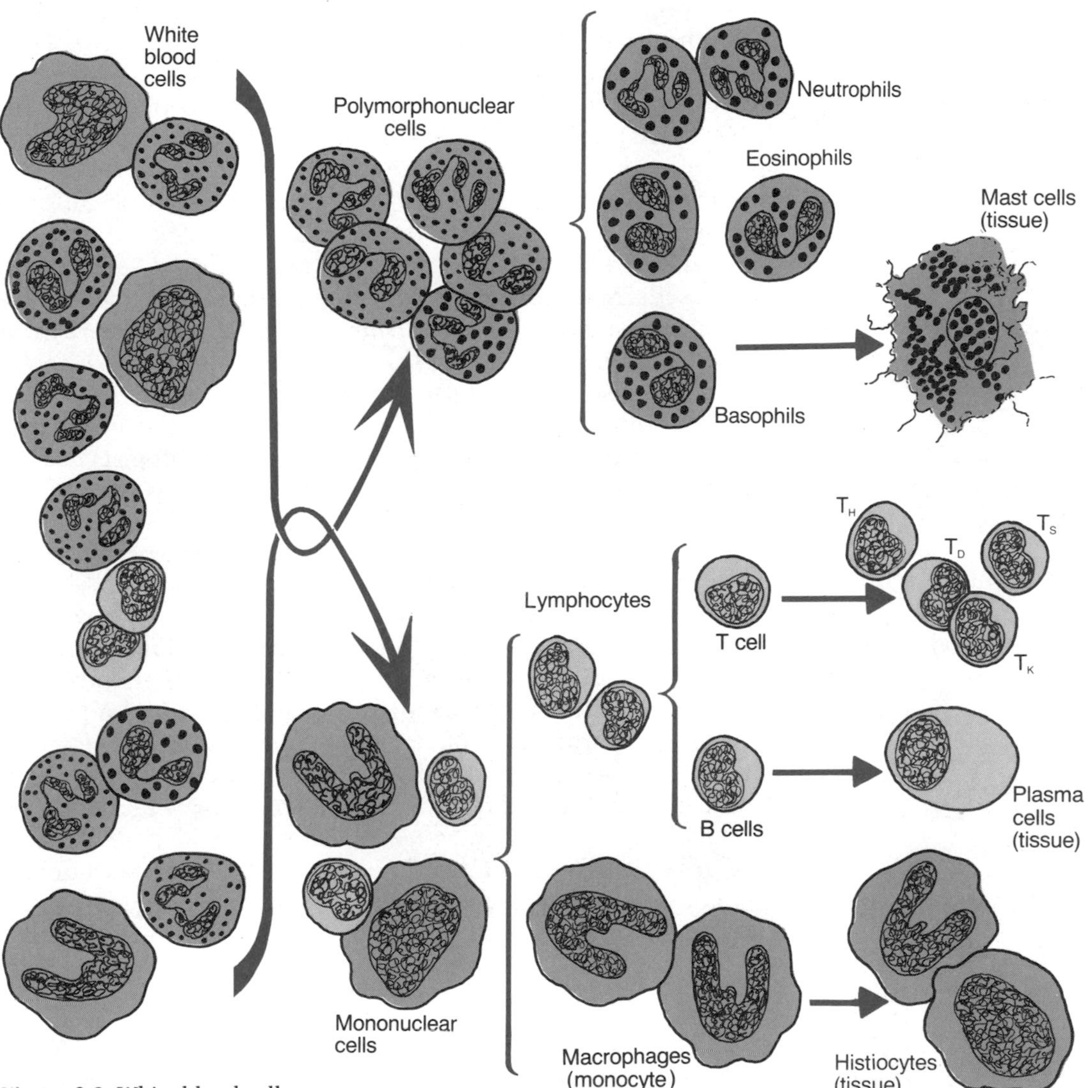

Figure 2-2. White blood cell nomenclature.

White blood cells (WBC) may be divided into two major populations on the basis of the form of their nuclei: single nuclei (*mononuclear* or *"round" cells*) or segmented nuclei *(polymorphonuclear)*. Mononuclear cells are further divided into large *(macrophage* or *monocyte)* and small *(lymphocyte)*. Lymphocytes may be further subdivided into two major populations, *T cells* and *B cells*, on the basis of function and cell surface phenotype (to be described later). B cells are the precursors of the cells that synthesize and secrete humoral antibodies. Subpopulations of T cells are responsible for a number of *cell-mediated* immune activities (see below). T cells and B cells cannot be differentiated on the basis of morphologic appearance, but do have different phenotypic markers. In addition, lymphocytes without distinguishing markers *(null cells)* are present in smaller numbers than T cells or B cells. Some null cells may *kill* certain other cell types in vitro (natural killer (NK) cells), and others may become "armed" by passive absorption of antibody (antibody-dependent cell-mediated cytotoxicity; killer (K) cells). The characteristics of these cells are presented in much more detail in a later chapter.

The large mononuclear cells (macrophages) are phagocytic cells. Macrophages in peripheral blood are termed *monocytes;* in tissues they are called *histiocytes.* Particular care must be taken in understanding *monocytes* and *mononuclear cells.* Hematologists use the term *monocytes* for the larger circulating mononuclear white blood cells found in the peripheral blood that are in the macrophage lineage. Pathologists use the term *mononuclear* or *"round" cells* for lymphocytes and macrophages seen in tissue, to differentiate them from polymorphonuclear cells. These similar terms must be carefully distinguished to avoid confusion.

Polymorphonuclear Leukocytes

Polymorphonuclear white blood cells are subdivided into three major populations on the basis of the staining properties of their cytoplasmic granules in standard hematologic blood smears or tissue preparations: neutrophil—pink, eosinophil—red, basophil—blue. Polymorphonuclear cells take part in both immune specific and nonspecific inflammatory reactions.

Neutrophils. Neutrophils (Fig. 2-3) are polymorphonuclear leukocytes (PMN) whose cytoplasmic granules do not take on strong acidophilic (red) or basophilic (blue) staining with the

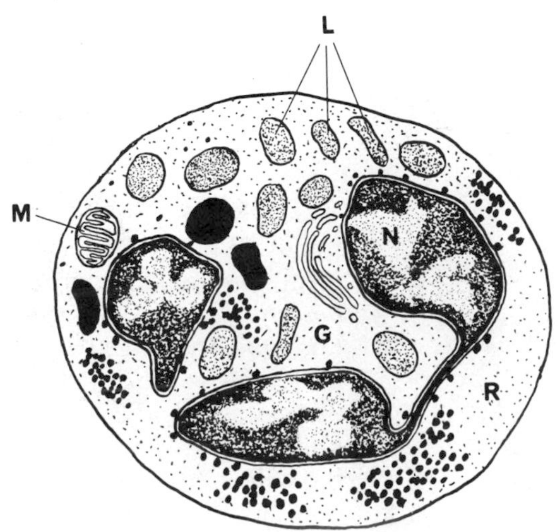

Figure 2-3. Neutrophil. The cytoplasm contains large numbers of membrane-limited bodies (lysosomes) that stain pale pink with the usual staining agents. The nucleus is divided into round or oval lobes connected to one another by thin strands of nuclear material. G, Golgi apparatus; L, lysosomes; M, mitochondrion; N, nucleus; R, ribosomes.

usual dyes used for blood smears, but show only a pale pink coloration. Such cells make up from 50 to 90% of the WBC of the peripheral blood and may be found scattered diffusely in many tissues. Like its relative, the macrophage ("large eater"), the neutrophil is active in phagocytosis and has been named by some a microphage ("small eater"). Neutrophils are rapidly migrating, phagocytic cells that appear in areas of infection or tissue damage. The nucleus of the neutrophil, characteristic of the polymorphonuclear leukocytes, is divided into round or oval lobes connected to one another by thin strands of nuclear material. The other outstanding feature of this type of WBC is the large number of uniform, membrane-limited granules. The granules of the neutrophil contain a wide variety of hydrolytic enzymes and are called primary lysosomes. These enzymes digest phagocytosed organisms. Neutrophils are the first wave of a cellular attack on invading organisms and are the characteristic cells of acute inflammation. The appearance of neutrophils in areas of inflammation may be caused by chemicals released from bacteria or factors produced nonspecifically from necrotic tissue, or may be directed by antibody reacting with antigen. The role of the neutrophil in acute inflammation is taken over by the macrophage in the chronic stage of inflammation (Chapter 12).

Eosinophils. Eosinophils (Fig. 2-4) are similar in appearance to neutrophils, except that they have prominent eosinophilic (red) granules that may contain rodlike crystalloid inclusions as viewed by electron microscopy. These eosinophilic granules are membrane limited and contain large amounts of hydrolytic enzymes, and thus are lysosomes. The granules differ from those of neutrophils in a high content of peroxidase, which is perhaps related to the crystalloid structure. The chemotactic

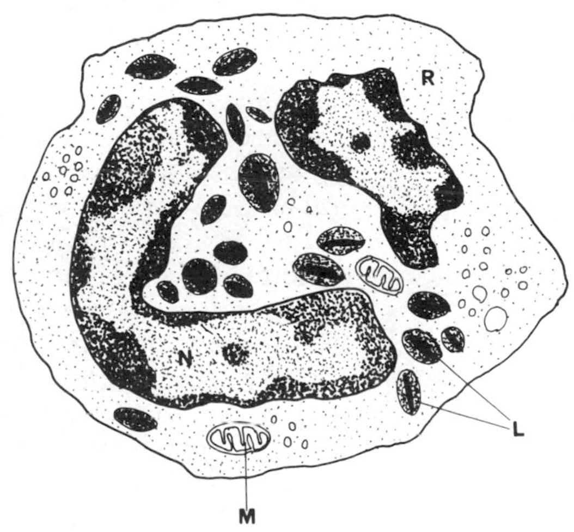

Figure 2-4. Eosinophil. Morphologically the cell resembles the neutrophil, but prominent cytoplasmic membrane-limited bodies (lysosomes) stain red with the usual staining agents and contain rodlike crystalloid structures as observed by electron microscopy. L, lysosomes; M, mitochondria; N, nucleus; R, ribosomes.

responses of the eosinophil are basically identical to those of neutrophils, but eosinophils are found in unusually high numbers around antigen–antibody complexes and parasites in tissues. Eosinophils appear to limit or modulate inflammation. Eosinophils make up from 1% to 3% of the circulating WBC.

Basophils. Basophils have prominent blue-staining cytoplasmic granules. Basophils located in solid tissue are called *mast cells,* and are found in loose (areolar) connective tissue. Blood basophils are rounded in appearance, whereas tissue mast cells may be elongated or irregular in cell outline. Blood basophils make up less than 1% of the peripheral WBC. Mast cell nuclei are round or oval, but circulating basophils have a lobulated form (polymorphonuclear). However, they, like the eosinophil, tend to have bilobed rather than multilobed nuclei. An outstanding feature of basophils is the abundance of oval basophilic (blue) granules with a finely granular or reticular ultrastructure. The predominance of granules overshadows other cytoplasmic structures: mitochondria, endoplasmic reticulum, ribosomes, and a Golgi apparatus. Basophil granules contain heparin, histamine, serotonin (5-hydroxytryptamine), membrane-like material that is metabolized to prostaglandins and leukotrienes, and a battery of hydrolytic enzymes. The presence of these pharmacologically active agents in mast cell granules and the prominence of mast cells in perivascular tissues suggest that the release of such agents would have a marked effect on the smooth muscles of arterioles and the permeability of capillaries. Release of these pharmacologically active agents by mast cells is the mechanism responsible for early inflammatory changes and for the unleashing of anaphylactic or atopic allergic reactions. Mast cell–generated factors also attract neutrophils and eosinophils to inflammatory sites.

Lymphocytes

Lymphocyte is a morphological term that includes a population of cells of similar appearance but with different immune functions. The lymphocyte is a small, round cell found in the peripheral blood, lymph nodes, spleen, thymus, tonsils, and appendix and scattered throughout many other tissues. In smears of peripheral blood, lymphocytes appear slightly larger (7–8 μm) in diameter than red blood cells (erythrocytes) and make up about 30% of the total white blood cell count. A typical lymphocyte has very little cytoplasm and is composed mostly of a circular nucleus with prominent nuclear chromatin (Fig. 2-5). The narrow rim of cytoplasm contains scattered ribosomes as well as a few ribosomal aggregates but, in unstimulated states, is virtually devoid of endoplasmic reticulum or other organelles. Although it was once believed that the lymphocyte was a short-

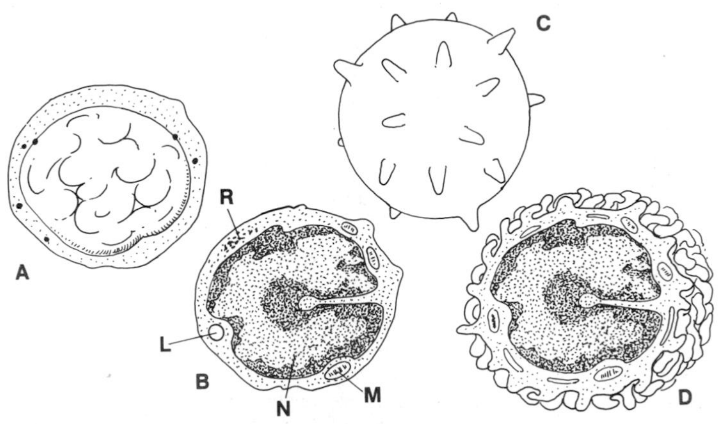

Figure 2-5. Lymphocyte. (a) Blood smear; (b) transmission electron micrograph; (c, d) scanning electron micrographs of two functional states of the lymphocyte surface: smooth (c) and hairy (d). Cell is composed mainly of a nucleus, with a paucity of cytoplasmic elements. A narrow rim of cytoplasm contains scattered ribosomes, a few membrane-limited bodies (lysosomes), and a few mitochondria. L, lysosome; M, mitochondria; N, nucleus; R, ribosomes.

lived "end" cell, it is now known that some populations of lymphocytes may survive for months or even years and recirculate from lymph nodes to lymph and blood.

The lymphocyte is responsible for the primary recognition of antigen and is an immunologically specific effector cell. Lymphocytes produce cell surface molecules that serve as receptor sites for reaction with antigen. The lymphocyte is the carrier of immunologically specific information. *Immunologically competent cell* and *memory cell* are functional terms for specialized cells that are found in immunized individuals and that are not morphologically distinguishable from other lymphocytes. The lymphocytes that interact during the production of circulating antibody have different functional and antigenic properties, but are structurally similar.

T cells. The term T cell is applied to the thymus-derived lymphocyte. T cell precursors (prothymocytes) are produced in the bone marrow and circulate to the thymus. Thymus-derived cells originate in the thymus from these precursor cells, are rereleased into the circulation, and subsequently localize in thymus-dependent areas of the other lymphoid organs. Thymus-derived cells may be identified by specific cell surface markers (see Chapter 4). Approximately 65% to 85% of lymph node cells and 30% to 50% of spleen cells are T cells.

In the human, T cells form *rosettes* with normal sheep erythrocytes (E rosettes). A rosette is composed of a central lymphocyte surrounded by a layer of four or more erythrocytes. B cells do not form rosettes with normal sheep erythrocytes but will form rosettes with sheep cells coated with antibody and complement (EAC) because of receptor sites for the third component of complement. In addition, as stated above, human B lymphocytes contain surface immunoglobulin that is detected by immunofluorescence. These techniques have been used to characterize human lymphoid cell populations. Ninety to one

Table 2-1. Some Properties of T and B Lymphocytes

Properties	T Cells	B Cells
Site of precursor	Thymus	Fetal liver, GI tract, bone marrow
Surface markers	T antigens	Surface Ig
Rosettes	E	EAC
Tissue distribution	Interfollicular (paracortical)	Follicles (cortical)
Percentage of lymphocytes in blood	80	20
Radiation inactivation	+	++++
Mitogen response	Con A, PHA	PPD, LPS
Function	Helper, suppressor, killer	Plasma cell precursor
Mixed lymphocyte reaction	Reactive cell	Stimulator cell

E, sheep erythrocytes; EAC, sheep erythrocytes coated with antibody and complement; GI, gastrointestinal; PHA, phytohemagglutinin; PPD, purified protein derivative; LPS, lipopolysaccharide.

hundred percent of human thymus cells form rosettes with unsensitized sheep red blood cells and no rosettes with EAC. Spleen, peripheral blood, and lymph nodes contain approximately 20% to 30% B cells and 60% to 75% T cells by rosetting analysis (Table 2-1).

T cells may be further divided into subpopulations on the basis of function and other phenotypic markers. Different T cell subpopulations function to help in antibody formation (T helper cells), to kill target cells (T cytotoxic cells), to induce inflammation (T delayed hypersensitivity cells), to inhibit immune responses (T suppressor cells), etc. (see Chapter 10). T lymphocytes activated by antigens produce effector molecules that activate or deactivate other lymphocytes (interleukins), contribute to immune-mediated inflammation (lymphokines), or interact with other cell types (Table 2-2). Not only does the T cell population contain a variety of effector cells, but T cells are also the master regulators of the immune system. As Richard Gershon said, "The T cell is the director of the immunological orchestra." T cells function to turn other cells in the immune system (T suppressors, T helpers, T contrasuppressors, and B cells) off or on.

B cells. B cells arise from precursors in the bone marrow and are the precursors of the cells that synthesize immunoglobulins (plasma cells). B cells contain readily detectable surface immunoglobulin (sIg), whereas T cells do not have surface immunoglobulin. When tissues are tested by fluorescent antiimmunoglobulin sera, 10% to 20% of lymph node cells, 20% to

Table 2-2. Some Factors Produced by Activated Lymphocytes[a]

PRODUCTS AFFECTING OTHER LYMPHOCYTES (INTERLEUKINS)
Helper factors
Growth promoting factors
Differentiating factors
Suppressor factor
Transfer factor
PRODUCTS AFFECTING MACROPHAGES (LYMPHOKINES)
Migration inhibitory factor
Activation factor
Chemotactic factor
PRODUCTS AFFECTING POLYMORPHONUCLEAR LEUKOCYTES (LYMPHOKINES)
Chemotactic factors
Histamine releasing factor
Leukocyte inhibitory factor
PRODUCTS AFFECTING OTHER CELL TYPES (LYMPHOKINES)
Cytotoxic factor
Growth inhibitory factors
Osteoclast activating factor
Interferon
Colony stimulating factor

[a] For more details see Chapters 10 and 13.

35% of spleen cells, and 0% of thymus cells contain surface immunoglobulin. The lymphoid cells in these organs that contain T cell antigen do not have surface immunoglobulin.

B cells develop from stem cells that originate in the fetal bone marrow or liver. The site of B cell differentiation may be in the fetal liver, the gastrointestinal lymphoid tissue, or the peripheral lymph nodes. After antigenic stimulation, B cells differentiate into antibody-secreting plasma cells (see below).

Null Cells. Some lymphocytes do not have detectable surface immunoglobulin or T cell markers. Such cells are termed *null cells* and are active in certain types of lymphocyte-mediated target cell killing (see Chapter 4).

Macrophages

The macrophage ("large eater"), the primary phagocytic cell, is the largest cell in the lymphoid system, ranging from 12 to 15 μm in diameter. Macrophages in the blood are called monocytes; those in tissue are called histiocytes. The macrophage nucleus usually has a bilobed kidney shape with considerable peripheral condensation of nuclear chromatin. The cytoplasm of the macrophage contains a great variety of organelles, including endoplasmic reticulum, a Golgi complex, mitochondria, free and aggregated ribosomes, and various membrane-limited phagocytic vacuoles (lysosomes, dense bodies, myelin figures, microbodies) (Fig. 2-6). The tissue macrophage

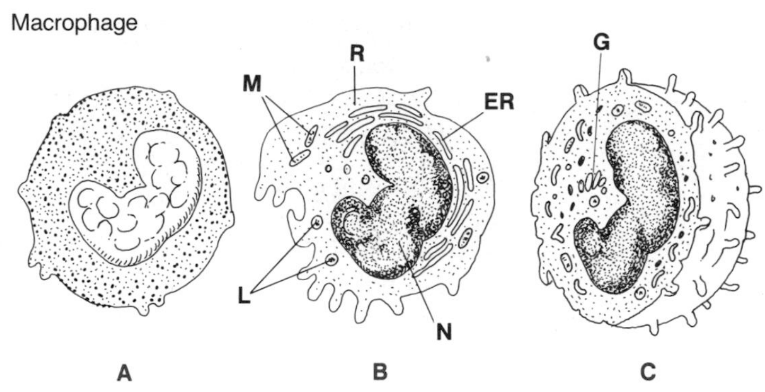

Figure 2-6. Macrophage. (a) Blood smear (monocyte); (b) transmission electron micrograph; (c) scanning electron micrograph. Large nucleus is centrally located and bilobed or kidney shaped. Cytoplasm is extensive and contains a wide variety of organelles. ER, endoplasmic reticulum; G, Golgi apparatus; L, lysosomes; M, mitochondria; N, nucleus; R, ribosomes.

or histiocyte is larger (15 – 18 μm) and may contain many more cytoplasmic vacuoles than do blood monocytes. Macrophages invade sites of inflammation after polymorphonuclear cells and serve to clear the site of necrotic debris. The digestive capacity of the macrophage is more effective than that of the polymorphonuclear cell. It appears that PMN get in quickly ("attack troops") to act on infecting organisms, but macrophages are needed to finish the job ("mop-up troops").

Role of Macrophages in the Immune Response. The uptake of antigens by macrophages is the first step in the processing of antigen leading to the production of circulating antibody. In such cases, antigen is not completely degraded by the macrophage but becomes bound to macrophage RNA or membrane. The macrophage is not the cell that recognizes antigen as foreign, but the macrophage nonspecifically processes the antigen so that it may be recognized by specific antigen reactive cells. Processed antigens are expressed on the surface of antigen-presenting macrophages in conjunction with self surface markers (class II major histocompatibility markers) that are recognized by T cell receptors for antigen and for self class II MHC. Further definitions of the role of the macrophage in the induction of immunity are discussed in Chapter 10.

The macrophage also plays a prominent role in the later stages of the inflammatory response and may accumulate in large numbers in sites of inflammation. The migration of macrophages (both blood and tissue) into inflammatory sites is generally believed to be non–antigen specific. Specifically sensitized lymphocytes may, upon reaction with antigen, release substances that attract and affect the migration of macrophages or products that increase the phagocytic or digestive capacity of macrophages (see Table 2-2).

Subpopulations of cells in the macrophage family may be recognized by a combination of cell surface markers, morphological appearance, and location in tissue (Table 2-3). Fixed histiocytes lining the sinusoids of the liver are given the special

Table 2-3. Macrophage Subpopulations

Macrophage Subpopulation	Organ	Presumed Function
Stem cell	Bone marrow	Precursor
Monocyte	Blood	Circulating macrophage
Fixed histiocyte	Reticuloendothelial cells	Phagocytic cells in tissue
Dendritic histiocytes	Lymphoid organs	Process antigen for B cells
Interdigitating reticulum cells	Lymphoid organs	Process antigen for T cells
Langerhans' cells	Skin, lymph nodes	Process antigen for T cells

name *Kupffer cells.* Factors are also produced by macrophages that contribute to induction and expression of immune responses as well as inflammation (see Chapter 12). One macrophage-derived factor, interleukin 1, plays a key role in induction of immune responses.

Langerhans' Cells. Langerhans' cells (Fig. 2-7) are a population of the macrophage series found within the mammalian epidermis and certain lymph nodes. They are derived from bone marrow macrophage precursors. They are able to present antigen to T cells in vitro and are believed to be important in promoting certain immune-mediated lesions, such as contact dermatitis. These cells are not usually visualized in hematoxylin and eosin (H&E)–stained sections but can be distinguished by the presence of class II markers of the major histocompatibility locus, by certain antigenic markers, and by the presence of Birbeck granules seen by electron microscopy.

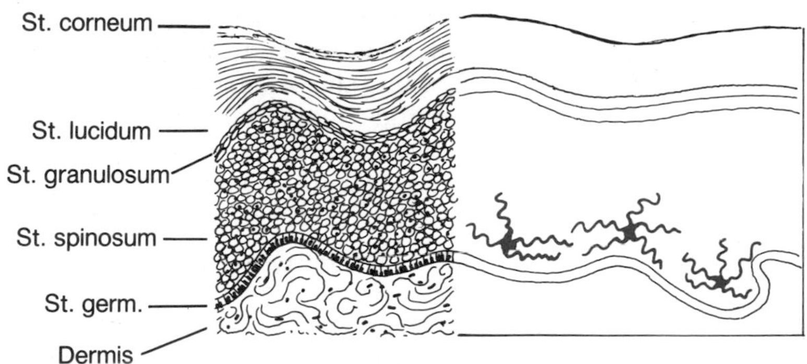

Figure 2-7. On the left is a drawing of the layers of the epithelium of the skin. On the right is depicted the location of Langerhans'cells as detected by special markers. Langerhans' cells are not distinguishable from epithelial cells by the usual methods used for staining tissue.

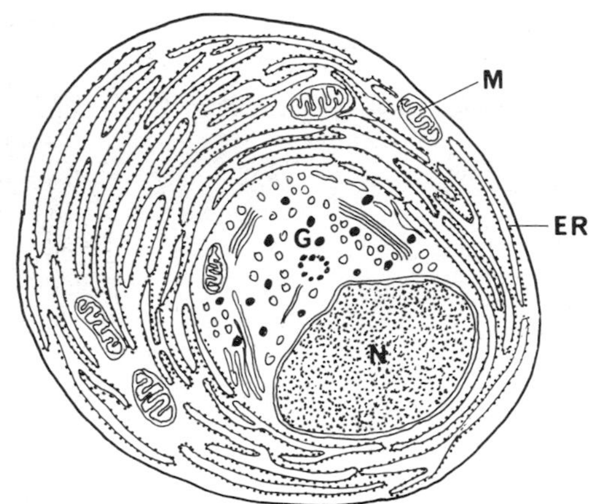

Figure 2-8. Plasma cell. Cell is composed of abundant cytoplasm containing mostly lamellar endoplasmic reticulum and a few other cytoplasmic organelles. Tissue sections show the polar location and the "cartwheel" appearance of the nucleus produced by the condensation of chromatin along the nuclear membrane. ER, endoplasmic reticulum; G, Golgi apparatus; M, mitochondria; N, nucleus.

Plasma Cells

The production of immunoglobulins (antibody) is the primary function of the plasma cell. Plasma cells differentiate from activated B cells (see Chapter 6). The plasma cell is a small, round or oval cell (9–12 μm in diameter) with a small, compact, dense nucleus located at one pole of the cell. Aggregation of the chromatin along the nuclear envelope gives rise to the characteristic "cartwheel" appearance of the plasma cell nucleus under the light microscope. The cytoplasm is dominated by rough endoplasmic reticulum organized in stacked laminae and a prominent Golgi apparatus (Fig. 2-8). The characteristic lamellar endoplasmic reticulum and the Golgi apparatus reflect immunoglobulin synthesis and rapid secretion. They are found in some other cells in which protein secretion is a major function (e.g., pancreatic acinar cells). Plasma cells are prominent in the lymph nodes, spleen, and sites of chronic inflammation. Plasma cells increase in number in lymphoid organs draining the site of antigen injection during the induction of antibody formation. Membrane-bound amorphous densities believed to contain stored immunoglobulins may be observed in more mature plasma cells (Russell bodies).

Blast Cells

A well-recognized feature of active immune responses is the presence of large *blast* cells. Blast cells are cells that are activated and are in the process of dividing. These cells have large nuclei containing finely divided chromatin and prominent nucleoli. The cytoplasm of blast cells is strongly basophilic and contains dense collections of free and aggregated ribosomes (Fig. 2-9). A variety of other subcellular organelles may be found in the cytoplasm, including a Golgi apparatus, varying amounts of endoplasmic reticulum, and mitochondria. Blast cells are found in lymphoid organs draining sites of antigen injection and in active inflammatory lesions (particularly those of delayed hypersensitivity reactions), and may be induced in vitro in pure cultures of lymphocytes by certain mitogenic

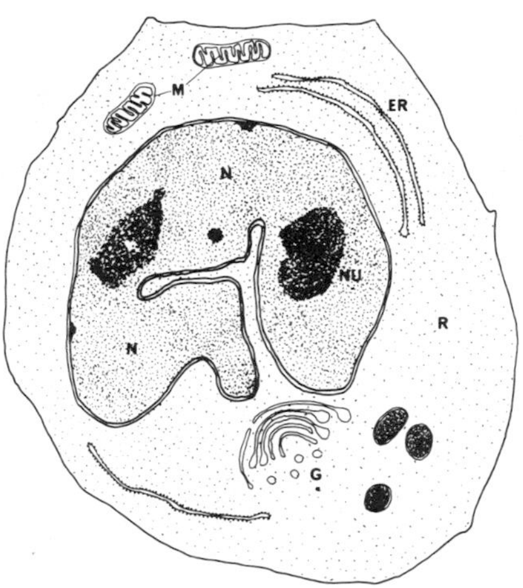

Figure 2-9. Blast cell. The blast cell has a large nucleus containing finely divided chromatin and prominent nucleoli. The cytoplasm stains blue with the usual staining agents and contains dense collections of ribosomes as well as other organelles. ER, endoplasmic reticulum; G, Golgi apparatus; M, mitochondria; N, nucleus; NU, nucleolus; R, ribosomes.

agents. Antigen-recognizing lymphocytes are stimulated by antigen to undergo transformation into blast cells that proliferate and differentiate into plasma cells or sensitized T cells.

Cellular Interactions in Immune Responses

At least three cell types are required for maximal antibody production to most antigens: T cells, B cells, and macrophages (Fig. 2-10). The characteristics and mechanisms of interactions of T and B cells in induction and expression of immune re-

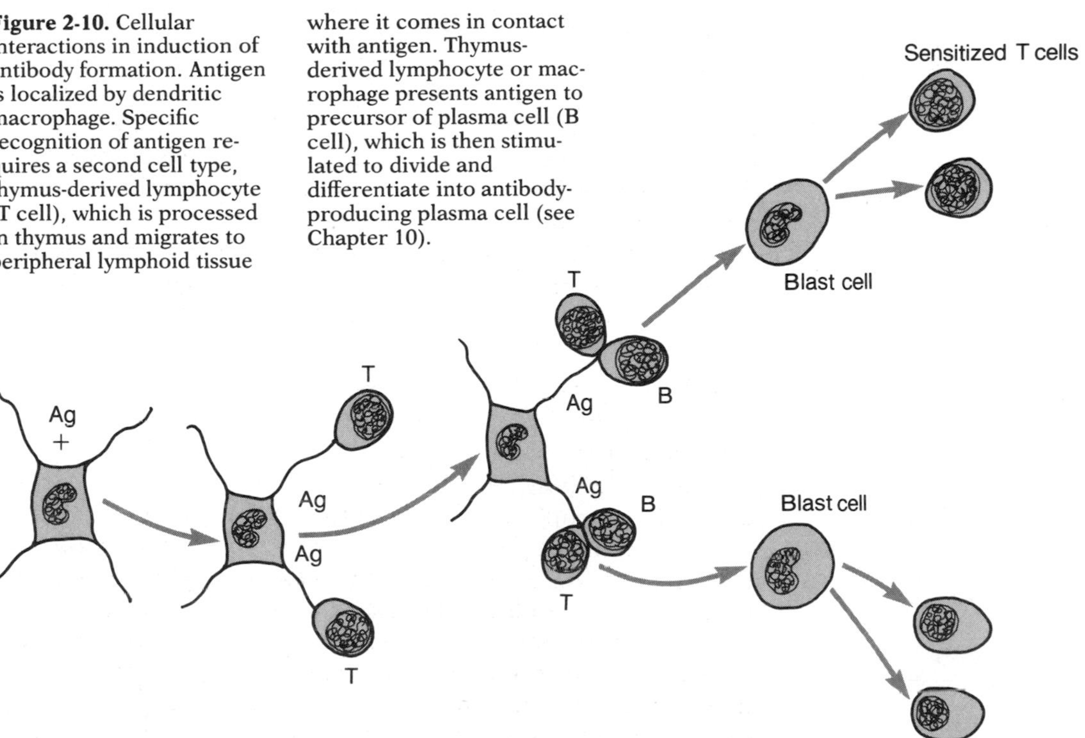

Figure 2-10. Cellular interactions in induction of antibody formation. Antigen is localized by dendritic macrophage. Specific recognition of antigen requires a second cell type, thymus-derived lymphocyte (T cell), which is processed in thymus and migrates to peripheral lymphoid tissue where it comes in contact with antigen. Thymus-derived lymphocyte or macrophage presents antigen to precursor of plasma cell (B cell), which is then stimulated to divide and differentiate into antibody-producing plasma cell (see Chapter 10).

sponse are discussed in more detail in Chapter 10. Specific recognition of most antigens requires the T cell. Macrophages process the antigen. T cells recognize self markers and antigen on macrophages and provide proliferation and differentiation signals to the precursors of plasma cells (B cells). The B cell is stimulated to divide and differentiate so that large numbers of specific antibody–producing plasma cells are produced. In some instances B cells can present antigen to T cells and bypass the macrophage requirement, or B cells may be stimulated directly.

Lymphatic Vessels

The lymphatic vessels retrieve fluid (lymph) and blood proteins that escape from blood capillaries and venules, and return them to the venous system. If this function of the lymphatic circulation is impaired, fluid will collect in the involved tissues (edema). The lymphatic vessels also permit wandering white blood cells in the tissues to return to the lymphoid organs. Lymphatic vessels drain every organ of the body except parts of the central nervous system, the eye, the internal ear, cartilage, spleen, and bone marrow (Fig. 2-11). The spleen and bone marrow have specialized capillary vessels that drain into the systemic vascular system directly and do not have lymphatics.

The fluid of the lymphatic circulation is made up of interstitial fluid drained from tissues or, in the gastrointestinal tract, fluid absorbed from the gastrointestinal contents. There is no pump for the lymphatic circulation corresponding to the heart for the systemic circulation. Lymphatic fluid is propelled by contraction of skeletal muscles or, in larger vessels, by smooth muscle cells that force the fluid from one level to another past valves that permit passage of fluid and cells only in one direction.

Lymphatic vessels drain from tissues through lymph nodes to larger *efferent* lymphatics that collect into larger lymph vessels, which drain into the thoracic duct or the right lymphatic duct. The thoracic duct is the largest lymph vessel in the body and joins the left subclavian vein. The right lymphatic duct joins the right subclavian vein. Seventy-five percent of body tissues are drained by the thoracic duct, and 25% are drained by the right lymphatic duct.

Lymphoid Organs

The cells of the lymphoid system are derived from blood cell precursors in the bone marrow and become organized in specialized organs of the body known as lymphoid organs. Lymphoid organs act as sites of immune responses, producing the products that provide specific adaptive immunity against a variety of infectious agents. Mature lymphoid organs are situated in the body in places where foreign material entering the body from the external environment will be brought into contact

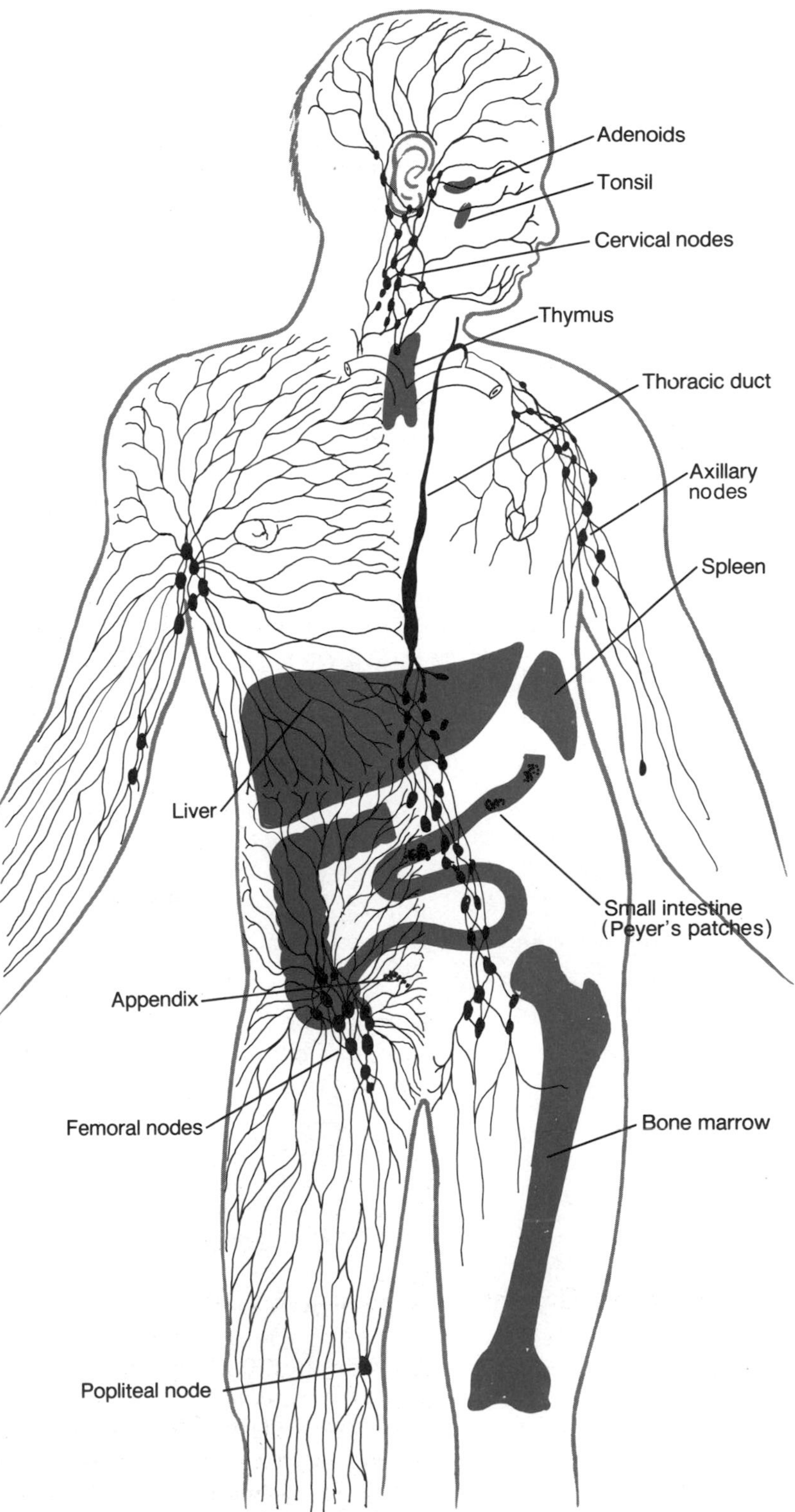

Figure 2-11. A diagram of the human lymphoid system. The system consists of circulating lymphocytes and the lymphoid organs, which include the tree of lymphatic vessels and the lymph nodes stationed along them, the bone marrow (in the long bones, only one of which is illustrated), the thymus, the spleen, the adenoids, the tonsils, the Peyer's patches of the small intestine, and the appendix. The lymphatic vessels collect the lymphocytes and antibody molecules from the tissues and lymph nodes and return them to the bloodstream at the subclavian veins.

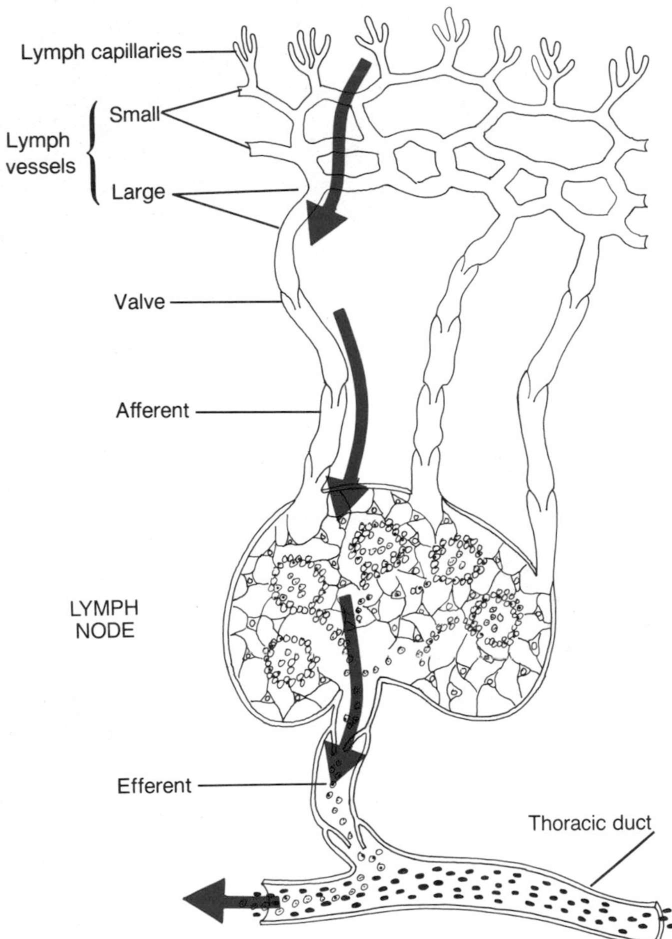

Figure 2-12. Lymphatic collecting vessels are similar to veins.

with lymphoid organs. Thus, lymph nodes are located along the course of lymphatic vessels that drain from the skin; gastrointestinal lymphoid organs are located along the absorptive areas of the gastrointestinal tract, where they act as filters of lymphatic fluids (Fig. 2-12). Lymphatic capillaries of the gastrointestinal tract are called *lacteals*. These capillaries absorb fats in the form of chylomicra. The spleen does not have lymphatics and serves as a filter for the circulating blood. The structure and function of the lymphoid organs are described in detail in the next chapter.

Summary

The lymphoid or immune system is made up of a number of organs connected by a network of vessels. The cells of the lymphoid system are the white blood cells. This chapter compares the structure and function of leukocytes (white blood cells). Mononuclear cells (lymphoid cells) include macrophages, lymphocytes (T cells, B cells, and null cells), and plasma cells. These cells are active in inflammation and in both induction and expression of immune responses. T cells, B cells, and macrophages cooperate in the induction of antibody responses to most antigens. Upon immune induction, T cells differentiate into specifically sensitized lymphocytes responsible for cellular immune reactivity, whereas B cells differentiate into antibody-secreting plasma cells. Polymorphonuclear cells and macrophages are active in the effector states of tissue inflammation in both a specific and a nonspecific manner.

References

More recent references on differentiation, identification of phenotypic markers, and genetics of the cells of the immune system are given in later pertinent chapters.

Polymorphonuclear Cells

Benditt BP, Lagunoff D: The mast cell: its structure and function. Prog Allergy 8:195, 1964.

Braunsteiner R, Zuker-Franklin D (eds): The Physiology and Pathology of Leukocytes. New York, Grune & Stratton, 1962.

de Duve C, Wattiaux R: Function of lysosomes. Annu Rev Physiol 23:435, 1966.

Oppenheim JJ, Rosenstreich DL, Potter M: Cellular Functions in Immunity and Inflammation. New York, Elsevier/North-Holland, 1981.

Spicer SS, Hardin JH: Ultrastructure, cytochemistry, and function of neutrophil leukocyte granules. Lab Invest 20:488, 1969.

Lymphocytes

Bianco C, Patrick R, Nuzzenzweig V: A population of lymphocytes bearing a membrane receptor for antigen–antibody complement complexes. J Exp Med 132:702–718, 1970.

Cooper HL: Studies on RNA metabolism during lymphocyte activation. Transplant Rev 11:3–38, 1972.

Gowans JL, McGregor DD: The immunological activities of lymphocytes. Prog Allergy 9:1, 1965.

Jondal M, Holm G, Wigzell H: Surface markers on human T and B lymphocytes. I. A large population of lymphocytes forming nonimmune rosettes with sheep red blood cells. J Exp Med 136:207, 1972.

Katz DH: Lymphocyte Differentiation, Recognition and Regulation. New York, Academic Press, 1978.

Miller JRAP, Osoba D: Current concepts of the immunological function of the thymus. Physiol Rev 47:437, 1967.

Moller G (ed): Lymphocyte immunoglobulin. Transplant Rev 14:1, 1973.

Moller G (ed): T and B lymphocytes in humans. Transplant Rev 16:1, 1973.

Raff MC: Surface antigenic markers for distinguishing T and B lymphocytes in mice. Transplant Rev 6:52, 1971.

Ross GD, Rabellino EM, Polley MJ, Grey HM: Combined studies of complement receptor and surface immunoglobulin-bearing cells and sheep erythrocyte rosette–forming cells in normal and leukemic lymphocytes. J Nat Cancer Inst 52:377–385, 1973.

Sell S, Asofsky R: Lymphocytes and immunoglobulins. Prog Allergy 12:86, 1968.

Macrophages

Anderson J, Sjoberg O, Moller G: Mitogens as probes for immunocyte activation and cellular cooperation. Transplant Rev 11:131–177, 1972.

Axline SG: Functional biochemistry of the macrophage. Semin Hematol 7:142, 1970.

Claman HN, Mosier DE: Cell–cell interactions in antibody production. Prog Allergy 16:40, 1972.

Cohn ZA: The structure and functions of monocytes and macrophages. Adv Immunol 9:163, 1968.

Fedorko ME, Hirsch JG: Structure of monocytes and macrophages. Semin Hematol 7:109, 1970.

Streilein JW, Bergstresser PR: Ia antigen and epidermal Langerhans cells. Transplantation 30:319, 1980.

Mitchison NA: The carrier effect in the secondary response to hapten–protein conjugates. II. Cellular cooperation. Eur J Immunol 1:18, 1971.

Miller JFAP, Basten A, Sprent J, Cheers C: Review: interactions between lymphocytes in immune responses. Cell Immunol 2:249, 1971.

Moller G (ed): Role of macrophages in the immune response. Immunol Rev 40:1, 1978.

Moller G (ed): Accessory cells in the immune response. Immunol Rev 53, 1980.

Lymphatics

Grey H: The lymphatic system. *In* Goss CM (ed): Anatomy of the Human Body, 29th ed. Philadelphia, Lea & Febiger, 1973, Ch 10.

Yoffey JM, Courtice FC: Lymphatics, Lymph and the Lymphomyeloid Complex. New York, Academic Press, 1970.

3 The Immune System II: Organs

A lymphoid organ is essentially a compartmentalized collection of lymphocytes and macrophages. Lymphoid organs have similarities as well as differences in structure. The prototype organ is encapsulated by collagenous connective tissue and divided into lobules by strands of connective tissue *(trabeculae)*. The "skeleton" of the organ is a network of interlocking reticular cells and fibers. By far the major cell type is the lymphocyte. Different populations of lymphocytes are found in different domains of a given lymphoid organ, forming functional microenvironments with macrophages of special types. The organ is supplied with blood by a single artery and, except for the spleen, is drained by both veins and lymphatics. The artery enters through an indentation in the capsule, called the *hilum,* and extends into the organ in the trabeculae. Smaller arteries and arterioles extend from the trabeculae into the parenchyma of the organ. Venous drainage begins in the parenchyma and flows out through veins in the trabeculae to the major draining veins, which exit at the hilum. The lymphatic drainage is different for each set of organs. Lymph nodes have both afferent and efferent lymphatics. The thymus has only efferent lymphatics and the spleen has no lymphatics.

Central Lymphoid Organs

The lymphoid cells in the bone marrow, liver, and thymus primarily serve as precursors for cells that develop further in other lymphoid organs; they are referred to as central lymphoid organs. The lymph nodes and spleen are classified as peripheral lymphoid organs. Gastrointestinal associated lymphoid tissue (GALT) and bronchus associated lymphoid tissue (BALT) have both central and peripheral compartments and functions.

Bone Marrow

The bone marrow is soft tissue found within the skeleton of the body in many bones. It contains fat cells and blood forming cells (hematopoietic tissue). The stem cells of all the blood elements, including the precursors of lymphoid cells, are located in the bone marrow. These stem cells and their progeny are organized into islands of cells within fatty tissue. In the bone marrow the cell types are admixed so that precursors of red blood cells (erythroblasts), macrophages, platelets (megakaryocytes), polymorphonuclear leukocytes (myeloblasts), and lymphocytes (lymphoblasts) may be seen in one microscopic field. It is impossible to differentiate stem cells for one cell line from those of another cell line by morphologic appearance alone. However, stem cells are usually surrounded by more mature cells of the same cell line, so that a given cell may be identified by the company it keeps. In normal bone marrow, the myelocytic series (polymorphonuclear cells) makes up approximately 60% of the cellular elements, and the erythrocytic series 20% to 30%. Lymphocytes, monocytes, reticular cells, plasma cells, and megakaryocytes constitute only 10% to 20%. Lymphocytes make up 5% to 15% of the cells of the normal adult marrow and 20% to 30% of a child's marrow. Normally, lymphocytes are mixed diffusely with the other cellular elements, but focal collections of lymphocytes may be seen in the marrow of elderly individuals. Plasma cells normally constitute fewer than 1% of the marrow cells but increase in percentage with age. Circulating blood enters via arteries that enter through the periosteum and pass through the compact bone in small canals. The marrow is drained by venous sinuses that collect mature blood elements for distribution into the peripheral blood. The mechanism whereby mature cells escape into the bloodstream while immature ones are held back is not known.

The bone marrow is not usually a site of reaction with, or response to, antigen. Marrow lymphocytes circulate from the marrow to other lymphoid organs and differentiate into lymphocytes capable of immune function. Cells originating in the marrow populate the thymus, where they may differentiate into T cells, whereas other marrow cells differentiate into B cells. An intriguing observation is that in the human, naturally occurring tumors of plasma cells that produce immunoglobulin (multiple myeloma) are often found in the bone marrow; an extramedullary location for multiple myeloma is much less frequent. This suggests that the precursors of plasma cells with malignant potential may be located in the marrow. In vitro studies of bone marrow after fractionation of the cells suggest that some immunologically reactive cells may be present in the bone marrow and are able to respond to antigenic stimulation. The contribution of bone marrow cells to the immune response of the whole animal remains unclear. However, the bone marrow may serve as a source of memory cells.

Liver

Early in ontogeny, the liver and yolk sac of mammals constitute the primary site of blood cell formation and, along with the bone marrow, may be the original site of maturation or production of B cells. The yolk sac and liver are closely related embryologically. The fetal liver is made up of immature liver cells (hepatocytes) surrounded by many islands of blood-forming cells containing essentially the same populations of hematopoietic cells as the bone marrow. Attempts to identify a tissue site for maturation of B cell populations have largely been influenced by the finding that the bursa of Fabricius, a gastrointestinal lymphoid organ of birds, is required for normal avian B cell maturation. A mammalian equivalent to the avian bursa in this regard has not been convincingly demonstrated. The mammalian gastrointestinal lymphoid tissue may also be a site for B cell development, but studies are inconclusive. Lymphocytes derived from mouse embryo liver develop surface Ig (B cells) when cultured in vitro. On the basis of this finding it has been suggested that the fetal liver of mammals is a major tissue site of B cell maturation. The yolk sac may also serve as a site for production of immature immune cells for the embryo.

Thymus

The thymus contains a cortical area of packed lymphoid cells, a medulla, a fibrous capsule, prominent trabeculae that divide the organ into lobules, and a hilum with entering arteries and draining veins and lymphatics (Fig. 3-1). The thymus differs

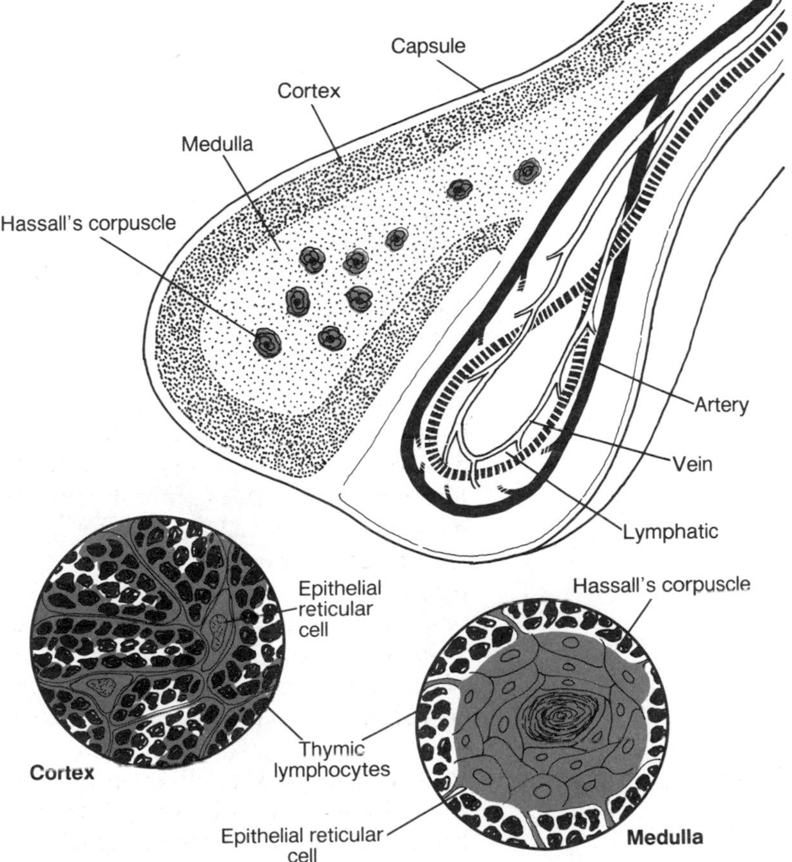

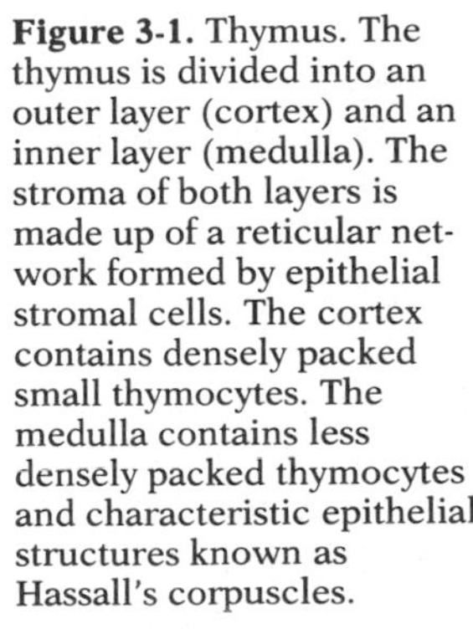
Figure 3-1. Thymus. The thymus is divided into an outer layer (cortex) and an inner layer (medulla). The stroma of both layers is made up of a reticular network formed by epithelial stromal cells. The cortex contains densely packed small thymocytes. The medulla contains less densely packed thymocytes and characteristic epithelial structures known as Hassall's corpuscles.

from the lymph nodes and the spleen in three important features: (1) Normally, there are no lymphoid follicles. The cortex consists of packed small lymphocytes and many proliferating cells in the T lymphocyte series. (2) The medulla contains remnants of epithelial islands that appear as concentric rings of eosinophilic tissue known as *Hassall's corpuscles.* (3) The medulla does not contain sinusoids but is a mesenchymal reticular network in which are found large numbers of lymphocytes. The cortex can be differentiated from the medulla because the lymphocytes are much more closely packed in the cortex. There are no afferent lymphatics in the thymus. The drainage of the thymus has not been well characterized; most drainage occurs through the vein, although significant lymphatic drainage has been claimed by some observers. The cortex is an area of active cell proliferation, with complete turnover of cells believed to occur every 3 or 4 days. The primary function of the normal adult thymus is the production of thymic lymphocytes (thymocytes). However, only about 1% of the lymphocytes produced ever leaves the thymus; the other 99% are destroyed locally. Cellular debris derived from this process is seen in the thymic cortex. The thymus is important for the development of immunity of the cellular type and for normal maturation of the paracortical areas of the lymph node and of the periarteriolar collection of lymphocytes in the white pulp of the spleen (see Lymph Node and Spleen, below). Essentially no B cells can be identified in the normal thymus.

Phenotypic characterization of both the thymocytes and stromal cells of the thymus reveals a complexity of cell types not apparent by morphology alone. The cortical epithelium is derived from an ectodermal branchial cleft, whereas the medullary epithelium is derived from the third pharyngeal pouch. The capsule is derived from mesodermal connective tissue (Table 3-1).

Table 3-1. Characterization of Thymic Stroma

Location	Tissue
Capsule	Mesodermal
Subcapsule	Endocrine epithelium
Cortex	Nonendocrine epithelium
Medulla	Endocrine epithelium

The medullary epithelial cells, including Hassall's corpuscles, represent stages of differentiation and express different phenotypes as differentiation from medullary endocrine epithelium to mature Hassall's corpuscles occurs. The differentiation parallels that seen in skin keratinocytes (Table 3-2).

Thymocytes also show differentiation-related phenotypic changes from cortex to medulla as defined by phenotypic

Table 3-2. Comparison of Differentiation Stages of Skin and Thymic Medullary Epithelium

SKIN						
Basal	→	Spinosum	→	Granulosum	→	Corneum
THYMUS						
Medullary endocrine epithelium	→	Epithelium around Hassall's bodies	→	Outer layer of Hassall's bodies	→	Inner layer of Hassall's bodies

markers identified by monoclonal antibodies. Most cortical thymocytes are surrounded by epithelial cell membrane extensions. These cortical epithelial cells, termed *thymic nurse cells,* may be responsible for early thymocyte differentiation. Further differentiation occurs after the cells leave the thymus (postthymic compartment). More details of the differentiation of thymocytes are presented in Chapter 4.

The term *T cell* refers to thymus-derived lymphocyte. Cells in the thymus are technically not T cells; T cells are cells that have matured in the thymus and are now present in other tissues (blood, lymph node, etc.). The role of the thymus in the development of other endocrine organs is not well known. Thymectomy leads to a reduction of pituitary hormone levels and atrophy of the gonads. Neonatal hypophysectomy results in thymic atrophy and wasting disease. Other evidence suggests that growth hormone may have an important effect on T cell maturation. Much remains to be learned about thymus–hypophysis interrelationships controlling T cell development.

Peripheral Lymphoid Organs

Lymph Node

Lymph nodes are located in areas of lymphatic drainage in the body and serve as filters for tissue fluid in lymphatic vessels (Fig. 3-2). The lymph node cortex contains nodules of lymphocytes (primary follicles), more loosely arranged nodules surrounded by a rim of tightly packed lymphoid cells (secondary follicles), and lymphocytes lying between germinal centers (paracortical areas) that extend irregularly as bulges into the medulla (deep cortex). Thymectomy of neonatal animals leads to a depletion of lymphoid cells in the paracortical and deep cortical zones; therefore, these zones have become known as the *thymus-dependent area.* On the other hand, depletion of the primary follicles and germinal centers occurs in birds upon removal of the bursa of Fabricius. The follicular areas are therefore termed *bursa dependent.* The medulla consists of a network of draining sinusoids formed by a meshwork of phagocytic reticular cells. The follicles are composed mainly of B cells *(B cell domain),* and the paracortical zone mainly of T cells *(T cell domain).* Specialized macrophages are also present in each of these domains (see Chapter 2). Afferent lymphatic vessels drain into a subcortical sinus; lymphatic sinusoids drain through the cortex around follicles and paracortical areas into the extensive sinusoidal network of the medulla. Some efferent

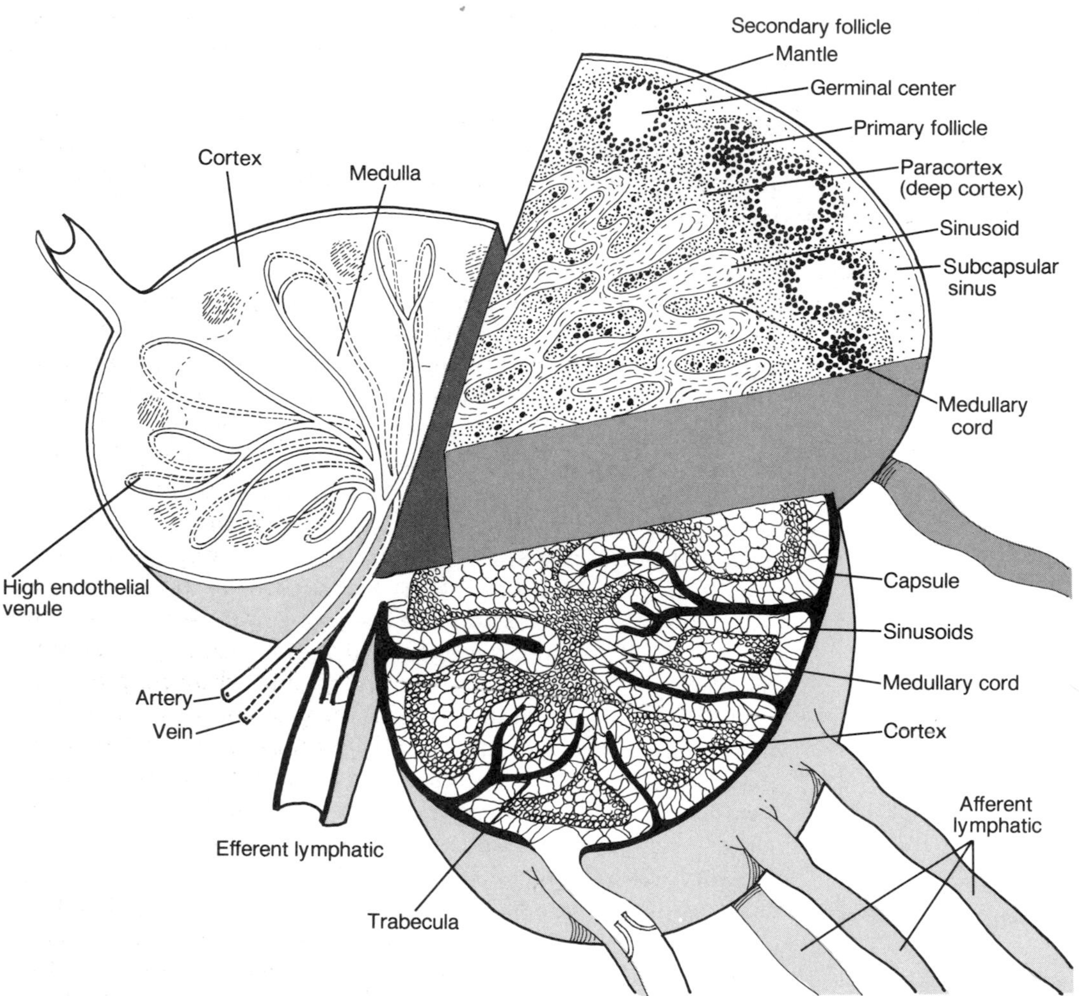

Figure 3-2. Normal lymph node. Nodes are made up of lymphoid cells contained in a meshwork of reticular fibers surrounded by connective tissue capsule. Most lymph nodes are bean-shaped, with an indented area known as the hilus. Cortex (outer layer) contains densely packed lymphoid cells and includes germinal centers responsible for production of antibody-synthesizing plasma cells and paracortical areas where lymphocytes are produced. Medulla (central area) consists of sinusoidal channels maintained by reticular cells. Columns of lymphoid cells are found between sinusoids in areas containing reticular macrophages. Afferent lymphatics drain through cortex around germinal centers into medullary sinusoids. Medullary sinusoids drain into efferent lymphatics and are collected by main efferent lymphatic that drains from the hilus. The main artery divides into capillaries supplying cortex. These capillaries drain into veins that follow trabeculae and exit at the hilus. (Modified from Bloom W, Fawcett DW: A Textbook of Histology, 9th ed. Philadelphia, Saunders, 1969.)

lymphatics arise at the junction of the paracortex and the medulla. It is here that T lymphocytes produced in the deep cortex enter the medullary sinusoids. The medullary sinuses drain into efferent lymphatics, which empty into the main efferent lymphatic vessel and exit through the hilum. The arteries divide into capillaries in the cortex. These capillaries drain into veins in the cortex, so that the cortex is supplied with circulating blood in a conventional manner, whereas the medulla is mainly supplied with lymph fluid by afferent and efferent lymphatics. Recirculating lymphocytes enter the lymph node via high endothelial postcapillary venules in the paracortex. B cells must pass through the T cell domain to home to the B cell domain (follicle).

Spleen

The lymphoid tissue of the spleen is analogous to that of the lymph node, but it is arranged differently (Fig. 3-3). Splenic lymphoid follicles are not demarcated into a cortical area as they are in the lymph node, but are scattered through the sinusoids. Lymphoid follicles and surrounding lymphoid tissue are called *white pulp*, and the sinusoidal area, which usually contains large numbers of red blood cells, is called *red pulp* because of the color seen on gross examination of the freshly cut organ. The white pulp is organized as a lumpy cylindrical sheath surrounding central arterioles. The arterioles curve back upon the white pulp to envelop it as the marginal sinus. The marginal sinus separates the white pulp from the red pulp. Circulating T and B cells enter the splenic white pulp by traversing the marginal sinus. T and B cells may be found mixed in the marginal zone, although B cells predominate. The B cells of the marginal zone appear to be in an activated state. It has been claimed that T-independent antibody responses may take place in the marginal zone. T cells are located in a tight sheath around the central arteriole called the periarteriolar lymphoid sheath; the B cell domain is the lumpy eccentric follicle of white pulp. These follicles may be primary or secondary (germinal center). There is a tightly packed zone of B cells surrounding splenic germinal centers, which is called the *mantle*. The mantle represents cells of the primary follicle pushed aside by formation of the germinal center. The spleen contains no lymphatic vessels. Blood enters through arteries running in trabeculae. The arteries branch and extend into the red pulp. The white pulp is positioned as a sleeve around the smaller arterioles. The arterioles continue out of the white pulp and supply the red pulp either by direct connection with the medullary sinusoids, by drainage into the intersinusoid reticular tissue known as the cords of Billroth, or by branching into specialized vessels of the marginal sinus before entering the sinusoids. Sinusoids have a basic structure similar to that of the lymph node, but drain into branches of the splenic vein and not into efferent lymphatics. There are three types of phagocytic–macrophage cells in the spleen: (1) cells lying free in sinusoids, (2) reticular cells lying between sinusoids that form a meshwork of reticular fibers, and (3) cells found in areas surrounding the white pulp (sometimes within the white pulp). The sinusoidal lining cells are of endothelial origin.

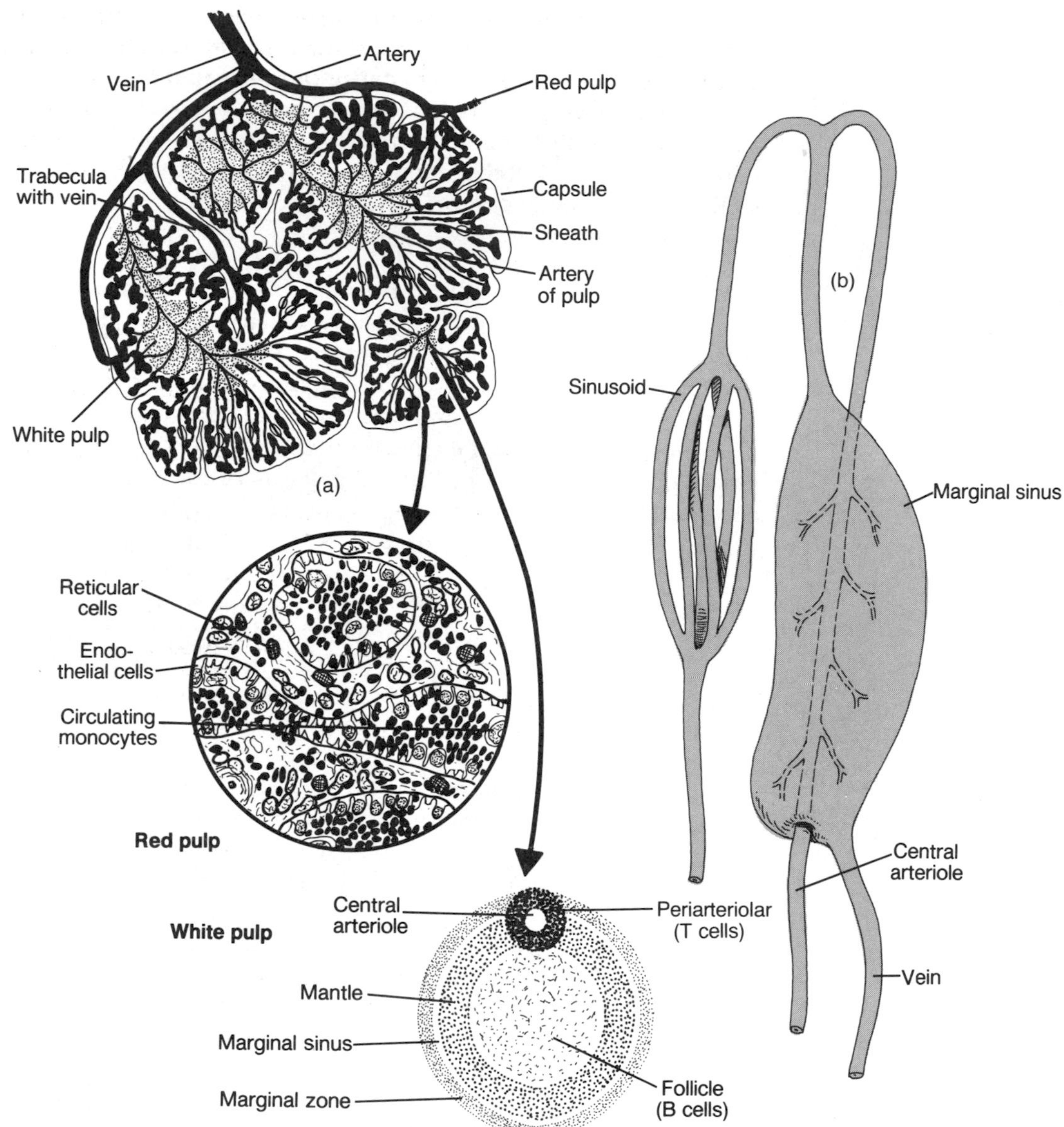

Figure 3-3. (a) Normal splenic lobule. Spleen is composed of a network of sinusoidal channels filled mainly with red blood cells (red pulp). There are no lymphatic vessels. Blood enters through arteries that may empty directly into splenic sinusoids or into reticular area between sinusoids. Sinusoids are drained by veins that exit via trabecular veins to a large vein that leaves spleen at the hilus. A zone of densely packed lymphocytes surrounding a central arteriole contains T cells (thymus-dependent area), whereas B cells are found surrounding the germinal center. The mantle surrounding germinal centers is composed mainly of B cells but also of T cells, believed to be pushed aside from the B cell zone by formation of the germinal center. Overlying the mantle is the marginal zone, containing venous capillaries that permit circulating cells to enter the white pulp. (b) The splenic microcirculation. Blood entering the spleen through central arterioles appears to circulate through either the white pulp or the red pulp. The central arteriole divides into two. One branch drains into capillaries that supply the white pulp, collects into the marginal sinuses, which surround the white pulp, and drains into the splenic vein. The other branch supplies the sinusoids of the red pulp and separately drains into the splenic vein.

It was once believed that the spleen was not an important organ for adaptive immunity; however, children who have their spleens removed surgically because of trauma, neoplastic disease, or hematologic disorders are subject to what is termed the *postsplenectomy syndrome*. Postsplenectomy syndrome is caused by bacterial sepsis, usually with large numbers of encapsulated bacteria (approximately 100 per milliliter). Thus the spleen does serve an important function in clearing the blood of infectious organisms.

Gastrointestinal and Bronchus Associated Lymphoid Tissue

Local collections of lymphoid tissue underlie the submucosa of many areas of the gastrointestinal tract and airways of the lung. In some areas, the collections become large enough to be identified individually. These areas are the tonsils (lingual, palatine, pharyngeal, and tubal) (Fig. 3-4), the appendix (Fig. 3-5), and Peyer's patches (Fig. 3-6). Different domains of lymphoid tissues may be identified in *gastrointestinal associated lymphoid tissue (GALT)*: the dome, the follicle, the thymus-dependent area, and submucosal IgA-containing areas. Similar collections

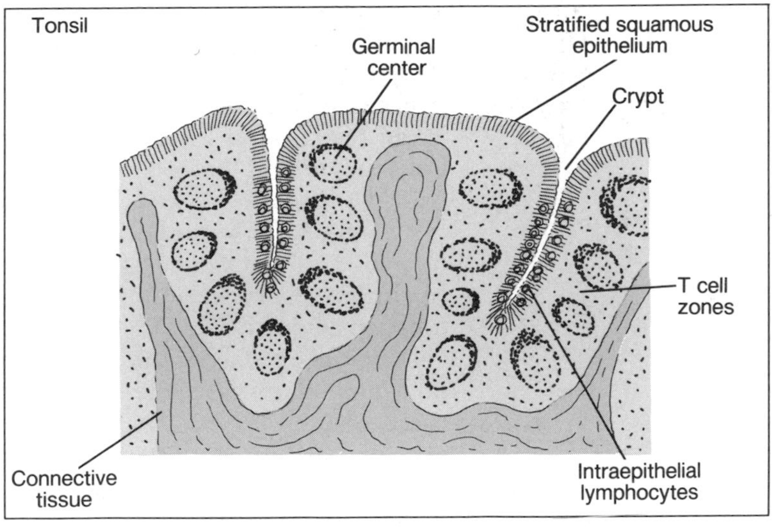

Figure 3-4. Tonsil. Tonsils are composed of a closely packed layer of germinal centers underlying epithelium. There are no afferent lymphatics, and efferent lymphatics are poorly defined. Overlying epithelium is characteristic of areas where tonsils are located (see Gastrointestinal and Bronchus Associated Lymphoid Tissue). Lymphoid cells produced by tonsil appear within overlying epithelium and are believed to emigrate into crypts.

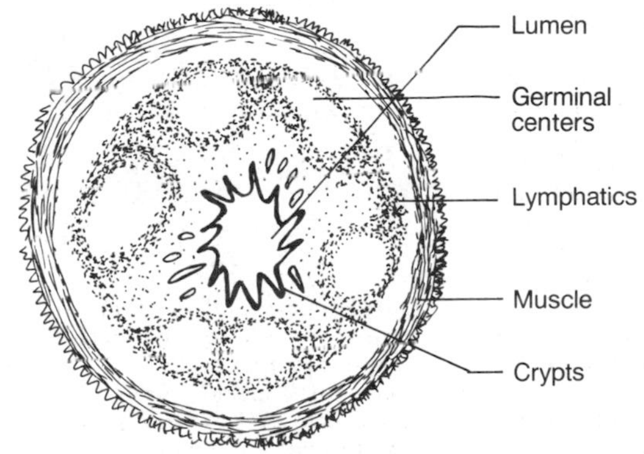

Figure 3-5. Appendix. Appendicular lymphoid tissue is composed of a layer of germinal centers underlying mucosa. Mucosa consists of crypts of goblet cells characteristic of this part of intestine. Many cells produced in appendix appear to be discharged into the lumen. Afferent lymphatics drain around germinal centers from origin in crypts; efferent lymphatics drain from germinal centers.

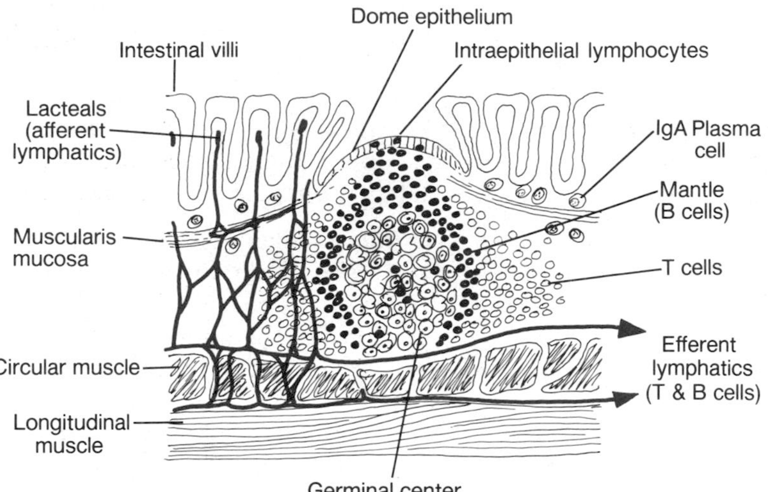

Figure 3-6. Structure of the Peyer's patch (see text).

of lymphoid tissue also occur under the epithelium of the bronchi of the lung (*bronchus associated lymphoid tissue* or *BALT*). The tonsils form a ring of lymphoid tissue at the base of the tongue and pharynx, known as *Waldeyer's ring,* which "guards" the passageway to the esophagus and trachea. The GALT is a major lymphopoietic organ in the adult and may be a source of T and B cells after thymic function declines with age. Antigen entering through the gut or lungs may stimulate cells in GALT or BALT that can then circulate to other tissues.

The overlying mucosa is characteristic of each location: lingual tonsil, stratified squamous; palatine tonsil, stratified squamous; pharyngeal tonsil, pseudostratified columnar; tubal tonsil, pseudostratified columnar; appendix, columnar goblet cells (crypts of Lieberkuhn); Peyer's patches, modified intestinal epithelium. The membranous epithelial cells overlying GALT contain less alkaline phosphatase and have shorter microvilli than adjacent mucosal cells. The GALT-associated mucosal cells are able to transport antigens and microorganisms selectively into GALT. In addition, afferent lymphatics in the form of lacteals deliver material absorbed through the intestine to the lymphatic tissue. The gastrointestinal lymphoid tissue is believed to be necessary for development of the antibody-forming organs (germinal centers, plasma cells) and to have a primary role in immunity to infectious agents entering the body through the mouth. Both immunoglobulin (antibody) and lymphoid T cells are produced by the gastrointestinal lymphoid tissue. These are delivered to the systemic circulation by draining lymphatics, but many of the proteins and cells produced are secreted into the gastrointestinal lumen.

The lactating breast is also a secretory lymphoid organ. Under the influence of prolactin, antibody-producing cells home to and proliferate in the breast, where they produce antibodies that are secreted into the milk. Upon suckling, these antibodies protect the newborn infant against diarrheal pathogens.

Comparison of Structures of Lymphoid Organs

A comparison of the characteristics of lymphoid organs is given in Table 3-3. The structure of each lymphoid organ is related to its functions, the most notable examples being:

1. The thymus, which does not normally respond to an antigenic stimulus, has no afferent lymphatics and no apparent structure associated with delivery of antigen to the organ. In addition, the thymus is the site of T cell development and does not normally contain B cell domains.
2. The lymph node, which serves as a filter for lymphatics, contains both afferent and efferent lymphatics. Both T and B cell domains are present, as well as a rapid delivery system for antibody and/or T cells into lymphatics.
3. The spleen, which is a filter for the blood and not the lymphatics, has no lymphatic vessels.
4. The bone marrow, which is the site of formation of blood cells, does not normally contain T or B cell domains.

Table 3-3. Some Characteristics of Lymphoid Organs

	Cortex	Medulla	B Cell Domain (Follicles)	Afferent Lymphatics	Efferent Lymphatics	Special Features
Thymus	+	+	0	0	+	Hassall's corpuscles, epithelial reticulum, no B cells
Spleen	0	0	+	0	0	White and red pulp, no lymphatics
Lymph node	+	+	+	+	+	Subcapsular sinus, prominent follicles, and paracortical zones
Gastrointestinal						
Tonsils	+	0	+	0	+	Zones of T and B cells, no prominent medulla or draining sinusoids, active mitoses
Appendix	+	0	+	±	+	
Peyer's patch	+	0	+	+	+	
Bone marrow	0	0	0	0	0	Hematopoietic cells in fatty tissue, few mature immune cells

+, present; 0, absent.

Lymphocyte Circulation

Histologic examination of the lymphoid organs provides a static view that belies the extensive recirculation of lymphoid cells. Lymphocytes, both T and B cells, leave their maturation sites, percolate through the lymphoid tissue, and enter other organs by circulation in the bloodstream. Entrance to the bloodstream occurs via either afferent lymphatics or draining veins. Mature lymphoid cells (memory cells?) as well as naive T and B lymphocytes may reenter lymphoid organs after circulating. Lymphocytes enter the lymph node by traversing specialized cortical capillary venules known as high endothelial venules (HEV), because of the thickness of endothelial cells. HEV have specific surface recognition sites for T and B lymphocytes, so that these cells traverse HEV located in different areas of lymphoid organs.

T cells and B cells enter at the same site but are able to go separately to their respective domains in the lymphoid organ. In the lymph node, B cells must traverse the T cell domain (paracortical zone) to reach the B cell domain (follicles). In the spleen, T cells traverse the B domain before reaching the T cell domain (periarteriolar lymphoid sheath). After traversing their respective domains, recirculating T and B cells enter the medullary or red pulp sinusoids before entering the efferent lymphatics. The lymphocyte fields of the lymph node thus contain slowly percolating masses of T and B cells, most of which are on their way from blood to lymph and back to blood. The ratio of the constitutive population of fixed cells to recirculating lymphocytes is not known. Stimulation with antigen results in a temporary increase in responding cells in lymphoid organs draining the site of antigen contact. There is some organ selectivity for lymphocyte localization, as lymph node lymphocytes preferentially localize to lymph nodes, whereas GALT lymphocytes preferentially localize to GALT (Fig. 3-7).

The GALT as well as bone marrow may be a major source of new lymphocytes in the adult animal. Both T and B lymphocytes are delivered from GALT via efferent lymphatics to the thoracic duct and to the systemic circulation. These cells may then localize in any lymphoid organ of the body (except perhaps the thymus) with preferential homing to mucosal lymphoid tissue (e.g., GI tract, lacrimal glands, mammary glands, BALT, and bladder) (Fig. 3-8).

The Effect of Antigens on Lymphoid Organs

The "normal" structure of the lymphoid organs depends upon antigenic exposure. In germ-free animals that have little antigenic contact, the lymphoid organs contain few primary or secondary follicles and sparse paracortical areas, and serum immunoglobulin levels are less than one-tenth those of ordinary animals. The medullary areas contain sinusoids relatively

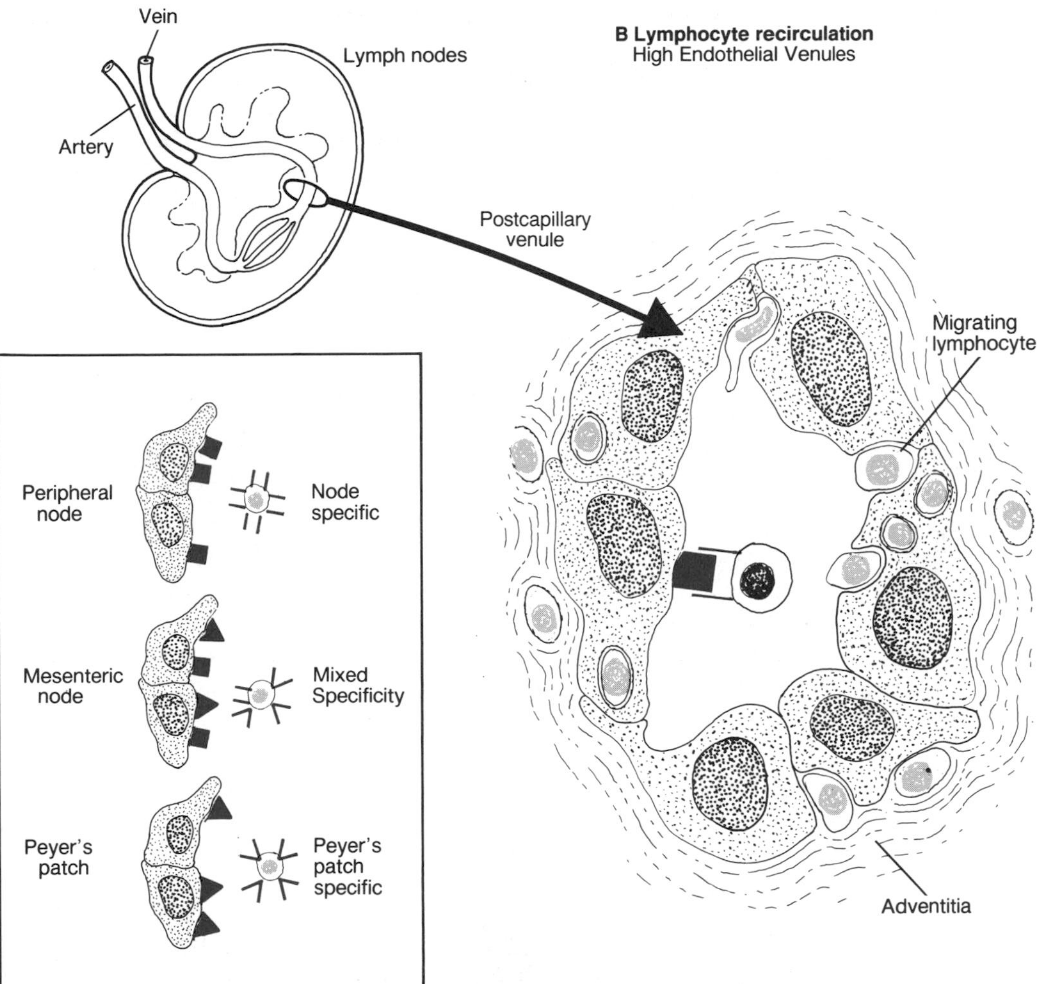

Figure 3-7. Diagram of model of B lymphocyte recognition and migration through high endothelial venules. Lymphocytes have receptors that serve to direct specific homing to lymphoid organs. Peyer's patch cells preferentially home to Peyer's patches; lymph node cells preferentially home to lymph nodes; T cells and B cells both home to the same venules, but with different preferences. In addition, T helper (H) and T suppressor cells also have slightly different homing preferences.

depleted of mononuclear cells or lymph fluid. If antigen is introduced, there is a marked increase in cortical follicles and paracortical tissue, and the serum immunoglobulin levels may increase to almost normal levels.

Antibody Production

Radiolabeled antigens that stimulate the production of both circulating antibody and nonantigens are taken up by the phagocytic cells (macrophages) of the medullary areas of lymph nodes and spleen (Fig. 3-9). However, they can also be

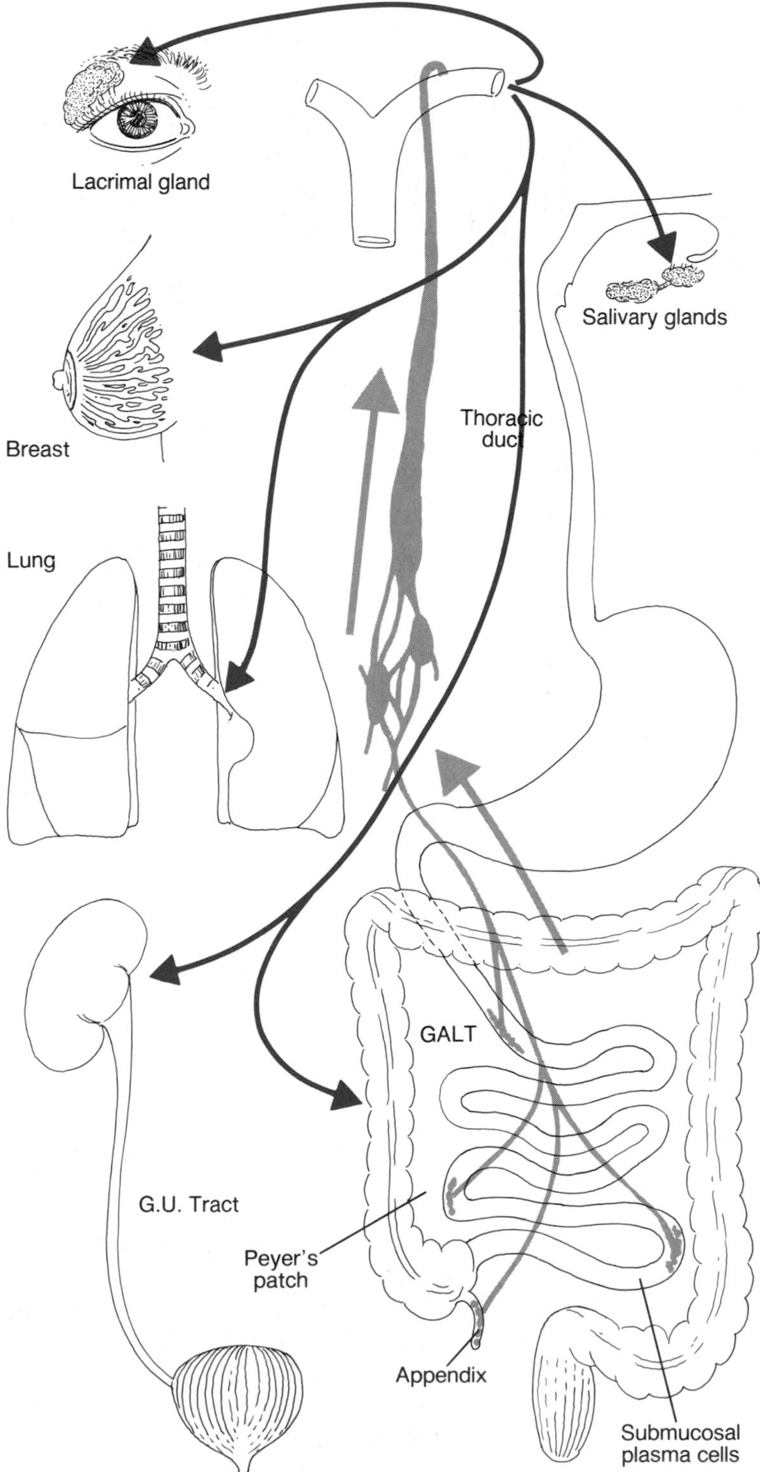

Figure 3-8. Cellular traffic in the secretory system.

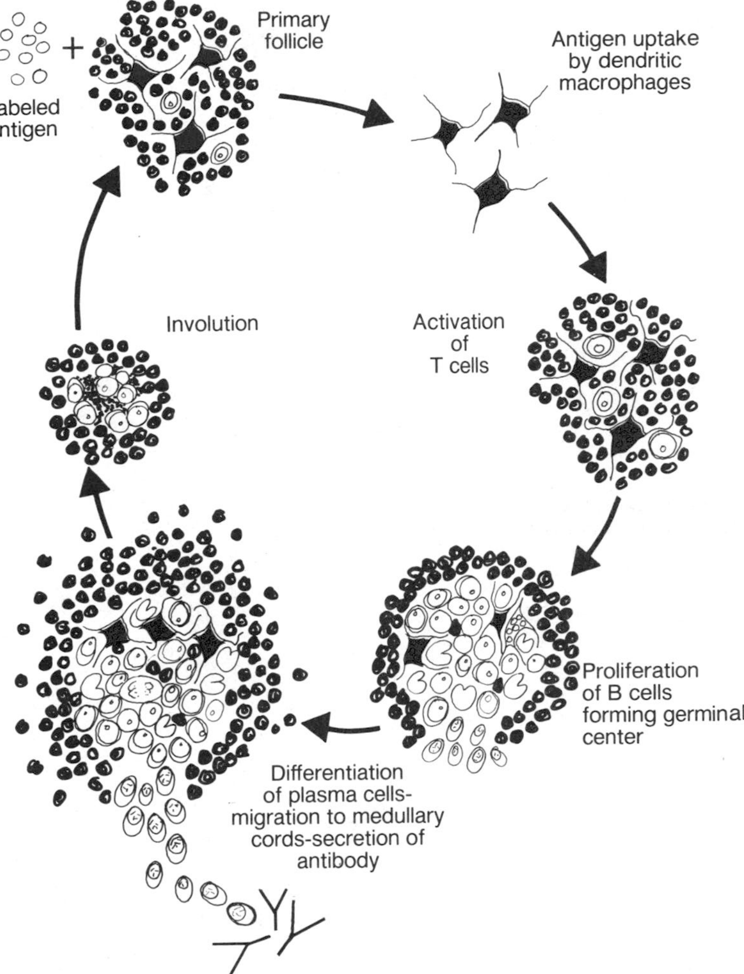

Figure 3-9. Germinal center formation. Localization of labeled antigen in lymph node following immunization demonstrates localization by Day 2 in dendritic macrophages in cortex. By Day 4, blast cells can be identified underlying the antigen-containing cells. These cells increase in number until typical germinal center (secondary follicle) is formed, with residual cells overlying an oval-shaped area of active proliferation (mantle). By Day 7 plasma cells appear deep in the germinal center. These cells then migrate into medullary cords. Germinal centers involute to primary follicles, which rapidly reactivate upon reexposure to the same antigen.

found in *dendritic* macrophages in the cortex or white pulp. Dendritic macrophages are elongated spindle-shaped cells with cytoplasmic extensions that are close to lymphocytes of the cortex or white pulp. Lymphoid follicles form around the dendritic macrophages containing the antigen. Cell proliferation leads to development of a nodule of cells *(follicle)*. The nonproliferating lymphocytes and antigen-containing macrophages are pushed aside to the periphery of the nodule to form a mantle around the follicle. Within 5 to 7 days after immunization, plasma cells appear below the germinal center and migrate into the medullary cords, where they produce and secrete immunoglobulin antibody that is released into the medullary sinusoids. Plasma cells may be observed in large numbers in the adjacent medullary cords or red pulp for periods of at least 10 weeks after immunization. The dendritic macrophages do not make antibody but interact with cells in the lymphoid series that are capable of responding (immunologically competent cells). Within 1 to 2 weeks after primary immunization, memory B cells can be identified in the lymph nodes draining the site of immunization; later, memory B cells are present in distal lymph nodes. After the active phase of antibody production the germinal center forms into a collection of lymphocytes in the cortex that is a primary follicle. Thus the primary follicles may be the location of memory cells. If this is the case, then the terms *primary* and *secondary* are inappropriate because a "primary" follicle may derive from a "secondary" follicle.

Germinal Center Cells

The morphology of cells in a germinal center is depicted in Figure 3-10. These cell types have been used to classify tumors arising from B cells.

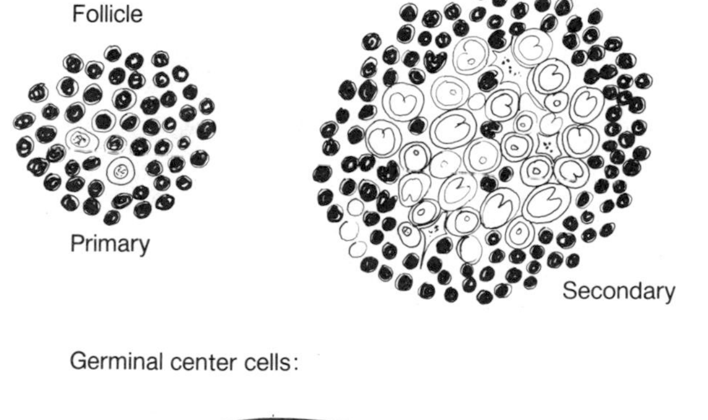

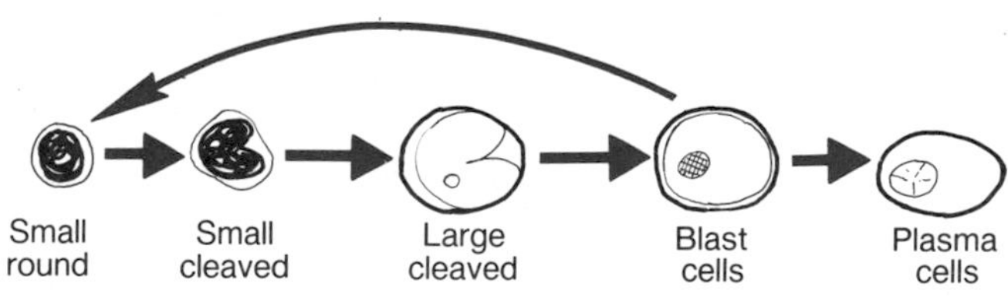

Figure 3-10. Germinal center cells. The cells seen in a germinal center range in size and shape from small round cells to large irregular "cleaved" cells on the basis of nuclear morphology. Primary follicles consist primarily of small round cells. Germinal centers contain a mixture of cells: small round, intermediate round, large round, small cleaved, medium cleaved, and large cleaved. Cleaved cells may represent "activated" B cells, with large round cells being "blast" cells that divide to form two daughter B cells that are small and round. These morphologic cell types have been used to classify tumors arising from B cells (B cell lymphomas). Small round B cell tumors have a good prognosis; large cleaved B cell tumors have a poor prognosis; cell types in between have an intermediate prognosis.

Delayed Hypersensitivity

The morphologic changes occurring in a lymph node during the development of specifically sensitized cells (delayed hypersensitivity) are different from those occurring during the production of circulating antibody (Fig. 3-11).

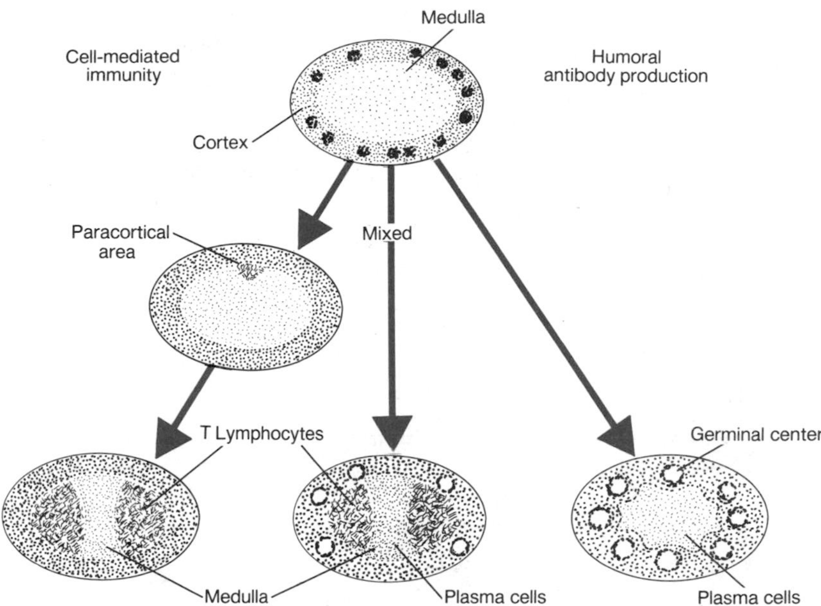

Figure 3-11. Morphologic response of lymph node to antigenic stimulus. Induction of essentially pure delayed hypersensitivity reaction leads to proliferation of lymphocytes in paracortical zone. Induction of pure humoral antibody formation results in germinal center formation and appearance of plasma cells in medullary cords. Immunization with most antigens produces both changes with enlargement of paracortical zones and production of germinal centers.

During the induction of delayed hypersensitivity, the proliferative changes in the lymph node do not occur in the follicles or germinal centers but in the other areas of the lymph node cortex that contain tightly packed T lymphocytes (the paracortical areas). Here, there is a population of macrophages known as interdigitating reticulocytes that are believed to process antigens in a manner similar to that of follicular dendritic macrophages, but to present the antigens to T cells. A few days after contact with an antigen, large "immature" blast cells and mitotic figures (dividing cells) may be recognized. A temporary increase in the number of small lymphocytes occurs in this area 2 to 5 days after immunization. It is likely that these are the specifically sensitized cells that are rapidly released into the draining lymph and disseminated throughout the body. It is not precisely clear how antigen is recognized during the development of delayed hypersensitivity. Lymphocytes may be able to recognize antigen at a site distant from the lymph node, where the sensitizing antigen is located, such as the skin. The reacting lymphocyte may return to the lymph node, lodge in the paracortical area, and undergo rapid replication, resulting in the formation of large numbers of sensitized cells that now may recognize and react with the sensitizing antigen.

In summary, different immune responses take place in different lymphoid tissue microenvironments (Table 3-4): specific T-dependent B cell proliferation in germinal centers; T cell proliferation in the paracortex or periarteriolar sheath; T-independent B cell proliferation in marginal zones; and antibody secretion in medullary cords. Memory B cells may differentiate in the mantle of germinal centers and be stored in primary follicles.

Table 3-4. Functional Lymphoid Organ Microenvironments

Microenvironment	Cells Present	Function
Germinal center	B cells, blasts, dendritic macrophages, T cells	T cell–dependent B cell proliferation and differentiation
Paracortex (lymph node), periarteriolar sheath (spleen)	T cells, interdigitating macrophages	T cell proliferation and differentiation
Marginal zones	Dendritic macrophages, B cells	T cell–independent B cell responses
Medulla (lymph node), red pulp (spleen)	Plasma cells, T cells, reticular cells	Rapid antibody production and release of sensitive T cells
Primary follicles	B cells, T cells, dendritic macrophages	Storage of memory cells
Mantle of germinal center	B cells	Memory B cell differentiation

Summary

The lymphoid cells responsible for specific immune responses are distributed in blood, lymphatics, and a number of tissues known as *lymphoid organs*. The morphologic characteristics and functional properties of lymphoid organs are different. Bone marrow serves as the major source of lymphoid stem cells. T cells develop from stem cells that migrate to the thymus and subsequently recirculate to home in thymus-dependent areas of other lymphoid organs: spleen, lymph node, and gastrointestinal tract. B cells mature in the bone marrow, liver, or gastrointestinal lymphoid tissue and migrate to B cell areas (follicles) of other lymphoid organs. Induction of antibody formation is associated with hyperplasia of follicles and plasma cell production, whereas cellular sensitivity is associated with hyperplasia of thymus-dependent areas.

References

Central Lymphoid Organs

Becker RP, DeBruyn PPH: The transmural passage of blood cells into myeloid sinusoids and the entry of platelets into the sinusoidal circulation: a scanning electron microscopic investigation. Am J Anat 145:183, 1976.

Cooper MD, Lawton AR III: The development of the immune system. Sci Am 231:58, 1974.

Cooper MD, Peterson RDA, South MA, Good RA: The functions of the thymus system and the bursa system in the chicken. J Exp Med 133:75, 1966.

Good RA, Gabrielsen AE (eds): The Thymus in Immunobiology. New York, Harper & Row, 1965.

McGregor DD: Bone marrow origin of immunologically competent lymphocytes in the rat. J Exp Med 127:953, 1968.

Melchers F: B lymphocyte development in the liver. II. Frequencies of precursor B cells during gestation. Eur J Immunol 7:482, 1977.

Metcalf D: The thymus: its role in immune responses, leukemia development, and carcinogenesis. *In* Rentchnick P (ed): Recent Results in Cancer Research, Vol 5. New York, Springer, 1966.

Miller JFAP, Marshall AHE, White RG: The immunological significance of the thymus. Adv Immunol 2:111, 1965.

Miller JFAP, Osoba D: Current concepts of the immunological function of the thymus. Physiol Rev 47:437, 1967.

Owen JJT, Cooper MD, Raff MC: In vitro generation of B lymphocytes in mouse fetal liver, a mammalian "bursa equivalent." Nature 249:361–363, 1974.

Waksman BH, Arnason BG, Jankovic BD: Role of the thymus in immune reactions in rats. III. Changes in the lymphoid organs of thymectomized rats. J Exp Med 116:187, 1962.

Peripheral Lymphoid Organs

Cantor H, Boyse EA: Lymphocytes as models for the study of mammalian cellular differentiation. Immunol Rev 33:105, 1977.

Fossum S, Ford WL: The origin of cell population within lymph nodes. Their origin, life history and functional relationship. Histopathology 9:469, 1985.

Goldschneider I, McGregor DD: Anatomical distribution of T and B lymphocytes in the rat. Development of lymphocyte specific antisera. J Exp Med 138:1433, 1973.

Makinodan T, Albright JF: Proliferative and differentiative manifestations of cellular immune potential. Prog Allergy 10:1, 1967.

Rocha B, Freitas AA, Coutinho AA: Population dynamics of T lymphocytes. Renewal rate and expansion in the peripheral lymphoid organs. J Immunol 131:2158, 1983.

Weiss L: The cells and tissues of the immune system. Structure, functions and interactions. *In* Foundations of Immunology Series. Englewood Cliffs, N.J., Prentice-Hall, 1972.

GALT–BALT

Archer OK, Sutherland DER, Good RA: Appendix of the rabbit: a homologue of the bursa in the chicken. Nature 200:337, 1963.

Brand A, Gilmour D, Goldstein G: Lymphocyte-differentiating hormone of bursa of Fabricius. Science 193:319, 1976.

Cooper MD, Lawton AR: The mammalian "bursa equivalent." Does lymphoid differentiation along plasma cell lines begin in gut-associated lymphoepithelial tissues (GALT) of mammals? Contemp Top Immunobiol 1:49, 1972.

Gallin JI, Fauci AS (eds): Advances in Host Defense Mechanisms, Vol 4, Mucosal Immunity. New York, Raven Press, 1985.

Glick B, Chang TS, Jaap RG: The bursa of Fabricius and antibody production. Poult Sci 35:224, 1956.

Nair PNR, Schroeder HE: Duct associated lymphoid tissue (DALT) of minor salivary glands and mucosal immunity. Immunology 57:171, 1986.

Waksman BH: The homing pattern of thymus-derived lymphocytes in calf and neonatal mouse Peyer's patches. J Immunol 111:878, 1973.

Waksman BH, Ozer H: Specialized amplification elements in the immune system: the role of nodular lymphoid organs in the mucous membranes. Prog Allergy 21:1, 1976.

Warner NL, Szenberg A: The immunological function of the bursa of Fabricius in the chicken. Annu Rev Microbiol 18:253, 1964.

Lymphocyte Circulation

Brahim F, Osmond DG: Migration of bone marrow lymphocytes demonstrated by selective bone marrow labeling with thymidine-H^3. Anat Rec 168:139, 1970.

Ford WL: Lymphocyte migration and immune responses. Prog Allergy 19:1, 1975.

Goldschneider I, McGregor DD: Migration of lymphocytes and thymocytes in the rat. I. The route of migration from blood to spleen and lymph nodes. J Exp Med 127:155, 1968.

Gowans JL, McGregor DD: The immunological activities of lymphocytes. Prog Allergy 9:1, 1965.

Marchesi VT, Gowans JL: The migration of lymphocytes through the endothelium of venules in lymph-nodes: an electron microscopic study. Proc R Soc Lond [Biol] 159:283, 1964.

Stamper HB, Woodruff JJ: An in vitro model of lymphocyte homing. I. Characterization of the interaction between thoracic duct lymphocytes and specialized high-endothelial venules of lymph nodes. J Immunol 119:772, 1977.

Stevens SK, Weissman IL, Butcher EC: Differences in the migration of B and T lymphocytes: organ selective localization in vivo and the role of lymphocyte–endothelial cell recognition. J Immunol 128:844, 1982.

Effect of Antigen

Movat HZ, Fernando MVP: The fine structure of lymphoid tissue during antibody formation. Exp Mol Pathol 4:155, 1965.

Nossal GJV, Ada GL: Antigens, Lymphoid Cells, and the Immune Response. New York, Academic Press, 1971.

Nossal GJV, Ada GL, Austin CM: Antigens in immunity. IV. Cellular localization of 125-I and 131-I labelled flagella in lymph nodes. Aust J Exp Biol Med Sci 42:311, 1964.

Schwartz RS, Ryder RJW, Gottlieb BAA: Macrophages and antibody synthesis. Prog Allergy 14:81, 1970.

Turk JL, Oort J: Germinal center activity in relation to delayed hypersensitivity. *In* Cottier H, Odortchenko N, Schindler R, Congdon CC (eds): Germinal Centers in Immune Responses. New York, Springer, 1967.

Unanue EA: The regulatory role of macrophages in antigenic stimulation. Adv Immunol 15:95, 1972.

Wortis HH: Immunological responses of "nude" mice. Clin Exp Immunol 8:305, 1971.

4 The Immune System III: Development of Lymphoid Organs (Ontogeny)

The most accepted model for the development of lymphoid organs is that proposed by Robert Good in the 1960s. According to this model, the precursor stem cells for all lymphoid cells are present in the bone marrow. During fetal development, the stroma for the peripheral lymphoid organs first develops in the absence of lymphoid cells and consists of epithelial or mesenchymal supportive tissue. T and B cells are derived from bone marrow precursors and acquire immune competence by maturation in inductive sites (Fig. 4-1).

T Cell Differentiation

T cell maturation involves stem cells produced in the bone marrow that circulate to and mature in the thymus (Fig. 4-2). The term *prothymocyte* is used for these cells, because they are characterized by homing to the fetal thymus. *Prothymocyte* is a functional term, as there are no phenotypic markers or other ways to identify this cell population. In the thymus these cells acquire T cell antigens such as the Thy and TL antigens found in the mouse. After proliferation in the thymus, some of the thymocytes migrate from the thymus and lodge in the thymus-dependent areas of spleen, lymph node, and other lymphoid organs. Developing thymocytes are also "educated" in the thymus to recognize self by developing receptors for self markers on the thymic epithelium (see Chapter 9). From this period on, thymocytes require recognition of self as well as foreign antigens in order to respond to an antigen. The large amount of proliferation and cell death in the thymus may be related to maintenance of tolerance to self (lack of an immune response to self antigens) through clonal elimination of self-reactive thymocytes. However, some lymphocytes must be able to recognize some self markers of the major histocompatibility system in order to function in helping B cells to respond to antigen (see Chapter 10). This type of self recognition is maintained and not eliminated during the maturation of thymocytes.

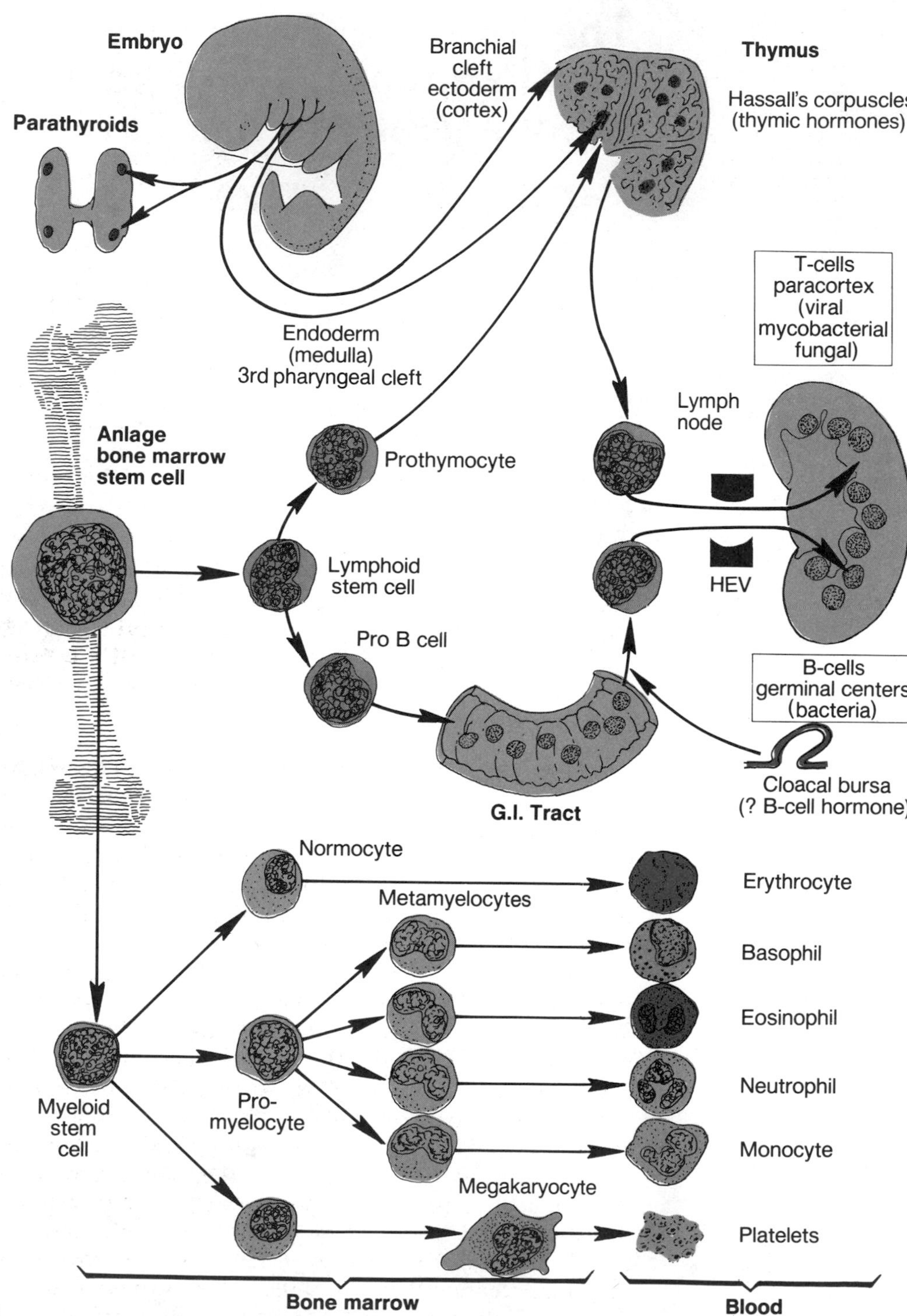

Figure 4-1. Maturation phases in the hematopoietic system. A common bone marrow hematopoietic stem cell gives rise to all elements in the blood and in the lymphoid system. In the stromal microenvironment of the lymphoid organs, specific differentiation of T and B cells occurs.

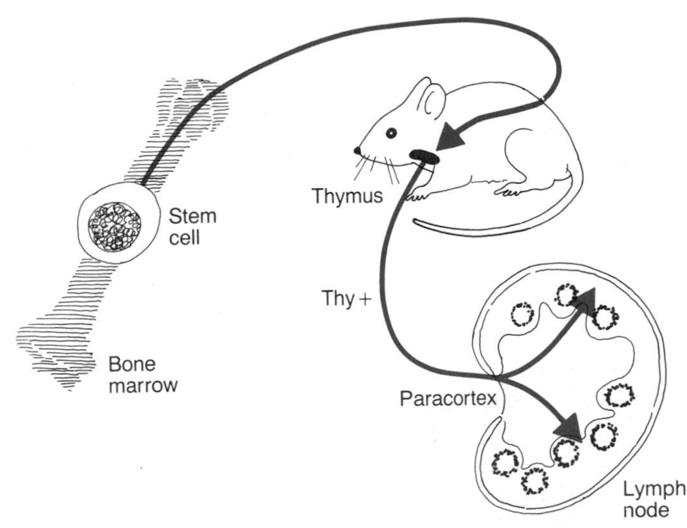

Figure 4-2. T cell differentiation (ontogeny). The model for T cell differentiation is as follows: Precursors of T cells (prothymocytes) arise from multipotent bone marrow stem cells and migrate to the thymus. In the thymic inductive microenvironment, these cells develop T cell characteristics, including the acquisition of T cell surface markers such as the Thy antigen. T cells that leave the thymus move to thymus-dependent areas, such as the lymph node paracortex, the periarteriolar sheath of the spleen, and thymus-dependent areas (TDA) of other lymphoid organs.

Thymectomy of newborn animals leads to an absence of T cells in the thymus-dependent areas of other lymphoid organs. The antigen receptor of T cells is fixed permanently in the thymus by rearrangement of genes coding for the T cell receptor. The expression of T cell receptor genes during development is presented further in Chapter 6.

Subpopulations of T Cells

In addition to providing help for T-dependent antibody production, T cells, as a class, have several other important functions. These include suppressor cells (T_S), which serve to limit or control immune responses; T cytotoxic or killer cells (T CTL or T_K), which are capable in vitro of lysing target cells to which they are sensitized; and T_D cells, which mediate delayed hypersensitivity in vivo through reaction with specific antigen and release of lymphokines (see Chapter 10). These functional subpopulations of T cells bear different cell surface markers. T cell surface markers are differentiation antigens that, for the most part, are found only on thymocytes or on cells derived from the maturation of thymocytes (T cells). As T cells differentiate into helper, suppressor, or killer cells, the expression of these markers changes (Fig. 4-3). There is also evidence for subpopulations of cells within these functional populations; that is, there may be at least two populations of T helper cells. In addition there is evidence for a population of T cells that counteracts the effect of T suppressor cells, called *T contrasuppressor cells* (see Chapter 10). The major phenotypes of mouse and human lymphocyte populations are given in Table 4-1. These phenotypes are based primarily on reactivity of monoclonal antibodies to different functional subpopulations of T cells. (For a discussion of monoclonal antibodies see Chapter 6.)

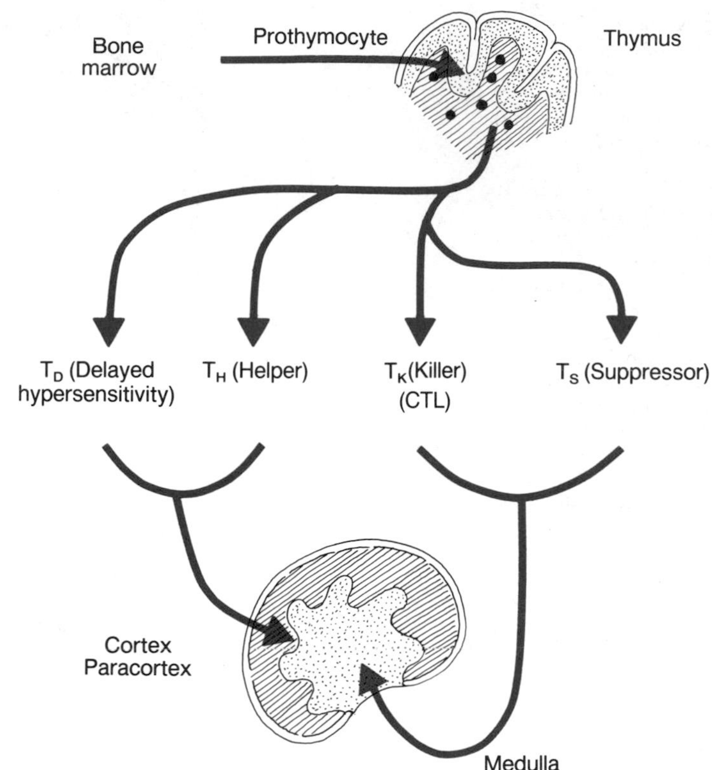

Figure 4-3. Functional differentiation of T cell subpopulations. T cells arise from prothymocyte precursors that pass through a developmental stage in the thymus. The T cell population may be identified by cell surface markers (see Table 4-1). Helper cells (T_H) are generally found in the paracortex of the lymph node, whereas T_K and T_S cells are found in the medulla.

Table 4-1. Phenotypic Markers for Major Lymphocyte Subpopulations

Human Marker[a]	Mouse Equivalent	Function
T_{11} (CD2)	Thy	Precursor
T_4 (CD4)	L3T4	Helper–inducer–DTH
T_8 (CD8)	Ly2	Suppressor, cytotoxic
9.3	—	(?) Killer

[a] See Appendix B: Cluster Designations.

Phenotypic Markers of Human T Cell Subpopulations

Human T cell differentiation markers are recognized by monoclonal antibodies (see Chapter 6) and are present on lymphocytes in different organs (Table 4-2, Fig. 4-4). The phenotypic specificities recognized by different monoclonal antibodies are now termed *cluster designations* (see Appendix). The CD4 and CD8 subpopulations in peripheral lymphoid organs generally correlate with the major functional populations of T cells, although the major difference between these two subsets is probably their ability to recognize self markers.

Two of the monoclonal antibodies listed (anti-TAC and anti-T_9) react with activated T cells. Anti-TAC recognizes the interleukin 2 (IL2) receptor (see Chapter 10), and anti-T_9 the transferrin receptor. The fact that anti-TAC does not react with activated B cells suggests that B cell activation requires binding of IL2 by a different receptor (see Chapter 10).

Table 4-2. Monoclonal Antibodies to Human T Lymphocyte Surface Antigens

Monoclonal Antibodies	Molecular Weight of Molecules (nonreduced)	Population Defined	Comments	Commercial Names	Cluster Designation[a]
PAN-T CELL					
Anti-T_1	69K	All mature T cells, medullary thymocytes, and at low density on cortical thymocytes	Homologue of murine Lyt1	Anti-T_{1_A}, Leu1, OKT1	CD5
Anti-T_3	20K	All mature T cells and medullary thymocytes	Modulates antigen-specific T cell responses; is mitogenic for resting T cells; is part of the T cell receptor complex	Anti-T_{3_A}, Leu4, OKT_3	CD3
Anti-T_{11}	55K	All thymocytes and T cells	E rosette associated protein; greatest density on thymocytes and suppressor T cells	Anti-T_{11}, 9.6, Leu5, OKT_{11}	CD2
T CELL SUBSET					
Anti-T_4	62K	Majority of thymocytes and 50–65% of peripheral T cells	$T4^+$ T cells contain most inducer helper functions; functions are class II MHC restricted	Anti-T_{4_A}, Leu3a,b, OKT_4	CD4
Anti-$T_8(T_5)$	76K	Majority of thymocytes and 25–35% of peripheral T cells	$T8^+$ peripheral T cells contain most suppressor functions; functions are class I MHC restricted	Anti-T_{8_a}, Leu2a,b, OKT_8	CD8
Anti-T_6	49K	70–80% of thymocytes	Specific for cortical thymocytes, β_2 M associated, homologous to murine TL	Anti-T_{6_A}, Leu6, OKT_6, Na1/34	CD1
INDUCIBLE ACTIVATION MARKER					
Anti-TAC	55K	5% of peripheral T cells, majority of activated T cells	Recognizes IL2 receptor; blocks proliferation and IL2 binding; inducible by antigen or mitogen		CD25
Anti-T_9	44K	10% thymocytes, majority of activated T cells	Transferrin receptor		None
CLONOTYPE MARKER					
Anti-Ti	92K dimer	Individual T cell clones in culture, 2–5% of T cells in vivo	Anti-variable region of T cell receptor		None

Anti-T designations are available through Coulter Electronics, Hialeah, Fla.; Leu designations through Becton–Dickinson, Mountain View, Calif.; OK designations through Ortho Pharmaceutical, Raritan, N.J.; Na1/34 through Accurate Chemicals, New Jersey.

[a] See Appendix: Cluster Designations.

Modified from Immunology Today, Sept 1982 (Reinherz E, Schlossman S, advisors).

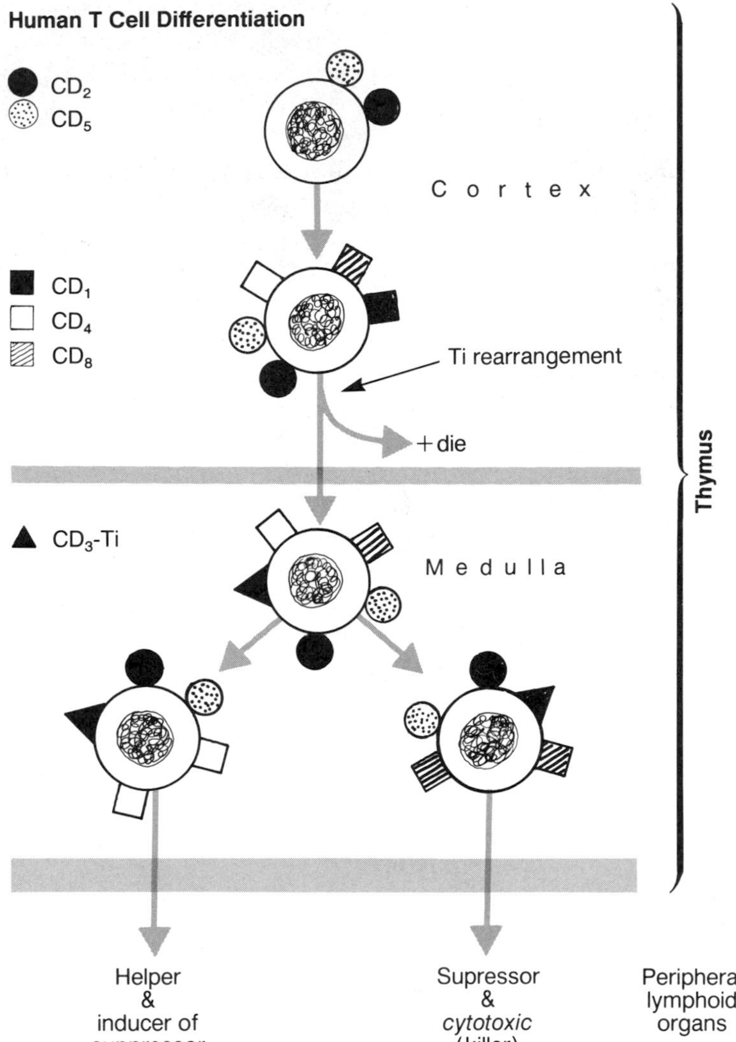

Figure 4-4. Differentiation markers of human thymocytes and T cells. *Thymocytes* refers to cells in the thymus, *T cells* to thymus-derived cells that have matured in the thymus and have migrated to peripheral lymphoid organs. The first identifiable marker is CD2; CD1, CD4, and CD8 are acquired as the cortical thymocytes mature. In medullary thymocytes, CD1 is lost and CD3 is acquired. As a final differentiation step before leaving the thymus, CD4 and CD8 segregate with two separate populations. CD4 denotes the helper–inducer population and CD8 the suppressor–cytotoxic population.

Thymic Hormones

Thymic endocrine epithelial cells produce factors known as *thymic hormones* that induce phenotypic maturation of thymocytes. Over 20 factors have been described; the four most extensively studied are listed in Table 4-3. Each of these factors added

Table 4-3. A Summary of Thymic Humoral Factor Effects

	T Cell Induction	B Cell Induction	Mitogenic	cGMP or cAMP	MLR[a]	Helper[b]	Suppressor[b]
Thymosin	+	0	+	cGMP	+	+	+
Thymopoietin	+	+	+	cGMP	+	+	+
Thymic humoral factor	+	+	+	cAMP	+	+	
Facteur thymique serique (thymulin)	+	+	0	cAMP	0	+	+

[a] MLR—induce ability to respond to mixed lymphocyte reaction.
[b] Helper, suppressor—induce these functions in thymocytes.

in vitro to thymus cells has the property of inducing the appearance of T cell differentiation markers, activating cyclic guanosine monophosphate (cGMP) or cyclic adenosine monophosphate (cAMP) and inducing mature T cell functions.

Natural Killer and Killer Cells

Natural cell-mediated cytotoxic activity is measured by lysis of selected tumor target cells (see Chapter 8). *Natural killer (NK)* cells share some properties of T cells and macrophages (Table 4-4). NK cells are nonadherent lymphocytes that reside in the spleen, peripheral blood, and lungs of most mammals. Much controversy has developed as to the lineage of these cells. Although NK cells are hemopoietically derived from the bone marrow, it is not known whether these cells differentiate from classic B or T cell precursors. Even though NK cells have been found to share several surface antigens with B cells, NK lymphocytes are not involved in antibody production. NK cells also

Table 4-4. Comparison of NK/K Cells with T Cells and Macrophages

Characteristic	LGL Property	Similar to	
		T Cell	Macrophage
Size	16–20 nm		+
Cytoplasmic/nuclear ratio	High ratio		+
Nuclear shape	Lobed or indented		+
Adherence	Nonadherent	+	
Phagocytosis	Nonphagocytic	+	
Nonspecific esterase	Absent	+	
Acid phosphatase	Present	+	+
α-Glucuronidase	In granules		+
Surface antigens	Several shared with other cell types		
Fc receptors for IgG	Shared with PMN		
Spontaneous reactivity	Present in vivo		+
Period to develop augmented effector activity	Short (minutes–hours)		+
Memory response	None		+
ADCC	Very effective		+
Activating factors	Interferon (α, β, γ)	+	+
	Interleukin 2	+	+
	Bacterial products		+
Inhibiting factors	Prostaglandin E	+	+
	Phorbol esters		+

PMN, polymorphonuclear leukocytes; ADCC, antibody-dependent cell-mediated cytotoxicity.
Modified from Ortaldo JR, Herberman RB: Annu Rev Immunol 21:359, 1984.

share some similar functional activities, such as their cytolytic mechanisms, with cytolytic T lymphocytes (CTL). What functionally distinguishes NK cells from CTLs is their capacity to lyse a variety of tumor cells without prior sensitization.

NK cells appear to have receptors that recognize target cells and have specificity for a given target cell, but the nature of the receptor is not known. By means of cross competition assays (cold target cell inhibition), it has been shown that suspensions of normal lymphocytes contain different subpopulations of NK cells specific for different target cells, and not all target cell lines are susceptible to NK cells.

Because of the presence of large cytoplasmic granules within NK cells these lymphocytes are referred to as LGL (large-granule lymphocytes). These cytoplasmic granules (lysosomes) of LGL contain enzymes and factors that cause lysis of target cells. Unlike that of T cells the cytotoxicity of NK cells is not MHC restricted. NK cells lyse a large variety of targets including leukemia cells, cells from carcinomas, and several types of normal cells. NK activity is increased by infections and IL2. NK cells activated by IL2 (lymphokine-activated killer cells, LAK) are now being tested for effects on cancer in humans. NK activity is regulated by suppressor cells, both T's and macrophages. The role of NK cells in vivo is not clear, but they are believed to have an important role in immunity to cancer as well as to certain viral infections.

NK cells were not recognized for some time because investigators considered the cytolytic activity of normal cell populations as background in their assays. For instance, comparisons of killing activity were made using lymphocytes from normal donors and lymphocytes from immunized donors. The lytic effect of the normal lymphocyte cell population, such as amount of ^{51}Cr release or inhibition of target cell growth, was considered background and subtracted from the effect of the immunized cell population. However, it was discovered that the effects of the nonimmune cells were due to a population of cells different from that of the immune cells, that is, null cells, not T cytotoxic cells.

Another population of *killer* cells (K cells) have receptors for the Fc or IgG and are able to bind IgG antibodies; they are directed to lyse target cells to which the antibody is directed (antibody-dependent cell-mediated cytotoxicity, ADCC). ADCC cells have been designated K cells, but it appears that NK and K cells may be the same, the difference being the direction of the killing activity by antibody (see Chapter 8).

B Cell Differentiation

Bone marrow stem cells are influenced by the environment of the bone marrow, liver, and gastrointestinal tract to differentiate into B cells, the precursors of plasma cells (Fig. 4-5). B cells differentiate into plasma cells after induction of specific

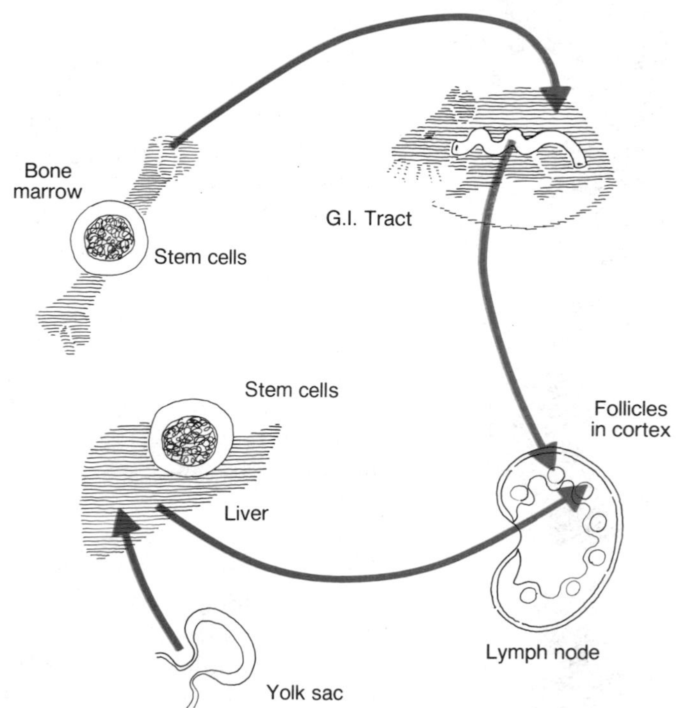

Figure 4-5. B cell differentiation. Precursors of antibody-producing plasma cells, B cells, arise from bone marrow or liver stem cells. For full development of B cells in birds, the inductive microenvironment of a gastrointestinal lymphoid organ, the bursa of Fabricius, is needed. In mammals this function may be provided by the liver or may occur in the bone marrow. B cells migrate to follicular areas of other lymphoid organs (i.e., lymph node cortex).

antibody responses by antigen. Thus, B cell differentiation is antigen independent, whereas plasma cell differentiation is antigen dependent. Differentiated plasma cells produce only one antibody of one specificity and immunoglobulin of only one class.

In mammals, the actual site of B cell differentiation remains uncertain. In birds, a special lymphoid organ, the bursa of Fabricius, located near the anus, is clearly responsible for B cell maturation. Surgical removal of the bursa at hatching leads to a lack of development of B cells and a deficiency in immunoglobulin production. In mammals, however, a clear-cut role for the gastrointestinal lymphoid tissue in B cell differentiation has not been demonstrated. There is evidence that B cells may arise in the fetal liver, or yolk sac, from stem cells that arise in the bone marrow and migrate to the liver, or from stem cells present in the fetal liver. The fetal liver and yolk sac are major blood cell–forming organs in fetal life and contain hematopoietic stem cells. Therefore B cells could arise directly in the liver in infants as well.

After B cells develop, they migrate to the B cell areas of other lymphoid organs. B cells are generally localized in lymphoid follicles of lymph node, spleen, and gastrointestinal lymphoid tissue. B cell maturation may depend on humoral factors produced by epithelial tissue in the inductive microenvironments. A factor extracted from the bursa of Fabricius of chicken, bursapoietin, apparently induces differentiation of bone marrow B cell precursors. Another factor, ubiquitin, may be extracted from thymus as well as other tissues. Ubiquitin induces differentiation of both T cells and B cells in vitro and may function as a receptor molecule for homing of circulatory lymphocytes. Again, the in vivo significance of these factors remains unclear. Attempts to restore immune competence in patients with immune deficiencies using such factors have not yet provided convincing beneficial effects. Maturation of B cells includes an antigen-independent stage and an antigen-dependent stage reflected by sequential immunoglobulin gene rearrangements and expression of cytoplasmic or cell surface immunoglobulins. Antigen-dependent B cell maturation is covered in Chapter 6.

Summary

A composite scheme of T and B cell development is shown in Figure 4-1. Both T and B cell precursors arise from a common lymphoid precursor. Lymphocytes that home to the thymus differentiate under the influence of thymic hormones produced by endocrine cells in the medulla. These cells leave the thymus as T cells (thymus-derived cells) and home via high endothelial venules to thymus-dependent pericortical zones in the lymph node. Phenotypic markers identified by monoclonal antibodies reflect T cell maturation. Functional T cells include T helper/inducer cells detected by the CD4 markers and T suppressor/cytotoxic cells detected by the CD8 markers. Functional T cells recognize antigen by a specific cell surface receptor. Cytotoxic cells without T cell or B cell markers are NK and K cells. NK cells kill certain target cells in vitro due to unstimulated recognition; K cells recognize target cells by passively absorbed antibodies (ADCC).

The site of B cell differentiation in mammals is not clearly defined. In birds, B cell maturation occurs in association with cloacal epithelium in the bursa of Fabricius. B cell maturation in mammals may occur in the gastrointestinal tract, fetal liver, yolk sac, or bone marrow.

In peripheral lymphoid organs T cells and B cells are located in different domains, but are able to cooperate in induction and control of immune responses (see Chapter 10).

References

T Cell Development

Auerbach R: Experimental analysis of the origin of cell types in the developing thymus. Dev Biol 3:336, 1961.

Cordier AC, Haumont SM: Development of thymus, parathyroids, and ultimo-branchial bodies in NMRI and nude mice. Am J Anat 15:227, 1980.

Goldstein G. Lymphocyte differentiations induced by thymopoietin, bursapoietin and ubiquitin. *In* Rutter WJ, Papaconstantinou J (eds): Molecular Control of Proliferation and Differentiation. New York, Academic Press, 1977.

Good RA, Gabrielsen AE (eds): The Thymus in Immunobiology. New York, Harper & Row, 1985.

Haynes BF: Phenotypic characterization and ontogeny of components of the human thymic microenvironment. Clin Res 32:500, 1984.

Komuro K, Boyse EA: Induction of T lymphocytes from precursor cells in vitro by a product of the thymus. J Exp Med 138:479, 1973.

Miller JFAP, Osoba D: Current concepts of the immunological function of the thymus. Physiol Rev 47:437, 1967.

Moller G (ed): Functional T cell subsets defined by monoclonal antibodies. Immunol Rev 74, 1983.

Moller G (ed): T cell antigens. Immunol Rev 82, 1984.

Owen JJT, Jenkenson EJ: Early events in T lymphocyte genesis in the fetal thymus. Am J Anat 170:301, 1984.

Romain PL, Schlossman SF: Human T lymphocyte subsets. J Clin Invest 74:1559, 1984.

Stutman O, Good RA: Thymus hormones. Contemp Top Immunol 2:299, 1973.

Tamaki K, Stingl G, Katz SI: The origin of Langerhans cells. J Invest Dermatol 74:309, 1980.

Tranin N, Small M: Thymic humoral factors. Contemp Top Immunol 2:321, 1973.

Turpen JB, Cohen N: Localization of thymocyte stem cell precursors in the pharyngeal endoderm of early amphibian embryos. Cell Immunol 24:109, 1976.

Turpen JB, Volpe EP, Cohen N: On the origin of thymic lymphocytes. Am Zool 15:51, 1975.

Van Ewjk W: Immunohistology of lymphoid and non-lymphoid cells in the thymus in relation to T cell differentiation. Am J Anat 170:311, 1984.

Natural Killer and Killer Cells

Herberman RB: Natural killer cells. Annu Rev Med 37:347, 1986.

Herberman RB, Callewert D (eds): Mechanisms of Cytotoxicity by NK cells. Orlando, Fla., Academic Press, 1985.

Herberman RB, Reynolds CW, Ortaldo JR: Mechanism of cytotoxicity by natural killer (NK) cells. Annu Rev Immunol 4:651, 1986.

Moller G (ed): Natural killer cells. Transplant Rev 44, 1979.

Ortaldo JR, Herberman RB: Heterogeneity of natural killer cells. Annu Rev Immunol 2:359, 1984.

Pross HF, Baines MG: Spontaneous human lymphocyte–mediated cytotoxicity against tumor target cells. Cancer Immunol Immunother 3:75, 1977.

Rosenberg EB, Herberman RB, Levin PH: Lymphocytotoxicity reactions to leukemia-associated antigens in identical tumors. Int J Cancer 9:648, 1972.

Timonen T, Ortaldo JR, Herberman RB: Characteristics of human large granular lymphocytes and relationship to natural killer and K cells. J Exp Med 153:569, 1982.

B Cell Development

Cooper MD, Peterson RDA, South MA, Good RA: The functions of the thymus system and the bursa system in the chicken. J Exp Med 133:75, 1966.

Cooper MD, Lawton AR: The development of the immune system. Sci Am 231:58, 1974.

Cooper MD, Lawton AR: The mammalian "bursa equivalent." Does lymphoid differentiation along plasma cell lines begin in gut-associated lymphoepithelial tissues (GALT) of mammals? Contemp Top Immunobiol 1:49, 1972.

Hamaoka T, Ono S: Regulation of B cell differentiation. Annu Rev Immunol 4:167, 1986.

Hanley-Hyde JM, Lynch RC: The physiology of B cells as studied with tumor models. Annu Rev Immunol 4:621, 1986.

Moller G (ed): Ontogeny of human lymphocyte function. Immunol Rev 57, 1981.

Moller G (ed): B cell differentiation antigens. Immunol Rev 69, 1983.

Moller G (ed): B cell growth and differentiation factors. Immunol Rev 78, 1984.

Sell S: Development of restrictions in the expression of immunoglobulin specificities by lymphoid cells. Transplant Rev 5:19, 1970.

Shields JW: Bursal dissections and gill pouch hormones. Nature 259:373, 1976.

5 Antigenicity and Immunogenicity

The unique feature of the adaptive immune system is its ability to recognize foreign molecules and produce new products (antibodies and cells) that react specifically with the foreign molecules (antigens). This process is called immunization. The essence of an immune or allergic response is the capacity to recognize and react to an antigen.

Antigens and Immunogens

An *antigen* is a molecular species capable of inducing an immune response and of being recognized by antibody and/or sensitized cells manufactured as a consequence of the immune response (Fig. 5-1). The ability of material to induce an immune

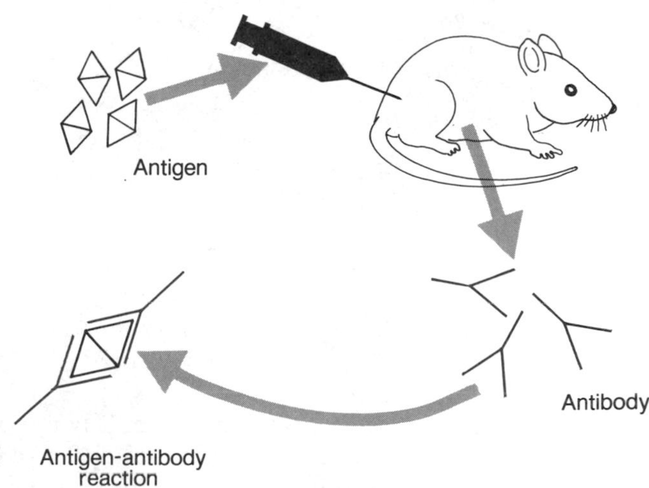

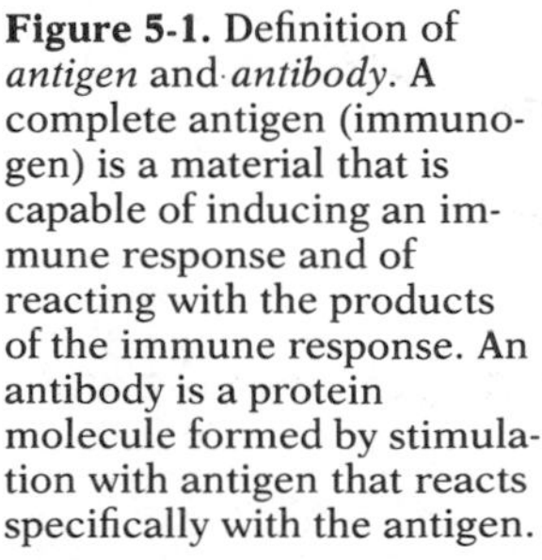

Figure 5-1. Definition of *antigen* and *antibody*. A complete antigen (immunogen) is a material that is capable of inducing an immune response and of reacting with the products of the immune response. An antibody is a protein molecule formed by stimulation with antigen that reacts specifically with the antigen.

response is referred to as *immunogenicity*, and such a material is called an *immunogen*. The ability of an antigen to react with the products of an immune response is referred to as *antigenicity*. The immune products in serum (blood without fibrin and cells) that react with antigen are *antibodies*. Antibodies join to antigen by noncovalent binding of sites that can be juxtaposed because of a physical "lock and key" relationship (see Chapter 7). Serum containing specific antibody activity is called *antiserum*.

Complete and Incomplete Antigens

A complete antigen is one that can both induce an immune response and react with the products of that response. An incomplete antigen (hapten) is a chemically active substance of low molecular weight that is unable to induce an immune response by itself but can, by combining with larger molecules (carriers), become immunogenic. A complete antigen is both an immunogen and an antigen, whereas an incomplete antigen is not an immunogen but is an antigen. For example, a chemically active small molecule such as dinitrophenol (an incomplete antigen) may combine with a protein of the host's such as serum albumin to form a complete antigen, so that sensitization occurs (Fig. 5-2). An individual thus sensitized reacts with the

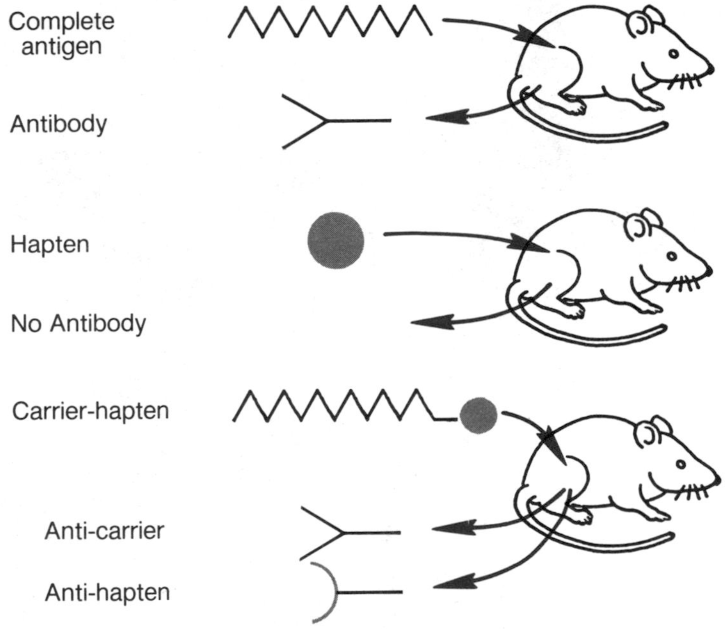

Figure 5-2. Carrier–hapten relationship in immunization. A complete antigen (immunogen) both induces an immune response and reacts with the antibody produced. Haptens are incomplete antigens. Incomplete antigens are *not* able to induce an immune response alone, but antibody can be induced if the hapten is complexed to a complete antigen.

dinitrophenol upon second contact with it because of the antibodies previously formed.

T-Dependent and T-Independent Antigens

Antibodies come from B lymphocytes, often with the help of T lymphocytes. In most hapten–carrier systems, B cells produce antibody specific for the hapten as well as the carrier, whereas T helper cells are specific for the carrier and do not recognize the hapten. Together T and B cells cooperate to induce a hapten-specific antibody response. Most protein antigens are thymus dependent.

Thymus-independent antigens, often polysaccharides, can elicit antibody production by B cells without T cell help.

Interaction of T-independent antigens directly with B cell surface receptors is sufficient to activate B cells directly.

The antibody molecules formed after immunization may express a variety of antigen-binding specificities, that is, recognize different structures on a complex multideterminant antigen. If the inducing antigenic specificity is limited to a small chemical group, the specificity of antibody binding may be exquisitely specific; if the immunogen is a large molecule, a large number of overlapping antigen-binding specificities may be represented in the antibody formed (see Chapter 7).

Epitopes and Paratopes

The parts of antigens bound by antigen-binding sites of antibody molecules (the antigenic determinants) are called *epitopes*.

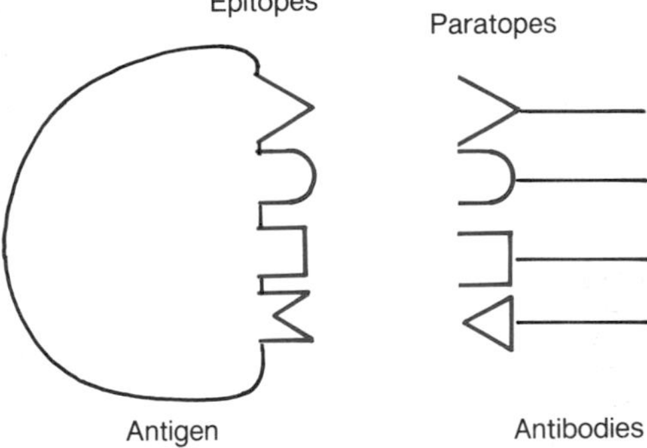

Figure 5-3. An antigen with four epitopes and antibodies with four different paratopes are represented schematically. The complexity of the antibodies is greatly increased by the fact that each epitope may be recognized from different structural aspects. Thus different antibodies with different paratopes could bind to the same epitope.

That portion of the antibody molecule that binds to the epitope is called the *paratope* (Fig. 5-3). Each antigen usually contains more than one epitope. Usually these are present on the surface of the antigen, but denaturation or unfolding of the antigen may reveal or create other epitopes. Most antigenic determinants (epitopes) are created by folding of the polypeptide chain to form overlapping antigenic surface domains (Fig. 5-4). Thus the epitopes of a protein may be sequential or assembled. Se-

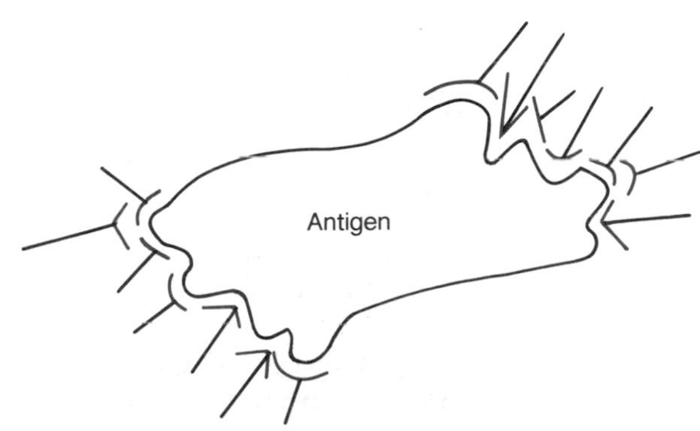

Figure 5-4. Schematic representation of antigenic determinants (epitopes) on a large antigenic macromolecule. Epitopes with which antibodies react are clustered at two "poles" of the molecule. Epitopes are determined by folding of the polypeptide chain to provide surface determinants. Amino acids distant in the linear sequence of the polypeptide chain are found together in the epitope.

quential epitopes are determined only by the amino acid sequence of the peptide sequence involved; assembled determinants are formed by bringing amino acids together by folding of the peptide chain of the molecule. Conformational folding brings together residues that are far apart in the primary sequence but end up close together on the folded protein. Most epitopes are conformational. Short polypeptides may inhibit binding of antibody to the complete native antigen but require a large molar excess to do so. Thus, these polypeptide fragments most likely contain only part of the epitope defined by the assembled determinant.

Chemical Nature of Antigens

Many different kinds of molecules may serve as antigens (Table 5-1). Heavy metals and small organic compounds may function as haptens, whereas most complete antigens are large molecules (macromolecules).

Table 5-1. Chemical Classes of Antigens

Type	Example
Metals	Nickel
Organic chemicals	Dinitrophenol, phenylarsonate
Proteins	Serum proteins, enzymes, microbial toxins
Lipoproteins	Cell membranes
Polysaccharides	Capsules of bacteria
Glycoproteins	Blood group substances (branched polysaccharides)
Polypeptides	Hormones (insulin), synthetic compounds (poly-L-lysine)
Nucleoprotein	Lupus erythematosus factor
RNA	Lupus erythematosus factor
DNA	Lupus erythematosus factor

Physical Properties of Antigens

Size, shape, rigidity, location of determinants, and tertiary structure affect antigenicity.

Size

Complete antigens (immunogens) usually have a high molecular weight (MW). Some naturally occurring immunogens may have a fairly low molecular weight, such as ribonuclease (MW 14,000), insulin (MW 6000), and angiotensin (MW 1031).

The size of an antigenic determinant or epitope may be estimated by determining the ability of a series of antigens of increasing molecular size to inhibit the reaction of antibody with the complete antigen of which the smaller compound is only a part. The smallest molecule that inhibits is considered to contain the complete epitope. Antibodies to dextran polysaccharide are optimally inhibited by six-unit saccharides (MW 990), and antibodies to polypeptides are optimally inhibited by four- to five-amino-acid oligopeptides (MW 650). Short polymers of amino acids are not usually immunogenic, but will function as haptens if added to carrier molecules such as a serum protein or if altered chemically to form a new antigenic site. Poly-L-lysine is not immunogenic, but the attachment of a dinitrophenyl (DNP) group to poly-L-lysine may establish immunogenicity of either the DNP or the poly-L-lysine. DNP-L-lysine$_7$ is immunogenic, but DNP-L-lysine$_6$ is not. In addition, L-lysine$_5$ inhibits the reaction of anti-L-lysine antibody with poly-L-lysine$_7$. Therefore a larger molecule is usually required to induce an immune response than is necessary to react with antibody. The more epitopes, the more likely that an antigen will be "complete," that is, immunogenic.

Shape

The shape of a determinant is important. Certain components, such as the DNP in DNP-L-lysine$_7$, give form to a molecule that is evidently not found in the homologous polymer. Copolymers of two amino acids may be immunogenic for some species, whereas polymers of one amino acid are not. The presence of more than one amino acid in a polymer results in a configuration not available in the polymer of a single amino acid. The location of a structure within a determinant may also be important.

The nature of antigenic determinants has been analyzed by study of the reaction of antibody with incomplete antigens (haptens). A hapten of known structure, such as *p*-azobenzoate, may be joined to an immunogen, such as bovine serum albumin. Immunization with bovine serum albumin chemically complexed with *p*-azobenzoate will stimulate antibodies to *p*-

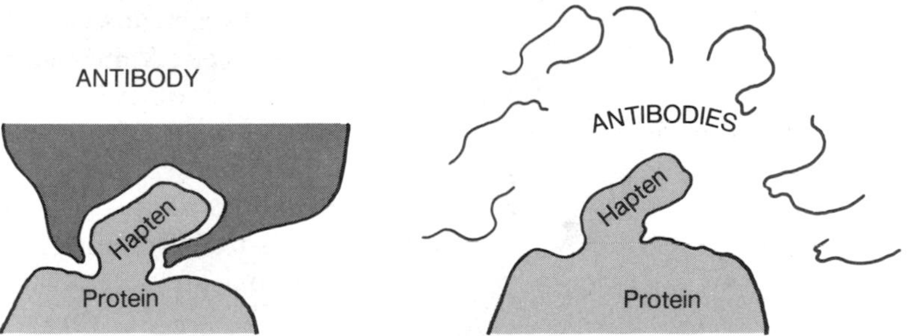

Figure 5-5. Heterogeneity of antigen-binding specificities of antibodies is demonstrated. In the serum of an animal immunized to a hapten, a mixture of antibodies with different specificities and avidities may be detected. The outline of the hapten represents van der Waal's outline of the haptenic group *p*-azobenzoate coupled to a protein carrier. The drawing on the left represents an idealized antibody for the hapten that would have a perfect fit for the haptenic determinant. Antibodies actually produced to such a hapten (right) consist of separate molecules that bind specifically to different parts of the hapten. Some antibodies bind to certain parts of the determinant and other antibodies to other parts, with varying degree of overlapping specificity. (Adapted from Kitagawa M, Yagi Y, Pressman D: J Immunol 95:455, 1965.)

azobenzoate as well as antibodies to the albumin. The heterogeneity of antibodies formed to *p*-azobenzoate is illustrated in Figure 5-5. As can be seen from this illustration, a large variety of antibodies with different binding specificities are produced. It is clear from the heterogeneity of antibodies to this relatively simple antigen that the antibodies formed to larger antigens such as the carrier albumin molecule may be extremely complex.

In many cases, immunizing with a complex antigen containing multiple epitopes leads primarily to production of antibody to one epitope, which is termed the immunodominant epitope of the antigen.

Rigidity

The role of rigidity and location of determinants in antigenicity is exemplified by the alteration in immunogenicity and antigenicity of gelatin by the addition of poly-L-tyrosine to the gelatin backbone. Gelatin, which may have a very high molecular weight, is almost completely nonimmunogenic. Addition of 1% tyrosine increases the immunogenicity and antigenicity of gelatin, and the specificity of antibody produced is directed toward the gelatin. Addition of tyrosine evidently makes the gelatin structure more stable or rigid. Addition of 3% to 10% tyrosine to gelatin changes the immunogenic capacity and results in the production of antibody with specificity directed toward the tyrosine; that is, all the antibody activity can be removed by absorption with poly-L-tyrosine and none by gelatin.

Determinant Location

Important antigenic determinants may be secluded inside large molecules and may be exposed by unfolding of the molecule. If the tyrosine is buried inside a tyrosine–gelatin molecule, it does not function as an antigen, but if the tyrosine is placed on the surface of the molecule, it is recognized. In addition, new determinants may be exposed by partial denaturation of proteins. Denaturation of a protein generally destroys its immunogenicity and antigenicity. However, partial denaturation may result in exposure of different configurations by altering the tertiary structure. This creates new antigenic determinants.

Tertiary Structure

Tertiary structure of proteins (spatial folding) is important in determining the specificity of an antibody response. Antibodies produced to the isolated alpha chains of insulin do not react with the intact molecule, which is an alpha–beta chain dimer. Reduction and reoxidation of ribonuclease under controlled conditions produce a mixture of refolded protein molecules differing only in tertiary structure. Some antisera to native ribonuclease are unreactive with these refolded, denatured molecules; other antisera to the native molecule do react with the refolded forms. Thus, the tertiary structure of antigens is recognized by antibodies and is important for affinity and specificity of binding.

Catabolism

The ability to catabolize or break down the antigen is important for the induction of an immune response. Catabolism of immunogens occurs in macrophages where they are complexed to self molecules. It is critical that the immunogen not be completely catabolized, or the antigenic determinants would be destroyed. L-Amino acid heteropolymers are catabolizable and are immunogenic, whereas D-amino acid heteropolymers are not catabolizable and are poorly immunogenic. The immunogenicity of D-amino acid polymers is dependent upon dose in mice and rabbits. The response to D-isomers exhibits a strong maximum at about 1 μg per mouse, but that to L-isomers is largely independent of dose. Therefore, the failure to detect responses to the poorly catabolized D-isomers may be due to selection of a nonimmunizing dose. Antibody formed to poorly catabolized immunogens may be difficult to demonstrate because of blocking or binding of the antibody formed with the noncatabolized antigen still present in the serum.

Partial antigen degradation or processing is a critical step in the cell–cell interactions between macrophages and T cells. Without antigen processing, T cells will not respond to the "carrier" determinants, leaving the B cells without T cell help.

Immunization

Immunogenicity is determined not only by the nature of the antigen, but also by the characteristics of the responding individual and the manner in which the antigen is presented. Contact between immunogens and responding individuals may occur by natural exposure to organisms, chemicals, or other immunogens in the environment, or may be artificially induced by controlled immunization. The following factors are involved in any controlled immunization and the detection of a subsequent immune response: (1) the source of the antigen, (2) the preparation of the antigen, (3) the form in which the antigen is given, (4) the route of immunization or anatomic location of initial contact, (5) the dose of antigen, (6) the time between the immunizing event and the testing for antibody or sensitized cells, (7) the number of immunizations given (primary or secondary response), (8) the type of test procedure employed, (9) the genetic makeup of the responding animal, and (10) the physiological condition of the responding animal (see Table 5-2). Given such a number of variables, some generalizations may be made, but in practice each immunizing situation must be evaluated individually.

Immunization is performed clinically to induce a protective response, as in vaccination with attenuated or avirulent polioviruses or diphtheria toxoid. Experimental immunization may be performed to explore immune reactions or to produce an antiserum that might be used as an immunochemical reagent. The reasons for performing a certain immunization determine, to a large extent, how it is given.

Table 5-2. Some Factors Determining Immunogenicity

Factor	Nature of Effect
ANTIGEN PROPERTY	
1. Source	Degree of foreignness; more evolutionarily distant source gives greater response
2. Preparation	Degree of purity determines extent of response and specificity
3. Form	More complex antigens are more immunogenic; particulate—DTH,[a] soluble—humoral antibody, adjuvants—enhance response
4. Route	Skin—DTH, intravascular—humoral antibody
5. Dose	Low-dose—DTH, high-dose—antibody, very low and very high doses—tolerance
6. Time	Antibody titer and type change with time after immunization
7. Number of exposures	Multiple exposures cause higher titers and sharpen specificity of response, but can also stimulate control pathways, decreasing response
8. Test procedure	Ability to detect immune products depends on sensitivity of test procedure
RESPONDER PROPERTY	
1. Genetics	High and low responders to certain antigens, genetically controlled
2. Physiological condition	Age, drugs, etc., affect response; nutrition, sex, pregnancy, hormones, stress, radiation, other infections

[a] DTH, delayed type hypersensitivity.

Source of Antigen

The source of antigen depends upon the purpose of the immunization. For protective immune responses, individuals may be immunized with living attenuated or killed infectious agents or with nontoxic extracts. In some cases, live attenuated vaccines are preferable, while in other cases, killed vaccines can immunize effectively. In experimental situations, an individual may be immunized with the serum proteins or tissues of another individual of the same or a different species, or with laboratory-synthesized material such as hapten-modified carriers or synthetic polypeptides.

As previously emphasized, one of the important features of reacting individuals is the ability to recognize foreignness. One of the ways to classify antigens is by the relationship of source of the antigen to the individual responding to the antigen. The classification given in Table 5-3 is used primarily for tissue transplantation but may be applied to all antigens.

In general the intensity of an immune response will be directly related to the degree of foreignness. Fortunately, autoimmune responses are of relatively low intensity as compared with immune responses to foreign antigens *(xenogeneic)*. An antigen that comes from the same individual or is present in that individual is an endogenous antigen; one that comes from outside the responding individual is an exogenous antigen.

Table 5-3. Source of Antigens

Source Term	Relationship to Responding Individual	Example in Humans
Xenogeneic (heterologous)[a]	Different species	Infectious organisms, animal graft
Allogeneic (homologous)	Same species, different individual	Tissue graft from another human, blood transfusion
Syngeneic (isologous)	Genetically identical individual	Tissue graft or transfusion from identical twin
Autologous	Same individual	Autoimmunity

[a] The terms in parentheses are those commonly employed in blood banks.

Preparation of Antigen

The final preparation of an antigen used for immunization depends upon the degree of specificity desired. For example, immunization of a rabbit with rat spleen produces an antiserum that reacts with various cell populations in the spleen (erythrocytes, lymphocytes, macrophages) and with as many as 30 different plasma proteins. By careful removal of the cellular elements or by immunization with rat serum (defibrinated rat plasma), a rabbit antiserum that reacts with rat serum proteins may be obtained (rabbit anti–whole rat serum). By chemical fractionation of the rat serum an antigen preparation may be obtained that contains only one serum protein. Immunization with this preparation will result in a protein-specific antiserum (rabbit anti–rat albumin). Further fractionation of an antigenic molecule may be accomplished by breaking the molecule into smaller units; an antiserum that reacts with only part of the molecule may thus be obtained.

Form in Which Antigen Is Given

The form in which an antigen is administered also may vary. A serum protein may be administered in soluble form. It may also be mixed with agents that will effectively increase the immune response (adjuvant). Precipitation with alum may result in a greater antibody response. An intense mononuclear infiltration at the site of injection is induced by injection of antigen incorporated into an oil-in-water emulsion. This greatly enhances the immune response. Many other variations may be employed to modify the nature and extent of the immune response. A partial list of adjuvants is given in Table 5-4.

Table 5-4. Some Commonly Used Adjuvants

Freund's complete adjuvant (emulsion of mineral oil, water, and mycobacterial extracts)
Freund's incomplete adjuvant (emulsion of water and oil only)
Aluminum hydroxide gels (alum)
Sodium alginate
Bordatella pertussis
Synthetic polynucleotide (poly(A:U))
Muramyl dipeptide

Route of Immunization

The routes of immunization of animals include intradermal, subcutaneous, intramuscular, intraperitoneal, intravascular, and intracranial injections, as well as injection into any organ. In addition, immunization may be accomplished by ingestion, inhalation, skin application, rectal infusion, or intratracheal infusion. The type of immune response elicited depends upon the route used. Those routes that lead to distribution in vascular spaces generally lead to the formation of humoral antibodies, whereas those routes that lead to focal deposition in peripheral lymphoid tissue (intradermal injection or application on the skin surface) tend to induce cellular sensitivity. Inoculation into organs of external secretion, such as salivary glands, breast, or nasal mucosa, may result in the production of antibodies of a different class of immunoglobulin (IgA) than would be found following intramuscular injection (IgG). IgA is the major class of immunoglobulin found in secretions. (For a discussion of immunoglobulin classes of antibody, see Chapter 6.)

Dose of Antigen

The amount of antigen given is extremely important, because too little or too much may result in a loss of immune responsiveness. One microgram of any antigen is usually enough to induce an immune response. Smaller amounts (as little as 1 ng) may actually induce tolerance (see Chapter 11), depending on the purity of the antigen. If a specific antiserum is desired, the purest possible antigen preparation should be used. Otherwise, trace contamination with undesirable antigens may result in the production of an antiserum with multiple specificities.

Interval between Immunization and Testing

In most controlled immunizations circulating antibody does not appear in significant amounts until 7 to 10 days after immunization. The immunoglobulin class of antibody produced also changes with time. Early antibodies are usually of the IgM class, whereas later antibodies are of the IgG class. Also, late antibodies may bind more strongly to antigens than do early antibodies (see Chapter 7). Usually after 3 to 5 weeks the amount of antibody produced starts to decline, so that later blood analyses give lower titers of antibody.

Immunization Schedule

The amount of antibody formed after the second injection of a given antigen (secondary or memory response) usually is much greater than that formed after one injection (primary response) (Fig. 5-6). If high-titered antiserum is desired, a series of injections is commonly given. However, after three or more injections, the titer of antibody may be smaller than that after only two injections. The antibody formed after a second injection of antigen (booster) tends to be of the IgG class and more avid (binding more strongly to antigen) than the antibody formed after one injection, which may be of the IgM class. Each bleeding of an immunized animal may yield antibody of different titer, of different avidity, and perhaps of different specificity. Each blood sample must be separately tested to ensure that results obtained with different bleedings can be compared. The remarkable adaptive response to produce higher-affinity antibodies is called *maturation* of the immune response and is due to the selective expansion of clones of B cells that produce antibody of the highest affinity.

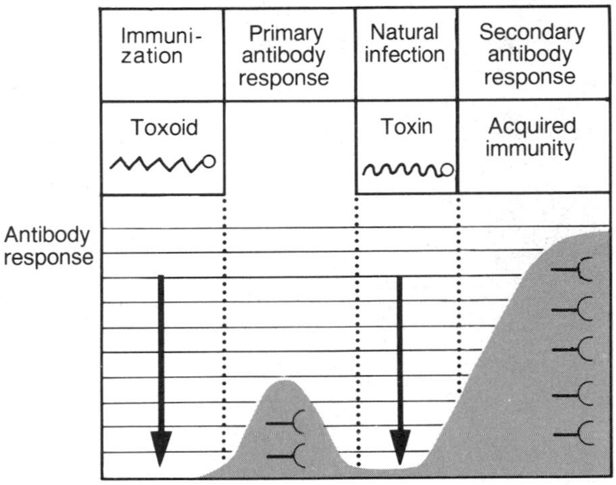

Figure 5-6. The principle of toxin immunization illustrated by the naturally induced secondary immune response to diphtheria infection following immunization with diphtheria toxoid. Diphtheria toxoid retains some of the epitopes of the diphtheria bacillus toxin, so that a primary antibody response to these epitopes is produced following vaccination with toxoid. In a natural infection the toxin restimulates B memory cells, which produce the faster and more intense secondary antibody response that neutralizes the toxin. In most individuals the circulating levels of antibodies to diphtheria and tetanus persist at high levels between exposures. (Modified from Roitt I, Brostoff J, Male D, Immunology. St. Louis, Mosby, 1985, p1.9.)

Tests for Antibody

The tests used for detection of antibody differ markedly in their ability to measure antibody activity (see Chapter 6). If a bactericidal or viral neutralization test is used, extremely small amounts of antibody may be detected within a few hours of immunization. If the double diffusion-in-agar technique utilizing a soluble protein antigen is used, a million times as much antibody may be needed for detection. In some situations antibody may be detected in vivo (by skin test or systemic anaphylaxis), while the in vitro test is negative. The procedures used for detection of antibody are discussed in more detail in Chapter 6. Whether or not antibody is found following immunization may well depend upon the test for detection.

Genetics of the Immune Response

The ability to produce an immune response and the type of response produced to some antigens are under genetic control. This subject is discussed in Chapter 9.

Condition of the Responding Animal

A wide variety of physiological factors may affect immune responses. For best results, young, healthy adult animals should be used. Very young or very old animals may not respond well to a given antigen. Diseases, immunosuppressive agents, and diet may alter immune responsiveness.

Antigenic Specificity

Chemical Specificity

The specificity of an antibody may be so exact that it can be directly related to a chemically definable structure. The specificity of the antibody may be used to determine, in part, the chemical structure of unknown antigenic molecules. Antibody to pneumococcal polysaccharide Type SII is specific for a D-glucose polymer joined in 1,4,6-linkages. Anti-SII antisera react to glycogens, glycogen-limit dextran, and amylopectins, all of which contain 1,4,6 glycoside linkages. The chemical structures of some unknown carbohydrates can be predicted on the basis of the finding that these unknowns react with anti-SII sera, and direct chemical analysis will demonstrate the presence of 1,4,6-linkages in the unknowns.

Type of Antigenic Specificities

Epitopes specific for different antigenic molecules may be classified on the basis of tissue of origin, species, molecular class, and subclass, and even for individual molecular species such as individual antibodies (Table 5-5).

Table 5-5. Classification of Antigenic Specificities

Type	Example
Organ	Thyroid antigens Serum albumin
Species (xenotype)	Human serum albumin
Individuals within a species (allotype)	ABO blood group antigens Immunoglobulin allotypes
Subfamily of related molecules (isotype)	Immunoglobulin classes
Individual molecular species (idiotype)	Specific antibody (monoclonal)

Organ Specificity

The same organs of different species share some common antigenic specificities. Thus, the thyroid antigens of one species are shared by the thyroid of another species; the adrenal or brain of one species shares specificity with the adrenal or brain of another species.

Serum proteins with different functional activities have different antigenic specificities, and serum proteins that perform similar functions in different species may share antigenic specificities. The albumins, α-globulins, and immunoglobulins of a given species possess different antigenic specificities. Rabbit anti-human albumin does not react with human immunoglobulins, and vice versa. However, the albumins of different species may contain common epitopes. Rabbit antiserum to human albumin will usually also react with bovine albumin, albeit more weakly.

Species Specificity (Xenotype)

Rabbit anti-human albumin reacts more strongly with human albumin than with the albumin of any other species. Human albumin contains some antigenic specificities unique for humans, but also contains some epitopes in common with the albumins of other species.

In some cases, for unknown reasons, an identical antigenic specificity is present in the tissues of different species. The classic example is the Forssman antigen. Anti-Forssman antibody is produced by injecting sheep red blood cells into rabbits. The resulting antiserum reacts with sheep cells, goat cells, guinea pig tissue, human type A red cells, certain bacteria, plants, and other animal or fish tissues. The Forssman antigen is a carbohydrate rich in galactosyl residues. Antibody to the Forssman antigen is clinically significant in that it appears in patients with infectious mononucleosis and was classically detected by the capacity of serum from an affected patient to bind to sheep red blood cells (Paul–Bunnell test). There is no known phylogenetic or functional relation for this antigenic specificity, only a chemical similarity. A similar relation exists between certain other organisms. For instance, the Weil–Felix reaction depends upon the fact that antiserum against *Rickettsia* reacts also with *Proteus* OX-19.

Allospecificity (Allotype)

Some individuals of a given species possess antigenic specificities not shared with other individuals of the same species. These specificities depend upon small structural differences and are best exemplified by ABO blood group specificities. Within the human species, the red blood cells of individuals of the same red blood cell group (A, B, AB, or O) have the same antigenic specificity, whereas the red blood cells of other individuals of a different blood group have different antigenic specificities. The same is true of serum proteins (immunoglobulins, α-lipoproteins) and solid tissues. The older terminology of blood group specificities referred to differences between individuals as isospecificities; the more recent terminology introduced to cover solid tissue transplantation antigens employs the term allospecificities. The attempt to identify and classify allospecific antigens in solid tissues is an important advance in human tissue transplantation, as perfectly matched donor organs have a good chance of functioning in the new host without undergoing graft rejection.

Isotypic Specificity (Isotype)

Some families of molecules contain subpopulations with different antigens. For example, the immunoglobulin family consists of five major classes (IgM, IgG, IgA, IgD, and IgE; see Chapter 6). The antigenic determinants that distinguish these classes are termed *isotypes.*

Idiotypic Specificity (Idiotype)

Idiotypes are antigenic specificities on antibody molecules that are limited to a unique antibody subpopulation. Each antigen-binding site of an antibody is different and may itself be recognized as a foreign epitope. Thus the paratope of an antibody is a unique antigen determinant called an *idiotope.* A cross-reacting idiotype is shared by a subset of antibodies, whereas an individual idiotype is unique for that molecule. Anti-idiotypes (antibodies to idiotopes) may react with the antigen-binding site of the antibody (antiparatope) or with conformational structures adjacent to the paratope. Idiotype-bearing antibodies also share common allotypic and isotypic antigens with other immunoglobulins, but have the unique idiotypic determinant as well. The regulatory role of anti-idiotypes will be discussed in Chapter 11.

Antigen Prevalence

Naturally, exposure to antigens is usually provided by contact with other organisms (bacteria, viruses, fungi). Experimental or therapeutic procedures provide opportunity for contact with other potential antigens, such as artificially produced macromolecules (drugs), serum proteins, blood cells, and tissues (grafts) from other individuals of the same species or of other species. A given individual does not usually make an immune response to his own tissues, although his own tissues contain many potential antigens recognized by other genetically different individuals in the same species. An individual may react against his own tissues *(autoallergic reaction)* if they are rendered antigenic by physical (heat, necrosis) or infectious processes, or if immune regulatory mechanisms break down.

Summary

The induction of an immune response is termed *immunization.* Immunization results in new products that recognize and react with substances that induce the response. A molecular species capable of inducing an immune response is termed an *immu-*

nogen. An *antigen* is a substance that can react with the products of an immune response. A complete antigen can both induce a response and react with the products; an incomplete antigen (hapten) cannot induce a response but can react with the products of the response. The site of the antigen (antigenic determinant) with which an antibody reacts is the epitope; the binding site of the antibody is the paratope. A number of variables concerning the nature of the antigen, the relationship of the antigen to the responding individual, the route and dose of the antigen, and the condition of the responding individual determine the nature and extent of the immune response.

References

Antigens and Immunogens

Atassi MZ, Young CR: Discovery and implications of the immunogenicity of free small synthetic peptides. CRC Crit Rev Immunol 5:387, 1985.

Benjamin DC, et al.: The antigenic structure of proteins: A reappraisal. Annu Rev Immunol 2:67, 1984.

Delisi C, Berzofsky JA: T cell antigenic sites tend to be amphipathic structures. Proc Nat Acad Sci USA 82:7048, 1985.

Heidelberger M: Lectures in Immunochemistry. New York, Academic Press, 1956.

Kabat EA: The nature of an antigenic determinant. J Immunol 97:1, 1966.

Kabat, EA: Structural Concepts in Immunology and Immunochemistry. New York, Holt, Rinehart & Winston, 1968.

Mauer PH: Use of synthetic polymers of amino acids to study the basis of antigenicity. Prog Allergy 8:1, 1964.

Mills JA, Haber E: The effect on antigenic specificity of changes in the molecular structure of ribonuclease. J Immunol 91:536, 1963.

Novotny J, et al: Antigenic determinants in proteins coincide with surface regions accessible to large probes (antibody domains). Proc Nat Acad Sci USA 83:226, 1986.

Sala M: Immunological studies with synthetic polypeptides. Adv Immunol 5:30, 1969.

Todd PEE, East IJ, Leach SJ: The immunogenicity and antigenicity of proteins. Trends Biochem Sci 7:212, 1982.

Yagi Y, Maier P, Pressman D: Antibodies against the component polypeptide chains of bovine insulin. Science 147:617, 1965.

Immunization

Freund J: The mode of action of immunologic adjuvants. Adv Tuberc Res 7:130, 1956.

Munoz J: Effect of bacteria and bacterial products on antibody responses. Adv Immunol 4:397, 1964.

Uhr JW: The heterogeneity of the immune response. Science 145:457, 1964.

Warren HS, Vogel FR, Chedad LA: Current status of immunological adjuvants. Annu Rev Immunol 4:369, 1968.

Antigenic Specificity

Jenkin CR: Heterophile antigens and their significance in the host–parasite relationship. Adv Immunol 3:351, 1963.

Landsteiner, K. The Specificity of Serological Reactions. New York, Dover, 1962.

See Chapter 7 for a more detailed discussion of specificity of antibody–antigen reactions, and Chapter 6 for a detailed presentation of idiotypes, allotypes, and isotypes.

6 Antibodies, Immunoglobulins, and Receptors

Antibodies belong to a group of structurally related glycoprotein molecules found in the blood and extracellular fluids and known collectively as immunoglobulins. Immunoglobulins are the products of plasma cells, which secrete these proteins into serum and tissue fluids. Each plasma cell synthesizes and secretes large numbers of a single antibody that has the same antigen-binding specificity. Whereas some immunoglobulins are produced at all times in most normal animals, specific antibodies are a unique subset of immunoglobulins produced in response to antigenic stimulation. Given the enormous number of antigen specificities (epitopes) identifiable, an individual must have the ability to produce a great variety of antibody molecules. Cell surface antibodies on B cells serve as specific receptors for antigen; T cells also bear receptor molecules similar to antibodies, but having different structural components.

Gamma Globulin

The first identification of antibodies among the serum proteins was accomplished by electrophoresis in 1938 (Fig. 6-1). It was

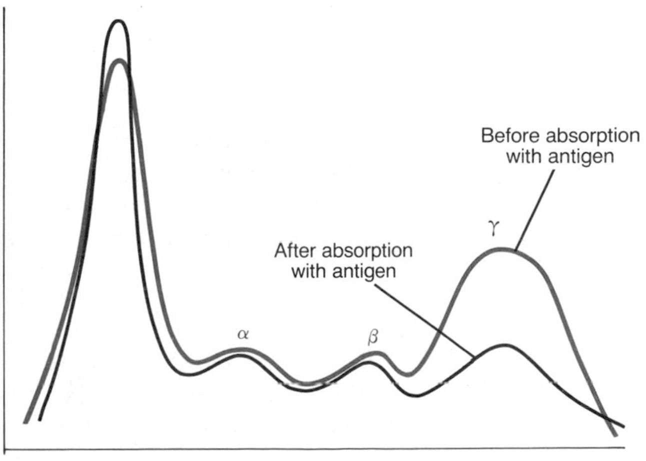

Figure 6-1. If serum is placed under an electric gradient, the proteins will migrate in the charged field produced. The solid line depicts the serum protein electrophoresis pattern produced after absorption of serum from a hyperimmunized animal with the immunizing antigen. The dotted line depicts the protein pattern before absorption. It was thus shown that antibodies are largely found in the gamma globulins (the least negatively charged serum proteins).

found that antibodies are part of the gamma globulin fraction of serum. With further characterization of antibody molecules, this class of proteins has been shown to be very heterogeneous and the term *immunoglobulin* has been applied to designate this group of serum proteins. Immunoglobulins possess a degree of structural heterogeneity not found in most other serum proteins, but at the same time immunoglobulins also have structural similarities.

Myeloma Proteins

The study of the structure, synthesis, and function of human immunoglobulins has been made possible by the production of homogeneous immunoglobulins by plasma cell neoplasms (multiple myeloma, macroglobulinemia). From the sera of individuals with such tumors, homogeneous proteins can be isolated. These homogeneous immunoglobulins (myeloma proteins) can then be studied and structural analysis made that is not possible using normal immunoglobulins because of the great heterogeneity of normal immunoglobulins.

Immunoglobulins

Classes (Isotypes)

Five major immunoglobulin classes have been identified in man. Some of the characteristics of these immunoglobulins are given in Table 6-1. The five classes include immunoglobulins G (IgG), A (IgA), M (IgM), D (IgD), and E (IgE). The basic structural unit of each immunoglobulin class consists of two pairs of polypeptide chains joined by disulfide bonds (Fig. 6-2). The disulfide bonds may be reduced by mercaptoethanol. In the presence of denaturing agent (e.g., acid, urea) four polypeptide chains, two L (light)- and two H (heavy)-chains, are liberated. Each antibody molecule contains two identical light chains and two identical heavy chains. The intact molecule may be digested by proteolytic enzymes to yield other fragments (Fc and Fab fragments; Fig. 6-3). The term *Fab* is used because it is this fragment that binds antigen. *Fc* was applied to a non–antibody-binding fragment of rabbit antibody that crystallized in the test tube. The Fc fragments of most antibodies do not crystallize. The L-chains are shared by immunoglobulins of the different classes and can be divided into two subclasses, kappa (κ) and lambda (λ), on the basis of their structures and amino acid sequences. A given immunoglobulin molecule is either type κ or type λ. Approximately 60% of the serum immunoglobulin molecules contain κ-type L-chains, and 40% λ-type L-chains. The H-chains are unique for each immunoglobulin class and are designated by the Greek letter corresponding to the capital letter designation of the immunoglobulin class (*α-chains* for the H-chains of IgA, *γ-chains* for the H-chains of IgG). IgM and IgA have a third chain component, the J-chain, which joins the monomeric units.

Table 6-1. Some Properties of Human Immunoglobulins

Property	Immunoglobulin Class				
	IgG	IgA	IgM	IgD	IgE
Serum concentration (g./100 ml.)	1.2	0.4	0.12	0.003	< 00005
Sedimentation coefficient (S)	7	7 (9,11,13)*	19 (24,32)*	7	8
Molecular weight	140,000	160,000Δ	900,000	180,000	200,000
Electrophoretic mobility	γ	Slow β	Between γ and β	Between γ and β	Slow β
H-chains	γ	α	μ	δ	ϵ
L-chains	λ or κ	λ or κ	λ or κ	λ or κ	λ or κ
Complement fixation	Yes	No	Yes	No	No
Placental transfer	Yes	No	No	No	No
Percent intravascular	40	40	70	—	—
Half-life (days)	23	6	5	3	2.5
Percent carbohydrate	3	10	10	13	10
Antibody activity	Most Ab to infections; major part of secondary response; Rh isoagglutinins; LE factor	Present in external secretions	First Ab formed; ABO isoagglutinins; rheumatoid factor	Antibody activity rarely demonstrated, found on lymphocyte surface	Reagin sensitizes mast cells for anaphylaxis

* Figures in parentheses indicates the existence of other molecular forms, such as polymers.
Δ Serum IgA 160,000 MW; secretory IgA 350,000 MW, may activate alternate pathway (see Chap. 10) (Modified from Fahey, J.L.: J.A.M.A. 194:183, 1966).

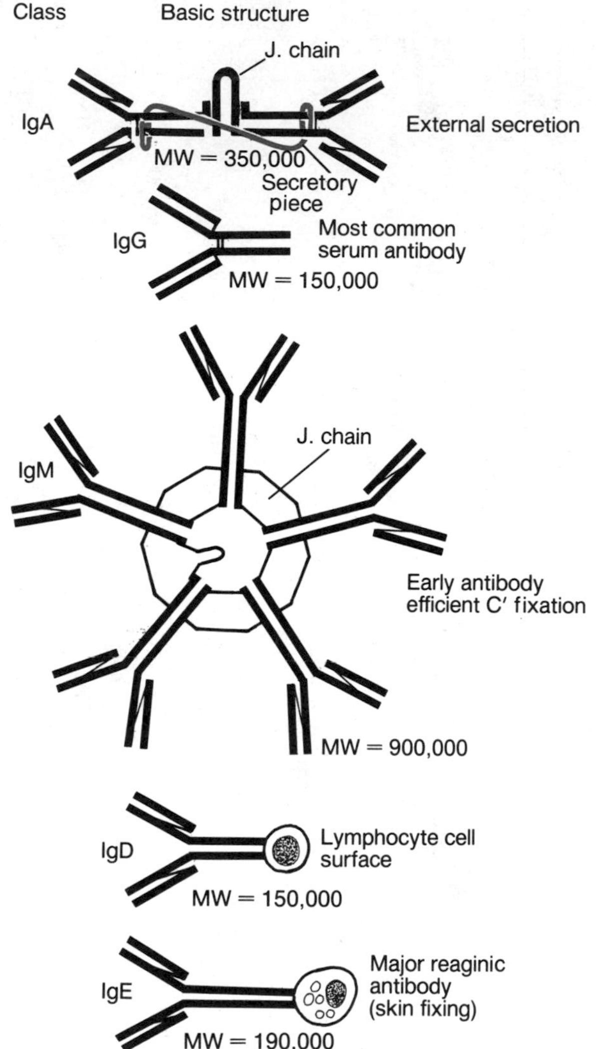

Figure 6-2. Human immunoglobulin classes. Human humoral (circulating) antibodies belong to five classes: IgA, IgG, IgM, IgD, and IgE. The basic unit of each immunoglobulin molecule consists of two pairs of polypeptide chains joined by disulfide bonds. All immunoglobulins have the same L (light)-chain components, identifiable antigenically as kappa (κ) or lambda (λ), with any given immunoglobulin molecule having two κ-chains or two λ-chains. No naturally occurring immunoglobulin molecule has one κ-chain and one λ-chain. H (heavy)-chains of each immunoglobulin class are unique for that class and determine its biologic properties. H-chains of each immunoglobulin class are designated by the Greek letter corresponding to the capital letter identifying the class.

Biological Properties of Immunoglobulins

The five classes of immunoglobulins have different biological properties and are distributed differently in the intact animal. The structure responsible for the biological properties of each immunoglobulin class is located on that part of the immunoglobulin molecule that is unique for each class (the Fc portion of the H-chain).

Each IgG molecule consists of one H_2L_2 unit with a molecular weight of about 140,000. Molecules of the IgG class are actively transported across the placenta and provide passive immunity to the newborn infant at a time when the infant's immune mechanisms are not developed. IgG is widely distributed in the tissue fluids and is about equally divided between the intravascular and extravascular spaces.

IgM is the first immunoglobulin class produced by the

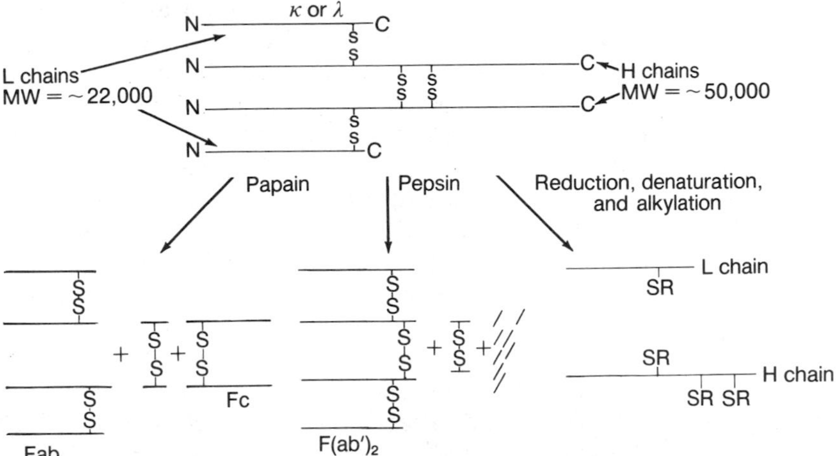

Figure 6-3. Human immunoglobulin fragments. The intact IgG molecule may be fragmented by different reagents into subunits. Digestion with papain occurs on the amino side of the interchain disulfide bond and results in three major fragments, two Fab and one Fc, and a minor fragment. Fab fragments consist of an L-chain and the amino half of an H-chain joined by a disulfide bond. The Fc fragment consists of the carboxy halves of H-chains joined by a disulfide bond. An additional small peptide from the middle of the heavy chains containing a disulfide bond is also produced. The Fab fragment contains an antigen-binding site and reacts with, but does not precipitate, antigen because it is monovalent. The Fc portion is responsible for biological properties such as complement fixation. Digestion with pepsin occurs on the carboxy side of the interchain disulfide bond and results in two F(ab') fragments joined by a disulfide bond because one of the disulfide bonds joining the H-chains is preserved. This fragment, $F(ab')_2$, reacts with and precipitates antigen because it is divalent (contains two antigen-binding sites). Additional peptide fragments, some containing disulfide bonds, are produced by the action of pepsin, presumably due to further digestion of the Fc fragment. Reduction of disulfide bonds, alkylation of free SH groups ($R = CH_2CONH_2$), and denaturation of ionic and hydrogen bonds result in liberation of polypeptide chains— two L-chains (MW 22,000) and two H-chains (MW 50,000). Each polypeptide chain contributes to the antigen-binding site of the intact Fab fragment. That portion of H-chain present in the Fab fragment is called the Fd piece.

maturing fetus and may be the first immunoglobulin class representing a given antibody specificity following immunization (primary response). IgM occurs as five H_2L_2 units joined to each other by disulfide bonds located on the Fc part of the molecule and to the J-chain; its molecular weight is 900,000. IgM is found mainly in the intravascular fluids (80%). It is also the most efficient class of immunoglobulin in fixing complement and therefore is highly active in cytotoxic and cytolytic reactions.

IgM does not normally cross the placenta from mother to fetus, but may be produced actively by the fetus prior to birth, especially if the fetus has been exposed to antigens by infection. Thus IgM antibodies in the cord blood of the fetus are evidence of fetal immunization by exposure to infectious agents.

IgA is found in relatively small amounts in serum and tissue fluids, but is present in high concentrations in external secretions such as colostrum, saliva, tears, and intestinal and bronchial secretions. The IgA molecules in these fluids exist as dimers (two H_2L_2 units) joined by a J-chain and bound to an extra protein (*transport piece*). This transport piece is produced by secretory mucosal or glandular cells and facilitates the secretion of the dimeric IgA into the external fluids. Because IgA antibodies are prominent in external secretions, such antibodies are part of the first line of defense against infectious agents.

IgE is present in very low concentrations in serum and tissue fluids, but binds to a specific cell surface receptor on tissue mast cells. These cells are so named because they contain cytoplasmic granules and appear to have eaten (German *Mast,* "forced fattening"). Mast cells are armed by IgE antibodies that are bound to their surface receptors. Each antigen to which an individual is allergic may interact with cell-bound IgE and trigger the release of the granules. This releases biologically active molecules, such as histamine and serotonin. Antibody with this biological property is termed *reaginic antibody* or *reagin.*

IgD is present in very low concentrations in the serum. IgD is found on the surface of a high proportion of immature human B lymphocytes, suggesting that IgD may serve as a cellular receptor for antigen. The same variable region is used for IgD on the cell surface and for the IgM, IgG, or IgA that will ultimately be secreted. Thus, when antigen binds the IgD receptor, it stimulates the cell to multiply and ultimately to differentiate and to secrete antibodies of other classes that will be specific for the antigen.

Subclasses (Isotypes)

In addition to the five major classes of immunoglobulins in humans, subclasses of IgG, IgA, and IgM have been recognized. For example, four subclasses of IgG may be identified. These subclasses are designated *IgG_1*, *IgG_2*, *IgG_3*, and *IgG_4*. The subclasses differ in the sequence of their heavy chain constant regions (Table 6-2). IgG_1 molecules predominate in normal serum (9 mg/ml). The serum content of IgG_2 is 2.5 mg/ml, and

Table 6-2. Biological Properties of IgG Subclasses

Property	IgG_1	IgG_2	IgG_3	IgG_4
Percentage of total IgG in serum	65	23	8	4
Complement fixation	++	+	+++	0
Placental transfer	+++	++	+++	+++
Passive cutaneous anaphylaxis[a]	+++	0	+++	+++
Receptor for macrophage	+++	0	+++	0
Reaction with staph protein A	+++	+++	0	+++
Prominent antibody activity	Anti-Rh	Anti-levan, anti-dextran	Anti-Rh	Anti-factor VIII

[a] Heterocytophilic antibody.

the serum content of IgG_3 and IgG_4 is 0.5 to 1.0 mg/ml. The biological significance of these immunoglobulin subclasses is not well understood. However, IgG_1 and IgG_3 are more active in fixing complement, whereas IgG_4 does not fix complement. IgG_2 predominates in the response to polysaccharide antigens and does not cross the placenta with the same efficiency as the other IgG subclasses. Therefore, the different IgG subclasses have different biological properties. In addition, the locations of the interchain disulfide bonds are different. IgA_1 and IgA_2 subclasses differ in sensitivity to bacterial proteases, and α_2 H and L chains are not joined to each other by disulfide bonds, as are α_1 chains, but are held together by electrostatic forces.

Antibodies

Primary Structure

The primary structure of a protein molecule is the sequence of amino acids that make up the light and heavy polypeptide chains (see Fig. 6-4). On the basis of antibody sequence data,

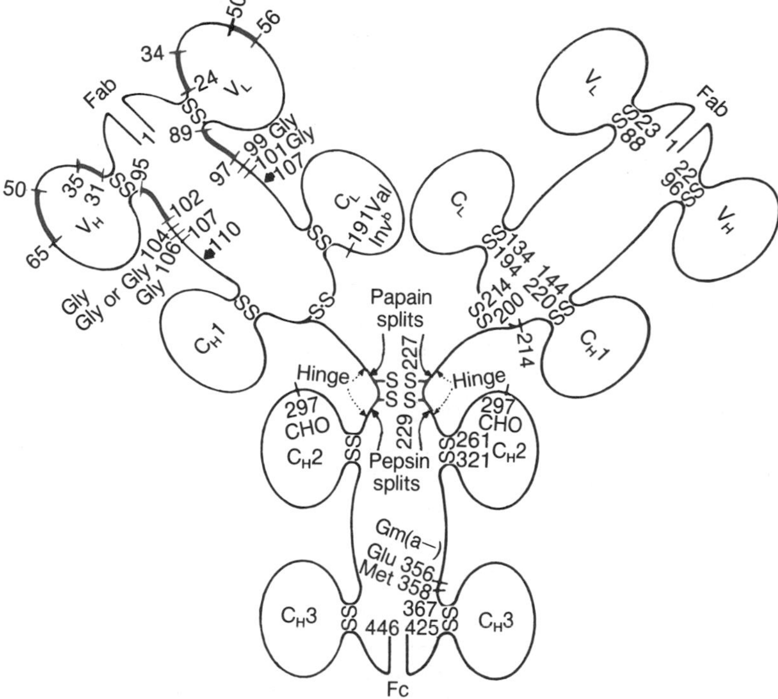

Figure 6-4. Schematic view of four-chain structure of human IgG molecule. Numbers on right side: actual residues of myeloma protein EU. Numbers of Fab fragments on left side aligned for maximum homology; light chains numbered as by E.A. Kabat (J Immunol 125:961, 1980). Hypervariable regions, complementarity-determining regions (CDR): heavier lines. V_L and V_H: light- and heavy-chain variable regions. C_H1, C_H2, and C_H3: domains of constant region of heavy chain. C_L: constant region of light chain. Hinge region in which two heavy chains are linked by disulfide bonds is indicated approximately. Attachment of carbohydrate is at residue 297. Arrows at residues 107 and 110 denote transition from variable to constant regions. Sites of action of papain before the hinge region and of pepsin after the hinge region show why papain produces Fab monomers and pepsin produces F(ab)2 dimers. Locations of a number of heritable allotypic differences (Gm, Inv) are given.

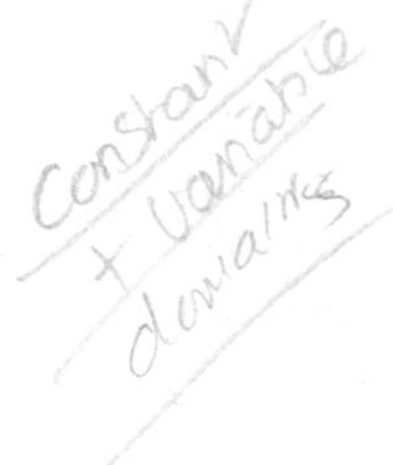

two L-chain regions have been identified. These are called *constant* (C_L) and *variable* (V_L). Of the total of 212 amino acids, those located at the carboxy terminal are virtually identical for each L-chain of κ type and each L-chain of λ type: the primary structure of the amino domain (that portion presumably containing the antigen-binding site) varies for each antibody studied. The H-chain consists of four or five structural domains, each containing about 106 amino acids in a folded β pleated sheet and a disulfide bond (Fig. 6-5). The amino-terminal struc-

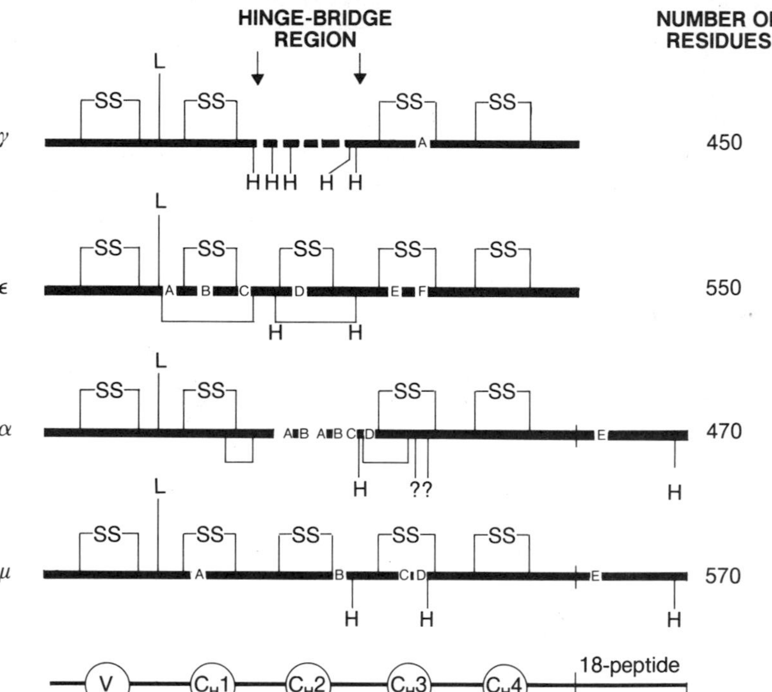

Figure 6-5. Diagrammatic comparison of the heavy chains of different immunoglobulin classes. The γ- and α-chains have three constant domains, whereas the μ- and ϵ-chains have four. γ- and α-chains have deletions resulting in loss of one of the domains. Other structural differences are indicated. These structural differences account for the biological properties of the different Ig classes. (Modified from Dorington KJ, Bennich HH: Immunol Rev 41:3, 1978.) The five different domains of the immunoglobulin heavy chains and the two domains of the light chains are related by homology and are believed to have evolved by gene duplication.

tural domain of the H-chain contains the H-chain variable region; the other three domains are constant for all H-chains of the same subclass. Therefore, a variable region of an immunoglobulin molecule consists of the amino terminal of the L-chain and the H-chain as they fold together to form a three-dimensional binding site for antigen.

Immunoglobulin molecules have a high degree of flexibility because of a "hinge" region between the first and second constant regions (between Fab and Fc) of the heavy chain. This section of the heavy chain is rich in proline residues, which interfere with the α-helical structure of the constant domains. The hinge region acts as a swivel allowing the Fab domain to assume angles that may vary between 0 and 180°. This permits the individual combining sites to move and assume different angles on reaction with antigenic sites. The length of the polypeptide chain between the last intra–H-chain disulfide bond and the first disulfide bond joining the L- and H-chains is not the same in each immunoglobulin class. The length of the "junction chain" determines the degree of flexibility of the antibody molecule and may influence whether or not reaction with antigen will affect the antibody structure so that functions such as fixation of complement are activated. Only IgM molecules do not have a hinge region.

The heavy chains of the different classes of immunoglobulin are not of the same length (Fig. 6-5). Deletions in the γ and α heavy chains are found in the hinge region. Thus a common ancestral heavy chain may have contained four constant domains. Deletion of some of the amino acids in one of these constant regions for IgG and IgA results in only three constant domains in γ and α heavy chains. An extra 18-amino-acid peptide is present on the carboxy-terminal end of the α and μ heavy chains. This peptide is involved in the formation of the polymeric forms of IgA and IgM molecules and of the cell membrane domain of IgM.

Antigen-Binding Sites (Paratopes)

The antigen-binding site of immunoglobulins (paratope) is located on the variable portion of the Fab of the antibody molecule (*Fab:* fragment that binds antigen). The ability to combine specifically with a given antigenic determinant (epitope) may be shared by immunoglobulins belonging to different classes. The actual site of antigen binding is small, but the complete paratope involves both the L- and the H-chains of a given antibody molecule (see Fig. 6-6). The primary structure responsible

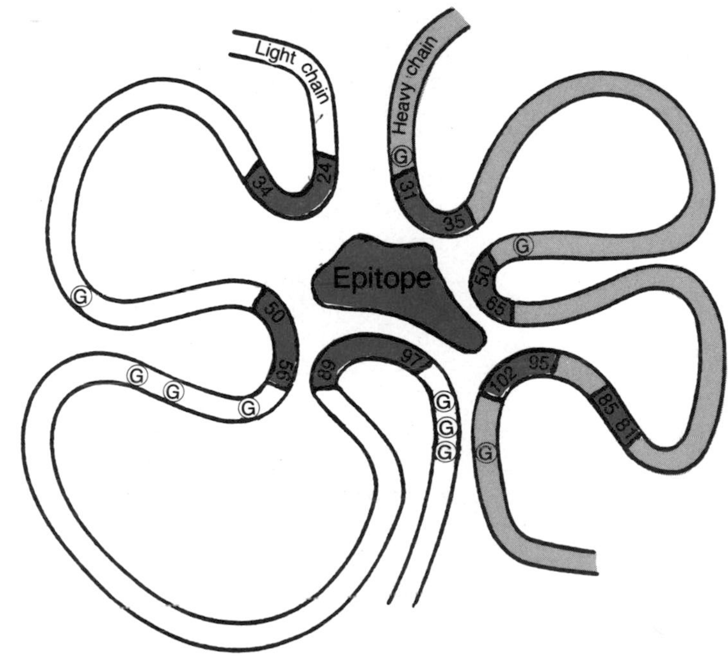

Figure 6-6. Formation of an antigen-binding site (paratope) by conformation of the hypervariable region (dark areas) on light and heavy chains. Numbers refer to amino acid residues. Glycine residues, which are always present at the positions indicated, are important in chain folding. The hypervariable amino acids occur at specific positions in the peptide chain of immunoglobulins. These "hot spots" lie relatively close together in the antigen-binding site and form a continuous surface capable of providing complementarity with a specific antigen. For a given antibody not all the hypervariable regions need be involved with binding of a given antigen.

for antigen binding is located in the variable portion of each chain. Within the variable portion are framework sequences (relatively constant segments) containing up to 30 amino acids and hypervariable sequences ("hot spots") of 4 to 7 amino acids where variability is marked (Fig. 6-4). Some amino acids not actually in the hypervariable segments may contribute indirectly to the conformational or contacting components of the site, by providing ancillary structural support. The "hot spot" segments of the variable region are folded to juxtapose in three dimensions in a manner that forms an appropriate pocket or groove for antigen to be bound (Fig. 6-6).

Biologically Active Sites

In contrast to the variable regions, found on the amino-terminal domains of the immunoglobulin chains, constant regions exist in the carboxy-terminal domains of the L-chain and the H-chain. This situation provides a structural basis for antibodies of different antigen-binding specificity (variable region) to have similar or different biologic properties due to shared constant portions. A variable region is needed to form antigen-binding sites of great diversity, whereas a constant region preserves the biological properties of each immunoglobulin class. The exact sites within the constant domains for biological properties have not been clearly identified. For instance, the site responsible for complement binding after reaction of antibody with antigen is believed to be in the C_{H2} region (see Fig. 6-5). The exact sites for placental transfer, skin fixation, or other biological functions are not known, but reside somewhere in the Fc domains of the appropriate immunoglobulin class.

The sharing of the same constant region among thousands of antibody molecules of different specificity and, hence, different variable regions presented an interesting theoretical question for molecular geneticists. The old theory of one gene–one protein required that the constant region be repeated thousands of times, contiguous with each variable region. Alternatively, immunoglobulins could be the first example of a protein that represented a composite of two genes brought together to form the V and C regions of a single portion. Then, the C region gene could be carried as a single copy on the genome but could be expressed along with any one of the thousands of V genes. This turned out to be the case, as discussed below.

Higher-Order Structure of Immunoglobulins

In addition to primary structure (amino acid sequence), immunoglobulins, like other protein molecules, have higher orders of structure: (1) *secondary*, the coiling of the individual polypeptide chains; (2) *tertiary*, the folding of the polypeptide coils; and (3) *quaternary*, the arrangement and association of the folded chains. Sedimentation, diffusion, and viscosity measurements indicate a tightly ordered structure for the polypeptide chains, with a considerable amount of helical coiling. The coiled chains of the immunoglobulin unit are folded together as well as connected by disulfide bonds. Reduction of the disulfide bonds does not separate the component chains until ionic bonds and hydrogen bonds are also broken, by denaturing agents, for example, acid, urea, or guanidine.

The folding of a constant domain of a heavy chain is illustrated in Figure 6-7. Four antiparallel chains form a β pleated

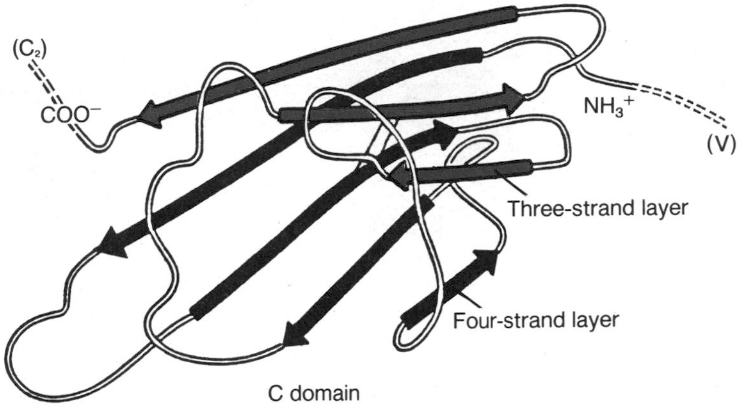

Figure 6-7. The basic folding pattern of the polypeptide chain in the constant (C) domains of an antibody molecule is cylindrical and has a sandwich-like structure: the top layer is composed of three adjacent strands of polypeptide chain (colored arrows) and the bottom layer of four (black arrows), with the two layers held together by a disulfide (sulfur–sulfur) bridge. Although the variable domain of both the light and the heavy chain has an additional loop, the overall folding pattern of the variable and constant domains is highly similar. This common domain structure is due to the presence, in the interior of both domain types, of hydrophobic amino acids that need to be protected from the aqueous environment.

sheet while three other antiparallel chain segments form another β pleated sheet. The two pleated layers enclose a hydrophobic interior and are held together by an intrachain disulfide bond as well as by hydrogen bonds. Nearly all the sharp bends in the polypeptide chains include glycine residues, which are essentially invariant. The structure of a complete light chain is depicted in Figure 6-8.

For the antigen-binding site of an antibody the hypervariable regions of the V_H and V_L domains are organized along a cylindrical surface known as "the binding site barrel." The V_L region β sheets form one side of the barrel, and the V_H β sheets the other. The hypervariable segments of the respective polypeptides are located at the free end of the barrel, forming the

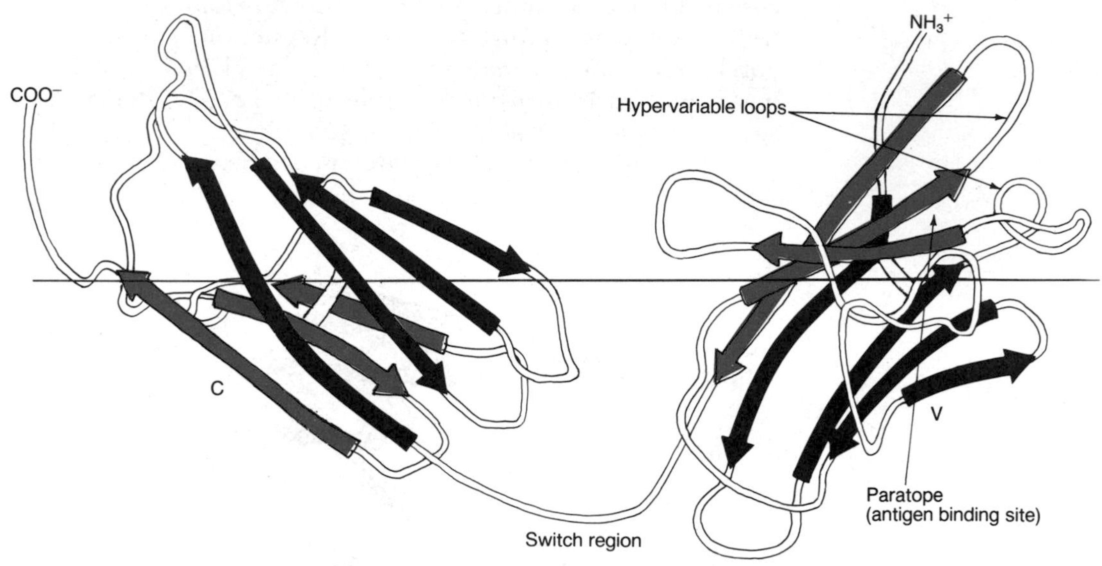

Figure 6-8. The light chain of an IgG molecule folds into a constant (C) and a variable (V) domain. The two domains are rotated 160° with respect to each other, so that their four-strand layers (colored arrows) face different directions. This rotation is accompanied by differences in the amino acid composition of the two domains that enable them to perform very different functions when they interact in pairs. For example, the association of two identical light chains in dimers forms a cavity (paratope) in which antigenic determinants (epitopes) bind. The dimers can thus be considered models for a primitive antibody. Three hypervariable regions located on three separate loops of the peptide chain lie close to one another, forming the L-chain portion of the antigen-binding site.

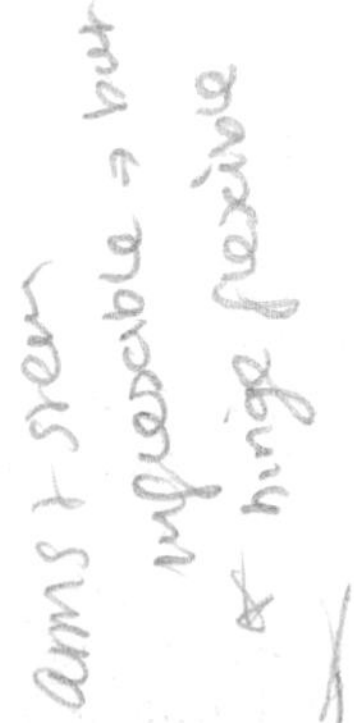

three-dimensional structure of the antigen-binding site. A three-dimensional model of human immunoglobulin G derived from crystallographic studies is shown in Figure 6-9.

Electron microscopic studies of IgG provide additional observations on the shape and form of the immunoglobulin molecule. IgG not bound to antigen is an irregular globular particle lacking a characteristic structure and with a maximum dimension of 120 Å. IgG antibody bound to antigen (virus particle, ferritin) appears as a Y-shaped molecule. Removal of the Fc piece of IgG causes loss of the stem of the Y. The structure identified has a thickness of 40 Å. Each arm of the Y is 65 Å long; the stem measures 50 Å. The arms and stem are inflexible, but the junction of the arms with the stem, the hinge region, is flexible. The angle between the arms may vary from 10 to 180°. The arms are the Fab pieces and contain the antibody combin-

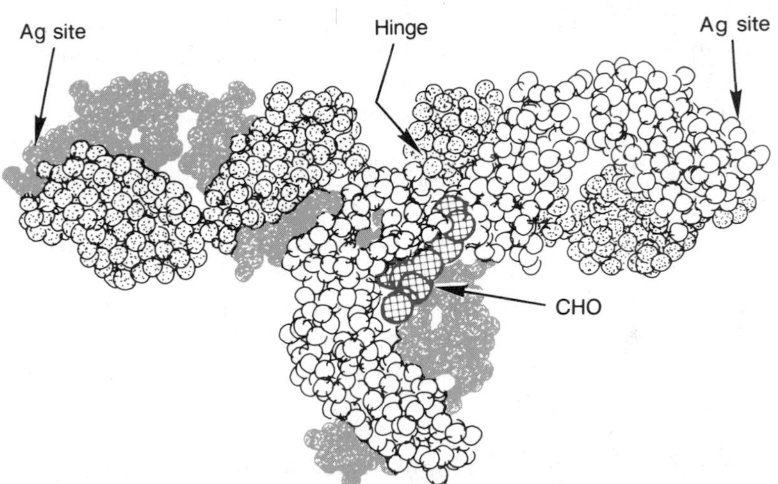

Figure 6-9. Three-dimensional structure of an immunoglobulin G molecule derived from the electron density map obtained by X-ray diffraction. One complete heavy chain is white and the other is light red. The two light chains are lightly stippled and the carbohydrate is crosshatched

ing site. Thus, the flexibility of the junction angle permits bridging of the antigen particles by binding sites that stretch between the antigen particles or looping and joining of two antigen sites on the same particle.

In fine structure, IgM consists of a central thin disk about 180 Å in diameter with five projecting arms measuring 35 × 125 Å; the entire molecule has a diameter of 270 Å. The structure is consistent with that postulated from chemical studies, that is, five MW 150,000 H_2L_2 units joined together. If each arm represents a Fab piece, the molecule would be expected to have 10 armlike extensions. Therefore, either each arm consists of two Fab pieces, or one of each pair of Fab pieces is incorporated into the central disk.

IgA also has a Y-shaped appearance, in which two basic units are superimposed on each other in a close-packed state. The additional fragment found in secretory IgA is located at the stem area of two Y-shaped units. This fine structure is consistent with that proposed from chemical studies.

Immunoglobulin Antigenic Specificities

The great variety of antigenic specificities that may be recognized on a given molecule is exemplified by the many specificities of antibodies that can react with immunoglobulins (anti-antibodies).

Species Cross-Reactivity

Antisera produced in distantly related species, such as rabbit anti-human immunoglobulin, not only recognize epitopes in human immunoglobulin but also react with immunoglobulin from other primate or mammalian species.

Species Specificity (Xenotypes)

The above antisera may also recognize epitopes present on essentially all human immunoglobulins but not on immunoglobulins from any other species.

Class Specificity (Isotypes)

Antisera may also recognize epitopes limited to a given immunoglobulin class, such as anti-immunoglobulin G, which does not react with IgA, IgM, IgD, or IgE. These are located on the constant domains of the heavy chains and are H-chain specific.

Subclass Specificity (Isotypes)

Antisera may specifically identify the IgG subclasses (IgG_1, IgG_2, IgG_3, IgG_4). Such antisera usually require absorption to remove IgG common specificities.

Fragment Specificity

Antisera may also be specific for the Fab, Fc, or Fd fragment of an immunoglobulin. This specificity may be so exact that it requires the fragment as antigen; reaction with native IgG does not occur.

Chain Specificity

Similar specificities may also be produced for L-chains only or H-chains only, because of epitopes determined by constant regions.

Allospecificity (Allotypes)

Immunoglobulins also carry genetically controlled antigenic specificities termed *allotypes*. Allotypes are epitopes that differ among individuals of the same species. Human immunoglobulin allotypes are discussed below.

Denatured Immunoglobulin Specificity

Antisera produced to heat-denatured or chemically denatured immunoglobulin may react only with denatured immunoglobulins and not with native immunoglobulins. Denaturation, if not extensive, causes the unfolding or refolding of the molecule so that determinants not present on the native molecule are revealed. Many rheumatoid factors react with denatured immunoglobulin epitopes.

Antivariable Region Specificity (Idiotypes)

An antibody that reacts with immunoglobulin is termed anti-immunoglobulin (anti-Ig). The varieties of anti-Ig may be exemplified by the antibody produced by immunizing an animal with an antibody–antigen complex. An animal so immunized may produce (1) antibody that reacts with the antigen; (2) antibody that reacts with the antibody, but also reacts with normal immunoglobulin, for example, anti-H, anti-L, or anti-Fc; (3) antibody that reacts with the antibody–antigen complex, but not with either uncomplexed antibody or antigen (anticomplex); and (4) antibody that reacts with the antibody itself in native form, but does not react with other normal immunoglobulins. This latter specificity, which is limited to single species of proteins (antibody) within a large population of molecules (immunoglobulins), is termed an *idiotype*.

Anti-idiotypic antibodies may react with three major components of an antibody species: (1) the antigen-binding site itself (complementary determining region), (2) variable region structures away from the antigen-binding site, or (3) a combina-

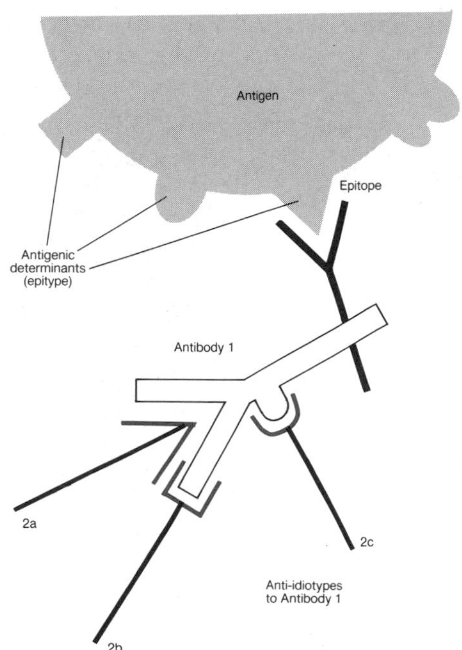

Figure 6-10. Anti-idiotypic antibodies to an antibody may react with the paratope (anti-idiotype 2a), with part of the paratope and part of the adjacent nonparatope variable region (anti-idiotype 2b), or with the nonparatope variable region (anti-idiotype 2c). The paratope of anti-idiotype 2a may mimic the antigen to which the original antibody reacts, and has been termed the *internal image* of the antigen. Anti-idiotype 2a will block the binding of the antigen to the antibody completely. Anti-idiotype 2b will block partially, and anti-idiotype 2c may not block at all unless the tertiary structure is changed by binding of anti-idiotype 2c.

tion of the two through an overlapping epitope (Fig. 6-10). The simplest explanation for the production of these anti-idiotypes is that anti-idiotypic antibodies are directed toward a site recognized as a foreign antigen because it is not present in detectable amounts in the normal immunoglobulin population. Sometimes different individuals will produce antibodies with the same idiotype when immunized with the same antigen (cross-reactive idiotype). Anti-idiotype to the antigen combining site (the paratope) will block reaction of the antibody with antigen and mimic the epitope of the antigen. Cross-reactive idiotypes often react with the antigen-binding site of the antibody. On the other hand, some anti-idiotypes do not interfere with the antigen-binding activity of the first antibody. Therefore, sites on the antibody not responsible for antigen binding but genetically codetermined with the antigen-binding site must be responsible (Fig. 6-11).

Complex Specificity

Anticomplex antibody is formed to new determinants revealed by alteration of the quaternary structure of the antibody, the antigen, or both as a result of formation of the antibody–antigen complex. This is similar to the determinants revealed by partial denaturation of immunoglobulins. Anticomplex antibody reacts with the antibody only when it is complexed with antigen. Anticomplex antibodies have been recognized that require the whole antibody molecule in complex form for reaction, whereas other anticomplex antibodies react with the Fab fragment of the complexed molecule.

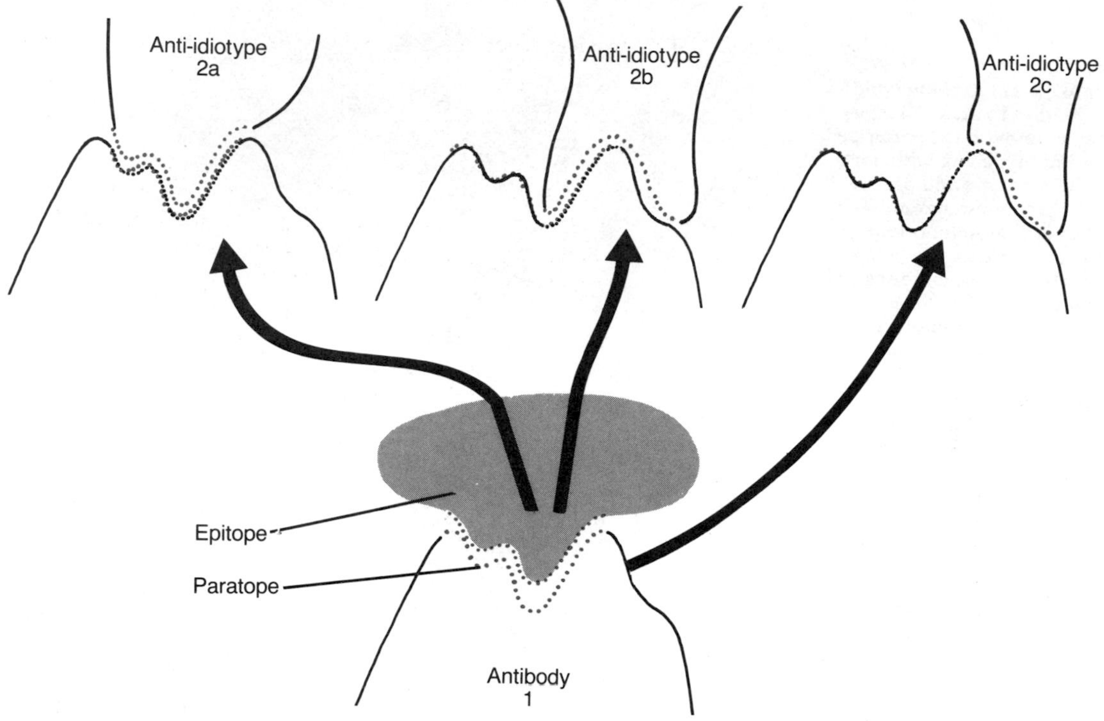

Figure 6-11. Paratopes, epitopes, and idiotopes. Depicted is an antibody combining site (paratope) and antigenic determinant (epitope) and types of anti-idiotypes. The antigen combining sites (paratopes) of anti-idiotypes are termed idiotopes. The idiotope of anti-idiotype 2a is essentially identical to the epitope of the antigen (molecular mimicry) and the mirror image of the paratope of antibody 1; the idiotope of anti-idiotype 2b shares some structures in common with the epitope, but not all; the idiotope of anti-idiotope 2c contains no structure in common with the epitope of the antigen, but contains mirror images of nonparatope regions of the antibody.

Human Immunoglobulin Allotypes

Immunoglobulin allotypes are genetic differences in the constant regions of H- or L-chains that are inherited in a codominant Mendelian pattern. Up to 30 different immunoglobulin allotypic specificities have been identified in humans. These are divided into three groups: the Gm, with up to 25 specificities; the Km, with three specificities; and allotypes restricted to IgA (Am) and IgM. The properties of these specificities are tabulated in Table 6-3. The Gm specificities are found only in IgG and are located on the γ-chain. Different specificities are found in the IgG subclasses and are inherited in fixed combinations. The Km specificities are located on the κ light chains of each immunoglobulin class and are determined by a single amino substitution at position 153 or 191 of the κ-chain.

Genetic Analysis of Human Gm Allotypes

Human immunoglobulin allotypic markers are highly specific, inbuilt, genetically determined labels that show strict adher-

Table 6-3. Some Representative Human Immunoglobulin Allotypes

Locus	Chain Location	Allotype	Amino Acid Residue
G1m	Cγ1 (CH1)	G1m (4)	Arg 214
		G1m (17)	Lys 214
	Cγ1 (CH3)	G1m (1)	Asp 356, Leu 358
		G1m (−1)	Glu 356, Met 358
G2m	Cγ2 (CH2)	G2m (23), G2m (23^-)	N.D.
G3m	Cγ3 (CH2)	G3m (5)	N.D.
		G3m (5^-)	N.D.
		G3m (15)	N.D.
		G3m (16)	N.D.
		G3m (21)	Tyr 296
		G3m (21^-)	Phe 296
	Cγ3 (CH3)	G3m (6)	N.D.
		G3m (11)	Phe 436
		G3m (11^-)	Tyr 436
		G3m (13)	
		G3m (14)	
G4m	Cγ4 (CH2)	G4m (4a)	Leu 309
		G4m (4b)	Gap at position 309
A2m	Cα2 (CH3)	A2m (1)	Phe 411, Asp 428, Val 458, Val 467
		A2m (2)	Thr 411, Glu 428, Ile 458, Ala 467
Km	Cκ	Km (1)	Val 153, Leu 191
		Km (1,2)	Ala 153, Leu 191
		Km (3)	Ala 153, Val 191

N.D., not determined.

ence to Mendelian law and are inherited as codominant alleles. The number of amino acid substitutions between two allelic allotypes is usually one, but at the most four. The known genetic markers are located on "constant" portions of the immunoglobulin chain. No human genetic marker has been found on the amino-terminal quarter of the H-chain or the amino-terminal half of the L-chain. Therefore, allotypic determinants are not involved in the antibody combining site.

The genes controlling Gm specificities are closely linked. Crossing-over between IgG genes has been directly observed in some family studies. The recombination frequencies have been estimated as follows: between IgG_1 and IgG_3, 1 : 1000 to 1 : 10,000; between IgG_1 and IgG_2, 1 : 100 to 1 : 1000. The higher frequency of recombinations suggests greater distance between the latter two loci. The IgG_4 gene may be next to that of IgG_2. This order is in agreement with linkage analysis and gene complexes in various population groups. The existence of a hybrid IgG_1-IgG_3 molecule in rare individuals is direct evidence for the existence of gene crossover or deletion.

Synthesis and Assembly of Immunoglobulins

Immunoglobulin molecules are synthesized, assembled, and secreted by plasma cells. This process is generally the same as synthesis of secretory proteins in other mammalian cells. Genetic information is encoded in DNA (deoxyribonucleic acid) of the nucleus and is transcribed into messenger RNA (ribonucleic acid). The messenger RNA molecules are released into the cytoplasm, where they become associated with a number of ribosomes to form a polyribosome. The polyribosome associated with rough endoplasmic reticulum is the basic unit of protein synthesis. The messenger RNA is translated, and the amino acids are linked into a polypeptide chain. When translation of the message is completed, the newly synthesized polypeptide is released into the lumen of rough endoplasmic reticulum, carbohydrate added, and the protein secreted.

The production of immunoglobulins by myelomas (plasma cell tumors) is the model system used to study immunoglobulin synthesis. L-chains and H-chains are produced on different-size ribosomes. H-chain polyribosomes contain 12–18 ribosomes, and L-chain polyribosomes 7 or 8. Newly synthesized L-chains enter a rapidly turning-over pool and then become associated with H-chains. Disulfide bonds usually form between free L-chains and H-chains still on the H-chain ribosome. However, assembly differs among different myelomas. In some cases, one L- and one H-chain are joined prior to formation of the inter-H-chain bond, whereas in others, the inter-H-chain bond forms first, followed by binding of the L-chains. Partially assembled molecules, such as half molecules of one L- and one H-chain joined together, may be formed, as well as L-chains alone (Bence Jones proteins) or H-chains alone (H-chain disease). However, normal lymphoid cells produce essentially equal numbers of L- and H-chains.

Immunoglobulin Gene Rearrangements

Synthesis of immunoglobulin by a given B lymphocyte is preceded by rearrangement of the immunoglobulin genes. In humans, H-chain genes are on chromosome No. 8, κ-chain genes are on chromosome No. 2, and λ-chain genes are on chromosome No. 22. The germ line DNA (Fig. 6-12) for the heavy and light chains of immunoglobulin contains multiple copies of variable region genes (V), joining region genes (J), and constant region genes (C). In addition heavy chain genes contain a diversity or "D" region. During B cell maturation, deletion of intervening sequences occurs between V and J or V and D and J, so the immunoglobulin-producing plasma cell contains DNA with juxtaposition of VJ or VDJ genomic regions required for encoding a given heavy or light chain. These rearrangements delete V region genes and J region genes that are not needed, and also bring together the V region promoter site and the J region enhancing site, which makes the new V–J–C

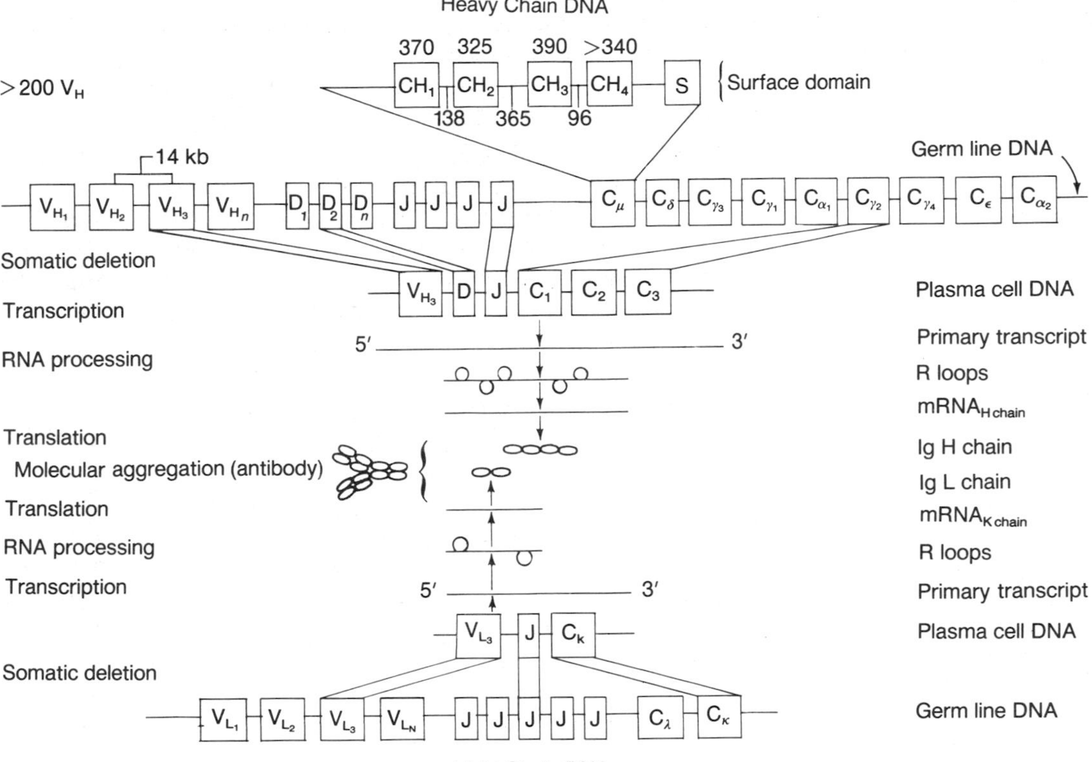

Figure 6-12. Immunoglobulin gene rearrangements associated with Ig synthesis by B cells. The example depicted has a γ_2 heavy chain and a κ light chain. The detailed genetic structure for the γ_2-chain constant regions, including four constant region domains and a sequence believed to be present on IgM molecules on the cell surface, is shown above the heavy chain germ line DNA. The numbers indicate the numbers of base pairs in each segment. The D region may also contribute to diversity by providing different sequences between V_H and J. During B cell development into an Ig synthesizing plasma cell the germ line DNA undergoes rearrangement so that one V_H region is combined with a set of constant region genes through deletion of the intervening sequences. The final mixture of mRNA is translated into the polypeptide chain including the short hydrophobic leader peptide responsible for transmembrane passage of the immunoglobulin, which is cleaved off during secretion.

transcriptionally active. Transcription of this genomic sequence results in production of a primary nuclear RNA transcript containing the base sequences necessary for translation into the protein chain (exons), separated by untranslated intervening sequences (introns). The introns are removed during RNA processing, resulting in a translationally active messenger RNA molecule. In a given plasma cell only one type of light chain and one type of heavy chain are synthesized. These then combine in the cytoplasm and are secreted as a four-chain immunoglobulin antibody molecule.

In order to attain a productive gene rearrangement DNA sequences between V and J must be removed. These sequences are flanked by a specific set of nucleic acids that match a homologous set of nucleotides (palindrome) to form a stem-and-loop:

-CACTGTG-
-GTGACAC-

A palindrome is a sequence that reads the same backward as forward (e.g., "Madam, I'm Adam"). Through this mechanism a loop of DNA is formed and chopped off (Fig. 6-13), which permits the splicing together of the DNA regions coding for V and J.

All immunoglobulin-producing B cells and plasma cells

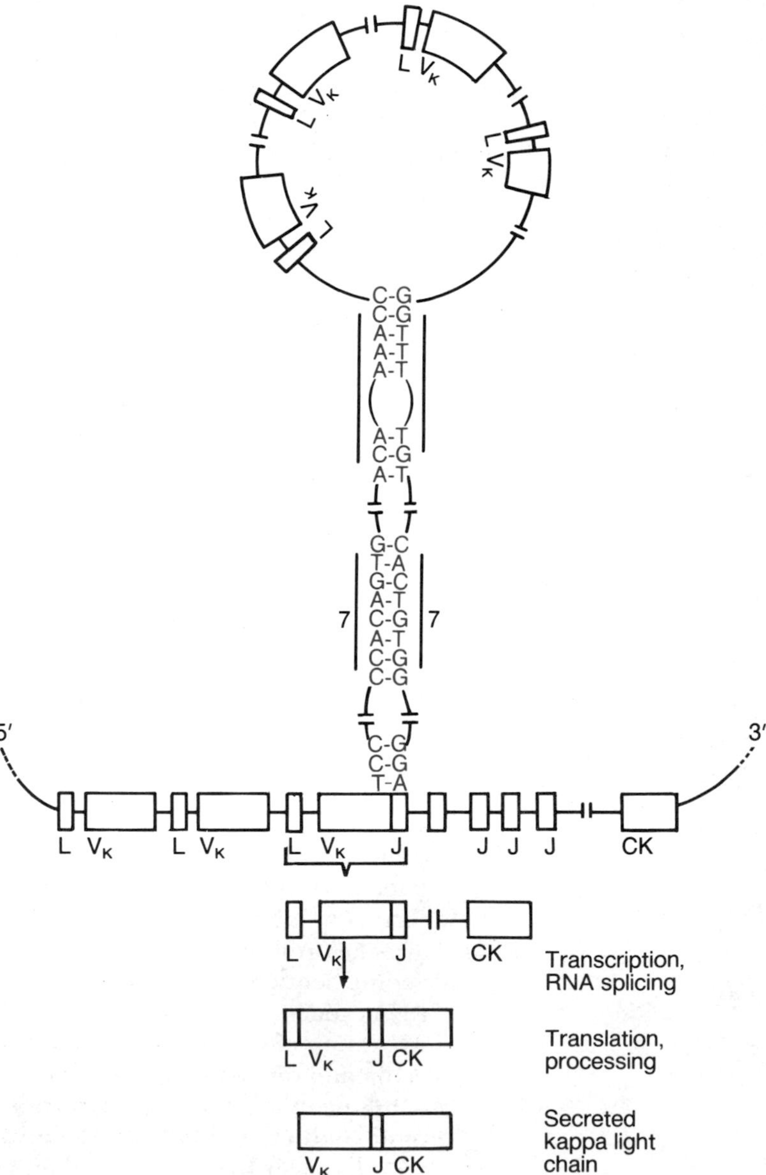

Figure 6-13. Model of V_H/J joining during immunoglobulin gene rearrangement. L = leader sequence, V_κ = kappa variable region, J = joining region, C_κ = constant region of κ light chains. Intervening L and V_κ regions are cut out as a loop formed from a stem structure of palindromic nucleotides on the 3′ end of the variable region that occur in reverse order on the 5′ end of the J region (red). DNA located between the V_κ and J region is deleted. Similar looping allows the J region to be spliced next to the C region so that the mRNA will be translated with the V_κ, J, and C_κ regions together.

must have rearranged immunoglobulin genes in order to produce immunoglobulins. To be productive the immunoglobulin genes must be rearranged correctly. In B cell differentiation, heavy chain genes appear to be rearranged before light chain genes and both κ genes appear to be rearranged before λ genes. If both κ genes are rearranged, only one will be a correct productive rearrangement (allelic exclusion). Each B cell usually produces one L-chain, which will be either κ or λ. The nonexpressed genes either will be in the germ line arrangement or will be aberrantly rearranged or deleted. The heavy chain genes are rearranged in a manner similar to the light chain genes. The heavy chains contain an additional region, the D region, which is incorporated into the V region of the heavy chain as V–D–J–C.

Cell Surface Immunoglobulin

In addition to serum antibodies, immunoglobulins also serve as cell surface antigen receptors for B cells. The mRNAs for the membrane and secreted forms of IgM are transcribed from the same gene, but the message for membrane IgM is processed differently, resulting in two additional carboxy-terminal exons coding for (1) a hydrophobic amino acid sequence that holds the molecule in the membrane lipid, and (2) a hydrophilic carboxy-terminal end on the cytoplasmic side (Fig. 6-14). The two

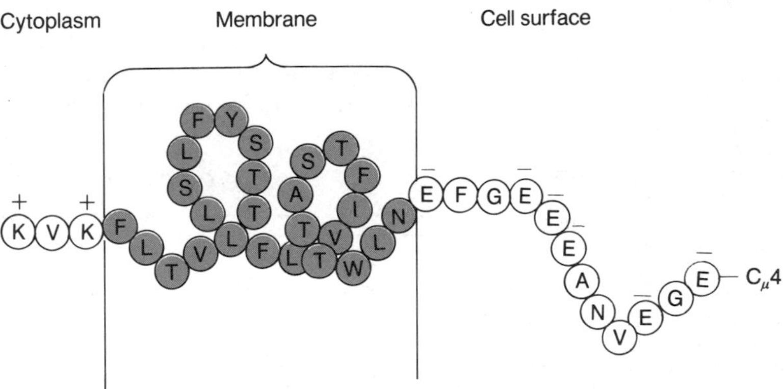

Figure 6-14. Configuration of the IgM membrane segment in the cell membrane. The μ chain is anchored in the cell membrane by the membrane (M) segment. The uncharged 26-residue sequence in the M segment is an α-helix spanning the membrane, depicted by the coiled segment in the diagram. Positive and negative charged residues that flank the transmembrane sequence are indicated.

forms of IgM are designated IgM_s (serum IgM) and IgM_m (membrane IgM) and the heavy chains μ_s and μ_m. The μ_m mRNA is assembled identically to the μ_s mRNA except that the additional coding segment containing the M polypeptide remains attached to the Cμ4 gene with an intervening sequence cut out during RNA processing (Fig. 6-15). This results in a mRNA for μ_m with an additional M polypeptide of 41 residues, 26 of which are uncharged and represent the hydrophobic membrane domain (Fig. 6-14).

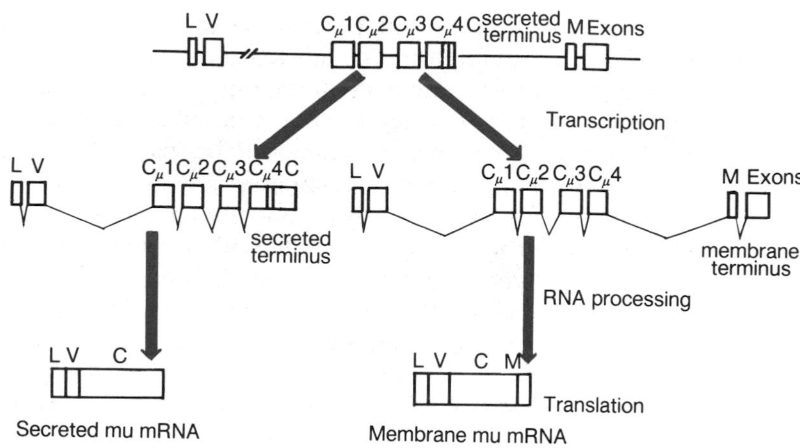

Figure 6-15. Splicing of μ_s and μ_m mRNAs. The expressed μ gene as shown has been constructed by a $V_H/D_H/J_H$ rearrangement. L = DNA coding for the signal (leader) peptide; V = V_H region; Cμ1, Cμ2, Cμ3, and Cμ4 = four constant coding segments; M = DNA for the membrane segment; Exons = 3′ untranslated sequence; CT = the terminal segment of μ_s. The choice of the 3′ coding segments to give μ_s or μ_m is made at the level of RNA transcription, processing, and splicing. The bent lines indicate RNA splicing between exons.

Differentiation of B Cells and Expression of Immunoglobulin

During antigen-driven maturation of B cells to plasma cells a switch in immunoglobulin class expression occurs. Most B cells express IgM and IgD on the surface. Antigen stimulation results in the appearance of B cells restricted to surface expression of one of the other immunoglobulin classes, IgG, IgA, or IgE. This is accomplished by recombination between repetitive DNA sequence elements (Fig. 6-16). Ig class switching occurs

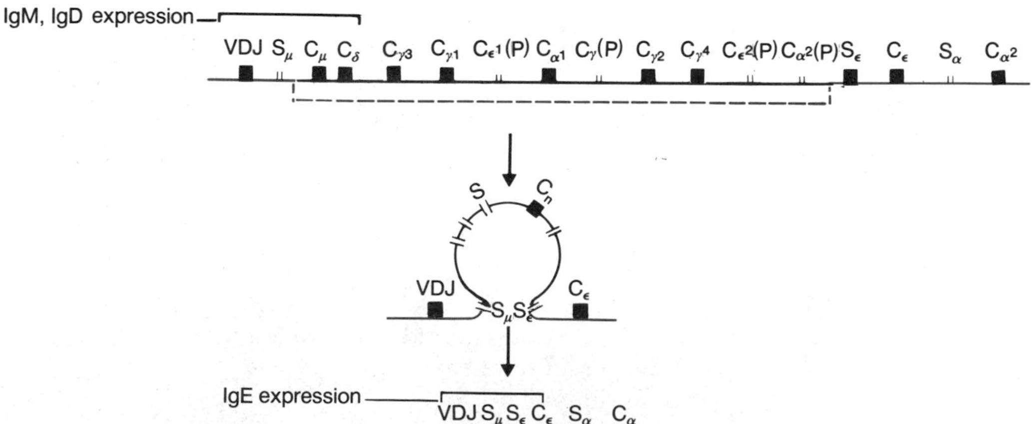

Figure 6-16. Immunoglobulin class (isotype) switching. Depicted is the sequence of constant gene regions of the immunoglobulin heavy chains of the human (Cμ, Cδ, Cγ, etc). In the B cell, IgM and IgD are expressed. This expressing correlates with the juxtaposition of the VDJ region next to Cμ and Cδ. When a cell line switches to IgE expression there is looping out between the switch regions of Cμ (Sμ) and Cϵ_1 (Sϵ_1) causing deletion of the intervening genes. (P) refers to pseudogenes.

by genetic recombinations between switch regions that lie in front of each constant region gene. The switch regions are as long as 1600 nucleotides and contain repetitive sequences that permit "looping out" of the intervening sequences by palindromic heterodimer formation. In B cell differentiation a switch from a pre-B cell expressing μ and δ to another class is accomplished by genetic recombination between the switch region lying before $C\mu$ and that lying before the $C\gamma$ or $C\alpha$ or $C\epsilon$ region to be expressed. The arrangement of the heavy chain genes also permits switching from one upstream C_H gene to another, for example, from $C\gamma 1$ to $C\gamma 2$ or from a $C\gamma 1$ to $C\epsilon$ with deletion of the intervening DNA. Two observations must be reconciled with this mechanism. First, occasional "back switching" may occur. In this situation a cell line expressing IgA may revert to expression of IgM. This may be explained by recombination of the other chromosome, by a mechanism that permits functional looping out without deletion and reestablishment of the original sequence, or by mRNA processing. Second, cells that express two or three isotypes at the same time are often found, usually μ and δ with another class. This may be explained by cells in transition from one class to another or by control of class switching during RNA processing.

A model for B cell maturation and generation of immunoglobulin class constant region (isotype) diversity is illustrated in Figure 6-17. There are two major phases of B cell develop-

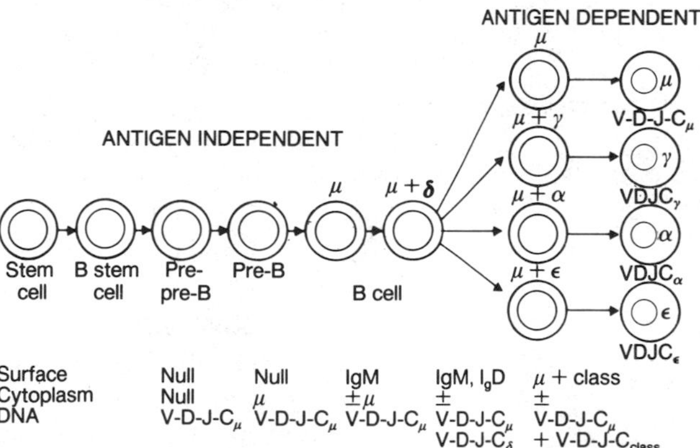

Figure 6-17. A model of B cell differentiation (for a description, see the text).

ment: antigen independent and antigen dependent. B cell maturation from a multipotent hematopoietic stem cell (see Fig. 4-1) to mature B cells expressing cell surface IgM and IgD is believed to be antigen independent. By rearranging a given V–D–J combination the antigen-recognizing specificity of the B cell may be determined at these steps before antigen enters the system. The first identifiable cell in the B cell lineage is the *pre-pre-B cell,* in which rearrangement of immunoglobulin heavy chain genes with juxtaposition of V_H–D–J–Cμ has occurred but rearrangement of the light chain genes has not. The pre-pre-B cell does not express either cytoplasmic or cell surface immunoglobulin. The next cell, the *pre-B cell,* expresses cytoplasmic μ-chains but not cell surface immunoglobulin and still has not rearranged or expressed light chain genes. Immature *B cells* have rearranged heavy and light chain genes and express both. They exist in two classes, those that express cell surface IgM only and those that express cell surface IgM and IgD. Upon antigenic stimulation and given appropriate signals from helper T cells (see Chapter 10), B cells proliferate to expand the clone and differentiate into plasma cells that express the same V–D–J combination as before but may now use a different constant region gene, which results in the same antigen recognition specificity but a different isotype (IgG, IgA, or IgE) or subclass of the secreted antibody molecule. Plasma cells have little surface immunoglobulin, but rapidly synthesize and secrete antibody of only one immunoglobulin class.

T Cell Receptor Expression

Similarities between T cell receptor domains and immunoglobulin domains indicate their common origin by duplication of a common ancestral gene. In contrast to antibody molecules as receptors for B cells, the receptor(s) on the T cell for antigen recognition has been difficult to characterize at the protein level. However, extensive structural studies of the T cell receptor have been possible through recombinant DNA methods. The specificity of recognition of antigen implies that the T cell receptor could be like an immunoglobulin molecule, but monoclonal antibodies to immunoglobulin epitopes do not react with T cells. In addition, T cells do not contain mRNA that hybridizes with cDNA probes for immunoglobulin. Three approaches have shed considerable light on the T cell receptor: (1) generation of T cell clones that produce homogeneous receptors, (2) production of monoclonal antibodies to T cell receptors, and (3) development of cDNA probes for the T cell receptor mRNA. Monoclonal antibodies have permitted isolation of an MW 80,000–90,000 heterodimer T cell receptor from T cell lines that contains an acidic (α) chain and a basic (β) chain (Fig. 6-18). Monoclonal antibodies to this receptor can activate T cells to proliferate. This receptor is quite variable among different T cell lines. It contains idiotypes and has constant and variable regions similar to those of immunoglobulin. The α and β chains are very different and are coded for by different genes. The DNA of T cells shows gene rearrangements in the genes for the T cell receptor that are characteristic of each T cell clone, similar to what occurs for immunoglobulin genes in plasma cells producing immunoglobulin. Sequence data from many clones have shown additional similarities be-

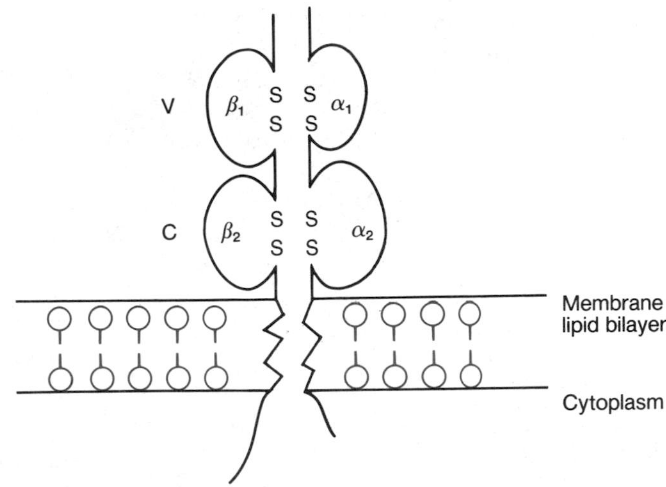

Figure 6-18. The T cell receptor contains extracellular, transmembrane, and cytoplasmic domains. It is a heterodimer of two polypeptide chains α and β. The β-chain contains variable and constant regions. The α-chain has not been well characterized.

tween B cell immunoglobulin expression and T cell receptor expression (Fig. 6-19). No clear correlation exists between T

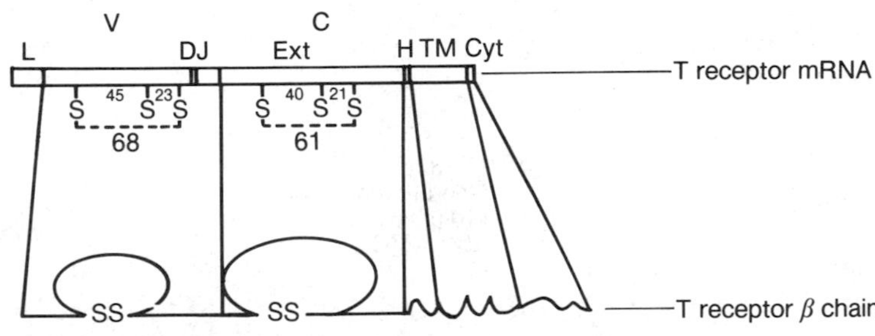

Figure 6-19. Gene rearrangements and predicted protein structure of the β-chain subunit of the T cell receptor indicate similarities to immunoglobulin gene expression. L = leader, D = diversity, J = joining, V = variable, C = constant, Ext = external, H = hinge, T_M = transmembrane, and Cyt = cytoplasmic. VDJ joining of genomic DNA and processing of transcripted RNA to form mRNA are similar to those of immunoglobulin genes. (Modified from Davis M, et al: Immunol Rev 8:235, 1984.)

cell receptor gene rearrangement and major histocompatibility complex (MHC) expression.

Origin of Immunoglobulin Gene Diversity

Two major mechanisms have been hypothesized to account for the great diversity seen in immunoglobulin molecules: germ line (evolution) and somatic mutation.

Germ Line

On the basis of comparison of the immunoglobulins of different species, it is postulated that a primitive immunoglobulin gene coding for a peptide chain equal in length to one-half of an L-chain developed in the prevertebrate era. The most primitive immunoglobulins yet found in vertebrates consist of fully developed L- and H-chains. The genes responsible for fully developed chains are believed to have evolved through gene

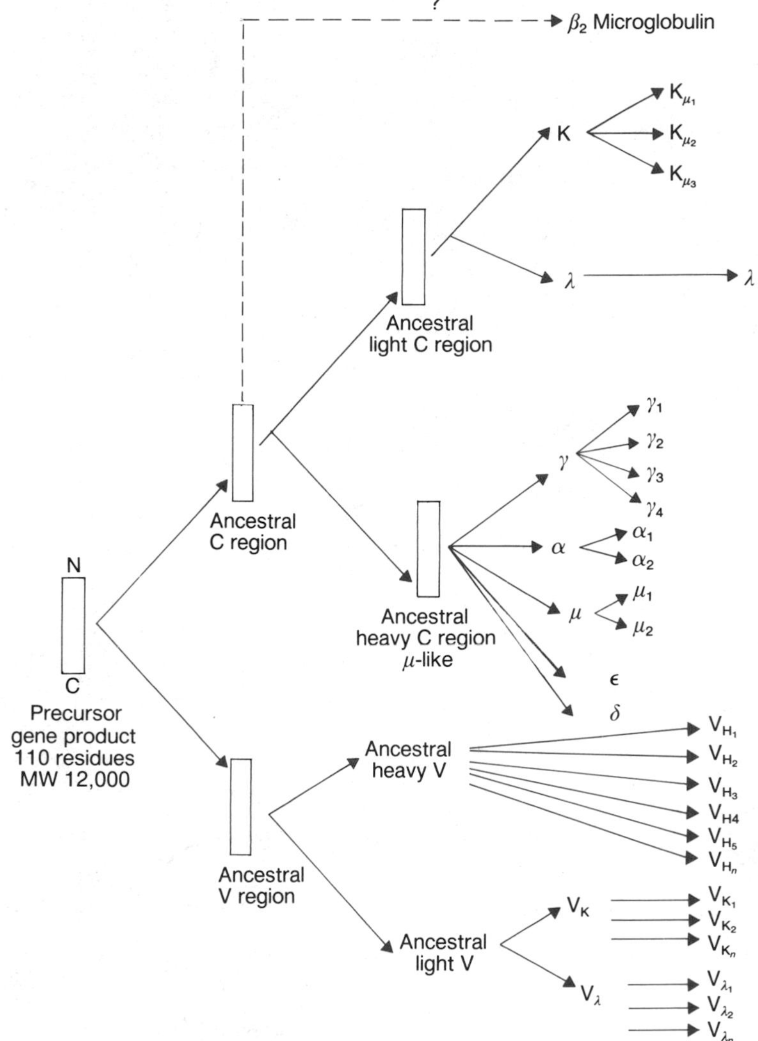

Figure 6-20. Immunoglobulin genes may have evolved from a single precursor gene by duplication and mutation. This has resulted in multiple V_H, V_κ, and V_λ genes in the different chromosomes that combine with a limited member of C_H, C_κ and C_λ genes to form the transcribed gene for the immunoglobulin mRNA.

duplication (Fig. 6-20). One duplication would result in a gene for a complete L-chain (constant and variable regions). Additional duplications would be required for production of a polypeptide chain the length of the H chain (four primitive units). A subsequent duplication of the L-chain gene would result in two L-chains, κ and λ. The most primitive H-chain identified (cyclostomes) is homologous to the μ-chain of IgM. Further gene duplication and divergence in teleosts and amphibians resulted in a gene coding for a chain homologous to the γ-chain of IgG. The α-, δ- and ϵ-chains may have resulted from further duplication of the μ-like ancestral gene chain gene. Later duplication of the γ-chain resulted in evolution of the IgG subclasses. This scheme is highly speculative and is dependent mainly on the observation that the L-chain consists of two MW 12,000 units (variable and constant regions) and the H-chain consists of four

MW 12,000 units (one variable region similar to that of the L-chain and three constant regions). Thus duplication of a gene coding for a MW 12,000 polypeptide chain could account for the evolution of human immunoglobulins.

It is not clear, however, how such duplication could lead to the genetic information required for the vast numbers of V_H and V_L regions needed for the many antigenic building sites possible. To account for these many specificities, further gene modification by somatic mutation is postulated.

Somatic Mutation

According to the somatic mutation theories, a small number of germ line genes become highly diversified during development of the individual, resulting in the formation of a large number of differentiated immunocompetent cells capable of individually recognizing a variety of antigens. This may be accomplished by point mutations occurring successively, perhaps through the influence of antigenic contact or by recombination of inherited germ line V genes during somatic cell division. The basic genetic information is probably derived from germ line diversity developed during evolution, and additional diversity arises during somatic development.

The complexity of the immunoglobulin genes permits great potential for generation of diversity. For instance in the heavy chain three segments of DNA, V_H, D, and J, must be joined together to assemble a gene coding for the entire variable region of the heavy chain. The D (diversity) region segments frequently have more than one open coding frame permitting several amino acid sequences to be produced by a single gene sequence. The D_H sequence codes for a sizable part of the third hypervariable region of the V_H domain. In this position it plays a major part in antibody specificity and is often recognized as an idiotype. The three segments, $V_H/D_H/J_H$, can use several frames for recombination, providing a molecular basis for diversity.

Summary

Antibodies are glycoprotein molecules that have the capacity to bind specifically to an antigen. Antibodies belong to a group of structurally related molecules termed *immunoglobulins*. There are five major classes of immunoglobulins with different biological properties. The basic immunoglobulin molecule consists of two pairs of polypeptide chains joined by disulfide bonds. Each chain contains regions of variable amino acid sequences and regions of constant amino acid sequences. This provides the uniqueness required for binding to different antigens and the commonality needed for the biological function of each immunoglobulin class. The genes coding for the two chains of immunoglobulin (heavy and light chains) are located on different chromosomes. The variable region genes (up to 500) and constant region genes (1 per subclass of Ig) are rearranged during development of B cells so that one V_H and one C_H region are joined in a productive sequence. During antigen-stimulated B cell development the same variable region may be joined to different constant region genes—"isotype switching." T cells also have receptors whose expression is controlled by similar mechanisms. This permits great diversity in antigen binding. One V_H region may be joined to different C_H regions in different cells and V_H regions may be altered by the process of rearrangement to permit different amino acid substitutions.

References

General

Kindt TS, Capra JD: The Antibody Enigma. New York, Plenum, 1984.

Nisonoff A: Introduction to Molecular Immunology. Sunderland, Mass., Sinauer Assoc., 1982.

Immunoglobulins

Cohen S, Milstein C: Structure and biologic properties of immunoglobulins. Adv Immunol 7:1, 1967.

Committee on Nomenclature of Human Immunoglobulins: Notation for genetic factors of human immunoglobulins. Bull WHO 30:447, 1964.

Edelman GM, Cunningham BA, Gall WE, Gottlieb PD, Rutishauser U, Waxdal MD: The covalent structure of an entire γ-immunoglobulin molecule. Biochemistry 63:78, 1969.

Fahey JL: Antibodies and immunoglobulins. JAMA 194:141, 183, 1966.

Franklin EC: Immune globulins: their structure and function and some techniques for their isolation. Prog Allergy 8:58, 1964.

Halpern MS, Koshland ME: The stoichiometry of J chain in human secretory IgA. J Immunol 111:1563–1660, 1973.

Kabat EA: General features of antibody molecules. *In* Pressman D, Tomasi TB, Jr, Grossberg AL, Rose NR (eds): Specific Receptors of Antibodies, Antigens and Cells. Basel, Karger, 1973.

Merler E, Rosen FS: The gamma globulins. I. The structure and synthesis of the immunoglobulins. N Engl J Med 275:480–536, 1964.

Metzer H: The chemistry of the immunoglobulins. JAMA 202:129, 1967.

Osserman EF, Takatsuki K: Plasma cell myeloma: gamma globulin synthesis and structure. Medicine 42:357, 1963.

Painter RH: The C1q receptor site on human immunoglobulin G. Can J Biochem Cell Biol 62:418, 1984.

Rowe DS, Hug K, Forni L, Pernis B: Immunoglobulin D as a lymphocyte receptor. J Exp Med 138:965, 1973.

Scharff MD, Laskov R: Synthesis and assembly of immunoglobulin polypeptide chains. Prog Allergy 14:37, 1970.

Silverton EW, Navia MA, Davies DR: Three dimensional structure of an intact human immunoglobulin. Proc Nat Acad Sci USA 74:5140, 1977.

Speigelberg HL: D Immunoglobulin. *In* Inman FP (ed): Contemporary Topics in Immunochemistry. New York, Plenum, 1972, pp165–180.

Spiegelberg HL: Biological activities of immunoglobulins of different classes and subclasses. Adv Immunol 19:259, 1974.

Tomasi TB, Bienenstock J: Secretory immunoglobulins. Adv Immunol 9:1, 1968.

Thorebecke GJ, Leslie GA (eds): Immunoglobulin D: Structure and Function. New York, Academy of Science, 1982.

Wilkelhake JL: Immunoglobulin structure and effector functions. Immunochemistry 15:695, 1978.

Antibody Structure

Bernier GM: Structure of human immunoglobulins: myeloma proteins as analogues of antibody. Prog Allergy 14:1, 1970.

Capra JD, Edmundson AB: The antibody combining site. Sci Am 236:50, 1977.

Givol D: Structural analysis of the antibody containing site. *In* Reisfeld R, Mandy W (eds): Contemporary Topics in Molecular Immunology. New York, Plenum, 1973, p27.

Gottlieb PD: Immunoglobulin genes. Mol Immunol 17:1423, 1980.

Green NM: Electron microscopy of the immunoglobulins. Adv Immunol 11:1, 1969.

Kabat EA: Origins of antibody complementarity and specificity—hypervariable regions and the minigene hypothesis. J Immunol 125:96, 1980.

Marquart M, Deisenhofer J, Huber R, Palm W: Crystallographic refinement and atomic models of the intact immunoglobulin molecule Ko1 and its antigen binding fragment at 3.0 Å and 1.9 Å resolution. J Mol Biol 141:369, 1980.

Novotony J, et al: Molecular anatomy of the antibody binding site. J Biol Chem 258:14433, 1983.

Ohno S, Mori N, Matsunaga T: Antigen binding specificities of antibodies are primarily determined by seven residues of V_H. Proc Nat Acad Sci USA 82:2945, 1985.

Padlan EA: Structural basis for the specificity of antibody–antigen reactions and structural mechanisms for the diversification of antigen-binding specificities. Rev Biophys 10:35, 1977.

Svehag SE, Bloth B: Ultrastructure of secretory and high-polymer serum immunoglobulin A of human and rabbit origin. Science 168:847, 1970.

Talmadge DW, Cann JR: The Chemistry of Immunity in Health and Disease. Springfield, Ill., Thomas, 1961.

Allotypes and Idiotypes

Bankert RB, Bloor AG, Jou Y-H: Idiotypes, their presence on B- and T-lymphocytes and their role in the regulation of the immune response. Vet Immunol Immunopathol 3:147, 1982.

Brient BW, Nisonoff A: Quantitative investigations of idiotypic antibodies. IV. Inhibition of specific haptens of the reaction of antihapten antibody with its anti-idiotypic antibody. J Exp Med 132:951, 1970.

Davis J, et al: Structural correlates of idiotypes 4:147, 1986.

Fudenberg HH, Pink JRL, Stites DP, Wang A-C: Basic Immunogenetics. New York, Oxford University Press, 1972.

Kelus AS, Cell PGH: Immunoglobulin allotypes of experimental animals. Prog Allergy 11:141, 1967.

Kohler H, Urbain J, Cazenave P (eds): Idiotypes in Biology and Medicine. Orlando, Fla., Academic Press, 1984.

Grubb R: The genetic markers of human immunoglobulins. *In* Kleinzeller A, Springer GF, Whittmann HC (eds): Molecular Biology, Biochemistry, and Biophysics, Vol 9. Berlin, Springer, 1970.

Moller G (ed): Anti-idiotypic antibodies as immunogens. Immunol Rev 90, 1986.

Moller G (ed): Idiotype networks. Immunol Rev 79, 1984.

Natvig JB, Kunkel HG: Genetic markers of human immunoglobulins: the Gm and InV systems. Semin Hematol 1:66, 1968.

Natvig JB, Kunkel HG: Human immunoglobulins: classes, subclasses, genetic variants and idiotypes. Adv Immunol 16:1, 1973.

Rajewsky K, Takemori T: Genetics, expression and function of idiotypes. Annu Rev Immunol 1:569, 1983.

Rodkey LS: Autoregulation of the immune response via idiotype network interaction. Microbiol Rev 44:631, 1980.

Immunoglobulin Genes

Calame KL: Mechanisms that regulate immunoglobulin gene expression. Annu Rev Immunol 3:159, 1985.

Cushley W, Williamson AR: Expression of immunoglobulin genes. Essays Biochem 18:1, 1982.

Honjo T: Immunoglobulin genes. 1:499, 1983.

Hood L, Campbell JH, Elgin SCR: The organization, expression, and evolution of antibody genes and other multigene families. Annu Rev Genet 9:305, 1975.

Moller G (ed): Molecular aspects of V genes. Immunol Rev 36, 1977.

Moller G (ed): Control of immunoglobulin gene expression. Immunol Rev 89, 1986.

Seidman JG, Leder A, Nau M, Norman B, Leder P: Antibody diversity. The structure of cloned immunoglobulin genes suggests a mechanism for generating new sequences. Science 202:11, 1978.

Wall R, Kuehl M: Biosynthesis and regulation of immunoglobulins. Annu Rev Immunol 1:393, 1983.

Yancopoulos CD, Alt F: Regulation and expression of variable region genes. Annu Rev Immunol 4:339, 1986.

B Cell Differentiation and Ig Expression

Brandtzaeg P: Role of J chain and secretory component in receptor mediated glandular and hepatic transport of immunoglobulins in man. Scand J Immunol 22:111, 1985.

Cebra JJ, Komisar JL, Schweitzer PA: C_H isotype switching during normal B cell development. Annu Rev Immunol 2:493, 1984.

Moller G (ed): B cell differentiation antigens. Immunol Rev 69, 1983.

Nossal CJV, Szenberg A, Ada CL, Austin G: Single cell studies in antibody production. J Exp Med 119:485, 1964.

Parkhouse RME, Cooper MD: A model for the differentiation of B lymphocytes with implications for the biological role of IgD. Immunol Rev 37:105, 1977.

Sell S: Development of restrictions in the expression of immunoglobulin specificities by lymphoid cells. Transplant Rev 5:19, 1970.

Whitlock C, Denis K, Robertson D, Witte O: In vitro analysis of B cell development. Annu Rev Immunol 3:213, 1985.

T Cell Receptor

Binz H, Lindeman J, Wigzell H: Cell-bound receptors for alloantigens on normal lymphocytes. II. Antialloantibody serum contains specific factors reacting with relevant immunocompetent T lymphocytes. J Exp Med 140:731, 1974.

Cosenza H, Kohler H: Specific suppression of the antibody response by antibodies to receptors. Proc Nat Acad Sci USA 69:2710, 1972.

Delisi C, Berzofsky JA: T-cell antigenic sites tend to be amphipathic structures. Proc Nat Acad Sci USA 82:7048, 1985.

Kronenberg M, Siu G, Hood L, Shastri N: The molecular genetics of the T cell antigen receptor and T cell antigen recognition. Annu Rev Immunol 4:529, 1986.

Meuer SC, et al: The human T cell receptor. Annu Rev Immunol 2:23, 1984.

Moller G (ed): Idiotypes on T and B cells. Immunol Rev 34, 1977.

Moller G (ed): T cell receptors and genes. Immunol Rev 81, 1984.

Watts TH, Gariepy J, Schoolnik GK, McConnel HM: T cell activation by peptide antigen: effect of peptide sequence and method of antigen presentation. Proc Nat Acad Sci USA 82:5480, 1985.

Weiss A, et al: The role of the T3/Ti antigen receptor complex in T cell activation. Annu Rev Immunol 4:593, 1986.

Generation of Diversity

Burnet FM: The Clonal Selection Theory of Acquired Immunity. Nashville, Tenn., Vanderbilt University Press, 1959.

Cohen EP: On the mechanism of immunity: in defense of evolution. Annu Rev Microbiol (Stanford) 22:283, 1968.

Gally JA, Edelman GM: Genetic control of immunoglobulin synthesis. Annu Rev Genet 6:1, 1972.

Grey HM: Phylogeny of immunoglobulins. Adv Immunol 10:51, 1969.

Hood L, Talmadge DW: Mechanism of antibody diversity: germ line basis for variability. Science 168:325, 1970.

Matsunaga T: Evolution of antibody diversity. Somatic mutation as a late event. Dev Exp Immunol 9:585, 1985.

Milstein C, Pink JRL: Structure and evolution of immunoglobulins. Prog Biophys Mol Biol 21:211, 1970.

7 Antigen–Antibody Reactions

Antibodies are defined by their ability to react specifically with antigen. Antibody molecules are made up of constant parts, which are responsible for the biological properties of the different classes, and variable parts, which are responsible for the ability to react with and bind to antigen. The antigen-binding site or *paratope* is formed by the folding and special arrangement of hypervariable regions of the heavy and light chains of the immunoglobulin molecule. A molecular site (paratope) is formed, which permits close juxtaposition of amino acid chains and other short range reactions of the antigen-binding site of the antibody and the antigenic determinant *(epitope)* of the antigen. An antigenic determinant or epitope is defined as that part of the antigen molecule that reacts with antibody (see Chapter 5).

Polyfunctional Antibody (Cross-Reactions)

A single antibody species may be able to react with more than one antigenic determinant. This is possible if the configuration of the antigen-binding site has the flexibility or capability to fit, and bind, to small parts of structurally different antigenic determinants. The nature of polyfunctional antigen combining sites of antibody is depicted in Figure 7-1. The activity of polyfunc-

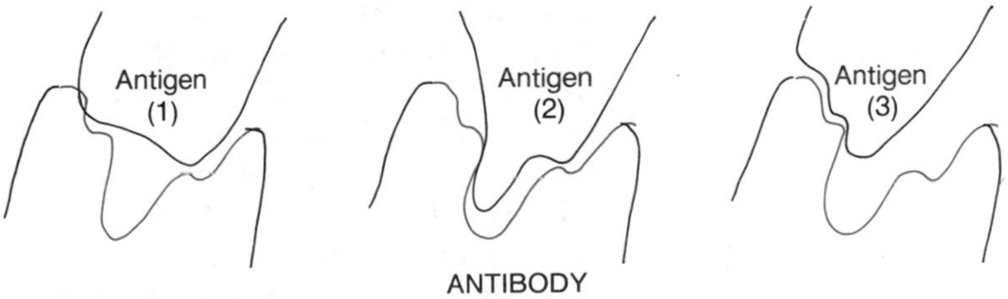

Antigen (1)
Antigen (2)
Antigen (3)
ANTIBODY

Figure 7-1. A single molecular species of antibody, termed *polyfunctional antibody,* may be able to react with seemingly different antigenic determinants that show some configurations recognizable by the antibody molecule. In this figure, antigens 1, 2, and 3 are different but each has a structure that is recognized by some part of the antigen combining site of the antibody (paratope, outlined in red).

tional antibodies helps explain the vast number of different antigens to which an individual can produce antibody. Antibody stimulated by one antigen may also cross-react with another antigen because of shared parts of the antigenic determinants or circumstantial fitting of the antibody-binding site to other antigens. Experimentally this is measured as the "cross-reaction" of the antibody with a seemingly unrelated second antigen.

Monoclonal Antibodies

The degree of complexity of the antigen-binding specificity of antibody is exemplified by the study of monoclonal antibodies (Fig. 7-2). Monoclonal antibodies may be produced by antibody-producing cells fused with tumors of plasma cells (myelomas). Most myeloma proteins do not react with known antigens. Monoclonal antibodies are engineered by fusion in vitro of lymphoid cells from an immunized animal with non-immunoglobulin-producing plasma cell tumor lines that have all the machinery necessary for antibody production and secretion, and also confer the ability for continuous growth in culture. Clones of hybrid cells are grown from single fused cells in vitro. Some of these cloned cell lines will retain the proliferative capacity of the tumor cell line and will also acquire the ability to produce specific antibodies coded for by the chromosomes of the cells from the immunized animal. Since each antibody-producing clone makes only one *(monoclonal)* antibody, characterization of the specificity of the reaction of a number of monoclonal antibodies to the same antigen leads to an understanding of the range of specificities produced by the

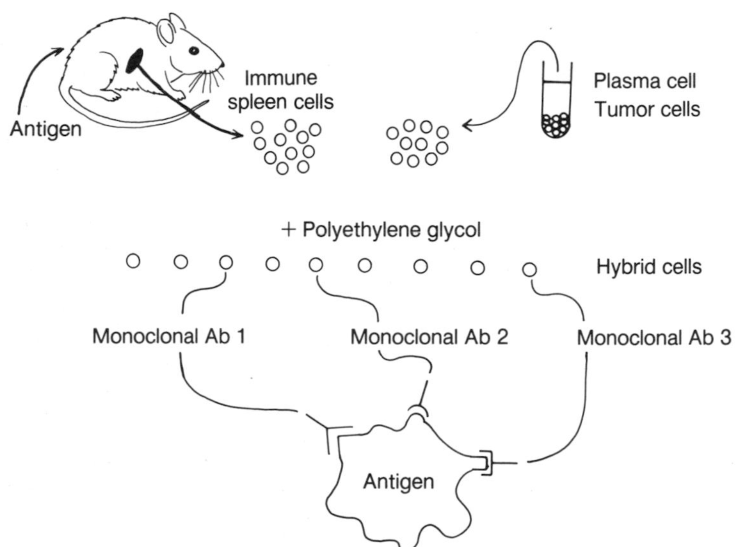

Figure 7-2. Each monoclonal antibody is the product of a single cell line produced by fusion of spleen cells from an immunized animal with cells from a plasma cell tumor. Hybrid cells with the capacity to produce and secrete a single molecular species of antibody can be produced, identified, isolated, and maintained in long-term culture. Since each individual antibody-producing hybridoma cell line produces antibody of only one specificity, more complete analysis of the possible antigenic determinant of an antigen is possible than with the mixtures of antibodies of different specificities produced by active immunization of the whole animal.

immunized animal. In this way, the number and relationship of the antigenic determinants of an immunogenic molecule may be more precisely determined than was previously possible with conventional polyclonal antisera.

Primary Antigen–Antibody Reaction

The combination of antibody with antigen to form an antibody–antigen complex is termed the *primary reaction*. The strength of the antibody–antigen bond is determined by the closeness of the geometric apposition of the antigen combining site with the antigenic determinant and the number and strength of bonds formed, including charge–charge, hydrogen, and hydrophilic bonds. The strength and specificity are determined by the complementarity of antibody and antigen. A tight fit is important because each bond acts at very short distance and is relatively weak, so that multiple bonds are needed to give a high-affinity interaction. The relationship between antibody and antigen has been likened to that of a lock (antibody) and key (antigen). The primary reaction of antibody (Ab) and antigen (Ag) may be expressed as an equilibrium reaction: $\mathrm{Ab} + \mathrm{Ag} \rightleftharpoons \mathrm{AgAb}$.

Affinity and Avidity

The strength of the noncovalent bond between the paratope of an antibody and the epitope of an antigen is termed *affinity;* the strength of the bond formed between a complete (divalent) antibody and antigen is termed the *avidity*. The presence of two or more antigen-binding sites on an antibody will increase the functional strength of its binding to antigen over a univalent antibody fragment; the avidity of an antibody is dependent on the affinities of its individual antigen-binding sites. Since most antigens have multiple determinants and both paratopes of an antibody may react with the antigen, it is difficult to measure affinity and avidity separately. This can be done using hapten antigens in excess (see below).

Equilibrium Dialysis

The actual affinity constant of an antibody can be measured by equilibrium dialysis (Fig. 7-3). Given the antibody–antigen binding equation

$$\mathrm{Ag} + \mathrm{Ab} \underset{K_2}{\overset{K_1}{\rightleftharpoons}} \mathrm{AgAb},$$

in which K_1 and K_2 are the rate constants for the association and dissociation of the antigen and antibody, the affinity constant K of equilibrium is

$$K_{\mathrm{A}} = \frac{[\mathrm{AgAb}]}{[\mathrm{Ag}][\mathrm{Ab}]} = \frac{K_1}{K_2},$$

where the brackets indicate the concentrations of the antigen [Ag], the antibody [Ab], and the complex [AgAb]. Since K is an

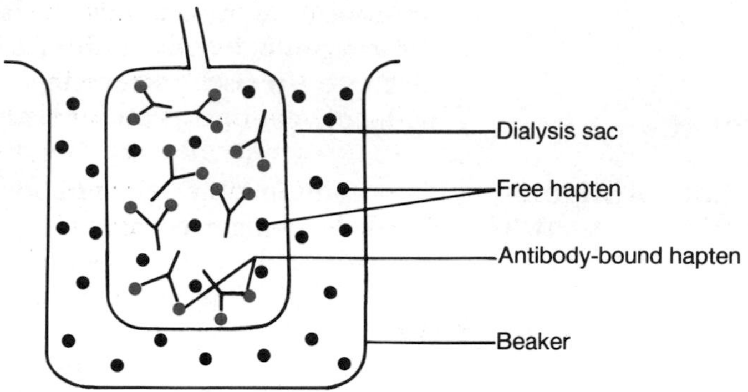

Figure 7-3. Equilibrium dialysis. A solution of antibody is placed inside a dialysis sac and the sac placed in a solution of free hapten. The dialysis sac is chosen to be permeable to the hapten but not to the antibody. Free hapten will dialyse into the sac where it will be bound by larger antibody. When the system reaches equilibrium the concentration of hapten inside the sac will be equal to the concentration of free hapten outside the sac, plus the concentration of the hapten bound to the antibody inside the sac.

"association constant," it will be a large number ($>10^5$) for high affinity complexes and a small number ($<10^3$) for low affinity complexes.

The affinity of antibody for monovalent antigens (haptens) is determined by equilibrium dialysis from the relationship

$$r = Kn - Kcr$$

where r is the ratio of moles of hapten bound to moles of antibody present, c is the concentration of unbound hapten, and n is the number of binding sides per antibody molecule. The moles of hapten bound are determined by subtracting the con-

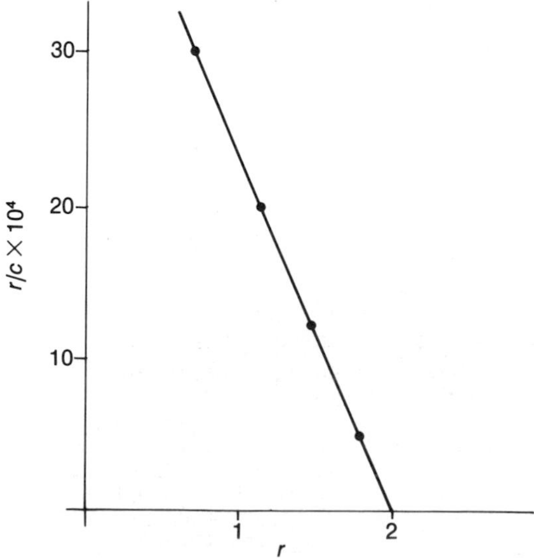

Figure 7-4. Plot of $r/c \times 10^4$ versus r for a monovalent hapten and a divalent IgG antibody. The r intercept is 2, the number of hapten molecules bound to each antibody molecule at infinite concentrations of hapten. The average association constant (K_0) = 3.5×10^5 liters/mole.

centration of hapten outside the dialysis sac from that within the sac containing the antibody. Since Kn is a constant, a plot of r/c versus r for different hapten concentrations (Fig. 7-4) will give a straight line with a slope of $-k$ and the valence of the antibody at the r intercept (infinite hapten concentration). Most antibodies have association constants from 10^5 to 10^{11} liters/mole, and most antibodies have a valence of 2.

The Farr Technique

A useful system for measuring the primary reaction of antibody and antigen was developed by Richard S. Farr. The principle of the Farr technique is the phase separation of bound antigen from free antigen. This assay forms the basis for many radioimmunoassays used for clinical and experimental quantification. The Farr procedure relies on the fact that the solubility properties of the AgAb complex may be different from those of the soluble antigen. The reaction used by Farr was that of bovine serum albumin (BSA) and rabbit antibody to BSA. The method relies on the fact that BSA is soluble in 50% saturated ammonium sulfate and that anti-BSA and BSA–anti-BSA complexes are not. The BSA is radiolabeled with ^{125}I or ^{131}I. The presence of radiolabeled BSA (*BSA) in the supernatant fluid or precipitate formed at 50% ammonium sulfate is determined by counting the radioactivity in each phase separately. Since the immunoglobulin antibody is precipitated at 50% ammonium sulfate normally, the *BSA bound to the antibody will precipitate along with the free antibody. The *BSA not attached to antibody, however, will remain soluble (Fig. 7-5). This method

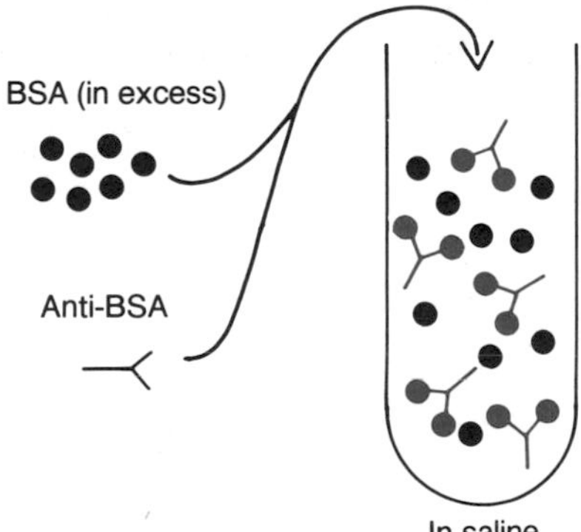

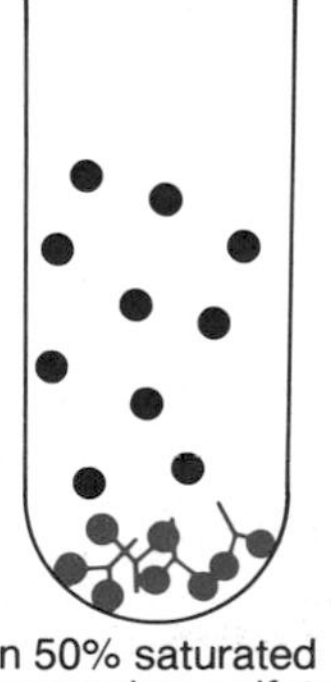

Figure 7-5. This figure demonstrates the principle of the Farr assay. The mixture of bovine serum albumin (BSA) and anti-BSA in saline (BSA in excess) results in complexation of all the antibody molecules to antigen. The free BSA molecules and the complexes are soluble in saline. However, if ammonium sulfate is added to form a half-saturated solution, the soluble antibody–antigen complexes become insoluble. By determining the distribution of radiolabeled BSA (in the supernatant fluid or in the precipitate), the amount of specific antibody can be quantified.

can be used to quantitate the binding capacity of an anti-BSA antiserum or the amount of competing, unlabeled BSA present in an unknown solution.

Antigen-Binding Capacity

One way to estimate the avidity of an antibody is based on the ability of antibody at different dilutions to bind antigen. Antibody of strong avidity is able to bind antigen at high dilutions, whereas the binding of a weak antibody is quickly lost upon dilution. In general, antibodies obtained early after immunization (2–4 weeks) do not have the ability to bind antigen at high dilutions, whereas antibodies collected late after immunization continue to bind antigen at high dilutions.

The antigen-binding capacity of an antiserum is determined by diluting the antiserum with normal serum until 33% of a constant amount of *BSA is precipitated as BSA–anti-BSA complexes in 50% ammonium sulfate. The antibody-binding capacity (ABC33) is calculated from the dilution of antiserum that results in precipitation of 33% of the *BSA. It is expressed as micrograms of BSA bound per milliliter of antiserum. To make this calculation, the radioactivity of the *BSA must be converted to micrograms of BSA. (The specific activity of the *BSA must be known.)

The strength of an antibody–antigen reaction also depends on the stability of the antibody–antigen bond after a complex has been formed. This property is a measure of the dissociation of antibody–antigen complexes or, in other words, the reaction to the left of the equilibrium reaction $Ag + Ab \leftarrow AgAb$.

This reaction can be measured by adding excess unlabeled antigen (BSA) to preformed complexes of antibody and labeled antigen (anti-BSA–*BSA). If the antibody–antigen complex is strong, a long time will be required for the radiolabeled antigen to appear in the supernatant fluid, whereas radiolabeled antigen will be rapidly displaced from the AgAb complexes by unlabeled antigen if the antibody–antigen complex is weakly bound.

Secondary Antigen–Antibody Reactions

After the binding of antibody and antigen in vitro, a number of different phenomena may be observed. These are termed *secondary reactions* and depend upon the nature of the antigen, the properties of the antibody, and the presence of other factors such as complement. Secondary reactions include precipitation, agglutination, cytolysis, complement fixation, immobilization, and neutralization (Table 7-1).

In the older literature, the secondary effect of the antibody–antigen reaction was used to apply a functional name to an antiserum. Thus, an antibody in a serum that caused precipitation upon reaction with a soluble antigen was called a *precipitin*. Other terms include *hemolysin* (lysis of red blood

Table 7-1. Examples of Primary and Secondary Antigen–Antibody Reactions

Primary Reaction Ag + Ab	$\rightleftharpoons$	Secondary Reaction Ag Ab
Antigen-binding assays (Farr)		Precipitation
Equilibrium dialysis		Agglutination
Radioimmunoassays		Complement fixation
		Neutralization
		Opsonification
		Hemolysis
		Toxin neutralization
		Bacteriolysis
		Immune labeling of tissues

cells), *agglutinin* (agglutination of particulate antigens), and *opsonin* (enhancement of phagocytosis of the antigen). The terms do not imply exclusive functions of an antibody. A precipitin may also be a hemolysin, an agglutinin, or an opsonin, depending upon the secondary reaction used to measure it. The antigen used to elicit a secondary response was given the suffix *-ogen*. For example, an antigen used to elicit precipitation is called a *precipitogen*, one that is used to produce agglutination an *agglutinogen*, etc.

Precipitin Reaction

The precipitin reaction depends upon formation of an insoluble antibody–antigen complex upon reaction of soluble antibody and soluble antigen. Most naturally occurring circulating antibody molecules (except for IgM antibodies) contain two antigen-binding sites of identical specificity (are divalent), and most antigens contain more than two antigenic determinant sites (are multivalent). Thus, when multivalent antigens are mixed in the proper proportions with divalent antibodies, each antibody molecule usually combines with two antigen molecules. As antibody molecules connect molecules of soluble antigen, a lattice-like conglomeration of antigen molecules connected by antibody molecules occurs. This results in the formation of large aggregates, which become insoluble, because of a decrease in affinity for water as a result of the interaction of the solubilizing polar groups of the antigen and antibody and an increase in density of the aggregates. If the antigen is soluble, this reaction with antibody results in precipitation of the complex, and visible precipitates may be observed when the appropriate amounts of antibody and antigen are mixed. If the antigen is particulate (large enough to be visible by itself), agglutination of the particulate antigen occurs as the individual particles of antigen are joined together by the antibody. Both precipitation and agglutination can be seen with the naked eye.

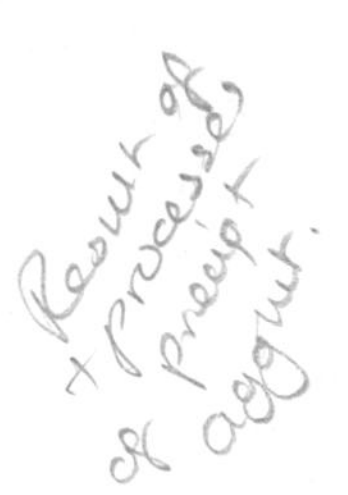

Soluble Antibody–Antigen Complexes

If the antigen is soluble and contains one or two determinant sites (is monovalent or divalent as opposed to multivalent), precipitation does not occur and soluble complexes are formed. Similar soluble antibody–antigen complexes are formed if the antibody is monovalent (Fab fragment) and the antigen multivalent. In these last two situations the number of combining sites of antigen or antibody is insufficient for a lattice-like structure to be built up.

Nonprecipitating (soluble) antibody–antigen complexes are also formed if the proportions of soluble antigen and specific antibody are such that a latticelike conglomeration of antibody and antigen is not formed. This situation exists in reactions where antigen or antibody is in excess. At antigen excess, each divalent antibody reacts with two separate multivalent antigen molecules, and there are not enough antibody molecules to form larger complexes. The complexes formed consist of only two antigen molecules and one antibody molecule. A complex of this size may not be large enough to be insoluble. Similarly, at antibody excess, each binding site of a multivalent antigen molecule is occupied by a separate antibody molecule, and not enough antigen sites are available for a divalent antibody molecule to join or bridge two antigen molecules. The resulting complex consists of one antigen molecule and the number of antibody molecules sufficient to cover its antigenic sites. Such a complex may not be of a form or size to be insoluble, and a soluble antigen–antibody complex is the result.

Quantitative Precipitin Reaction

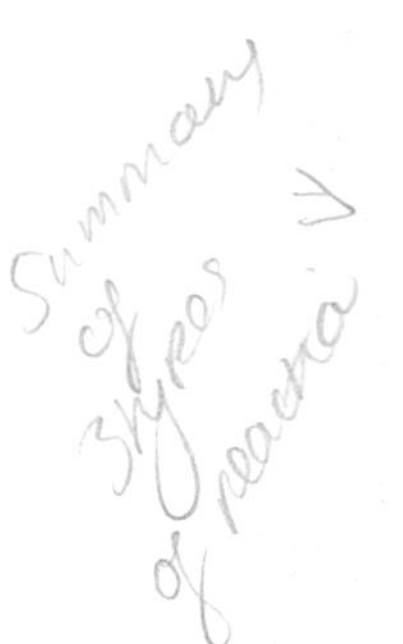

A precipitin reaction may be divided into three zones in relation to increasing amounts of antigen (Fig. 7-6): (1) zone of antibody excess—free antibody remains after all the antigen sites are covered by the antibody and soluble complexes are formed; (2) zone of equivalence—the amount of antigen is sufficient to bind all or most of the antibody so that the antigen–antibody complexes are insoluble and precipitate, with little or no unbound antibody or antigen remaining in soluble form; and (3) zone of antigen excess—the amount of antigen is sufficient to bind all the antibody to the extent that few, if any, antibody molecules can bind two antigen molecules together so that soluble complexes are formed.

Early tests for antibody activity depended upon effects such as neutralization of toxins, lysis, or agglutination of bacteria, which gave endpoints in the dilution of the antiserum that was still effective. The results of such tests were expressed as titers (dilutions). Expression of the activity of an antiserum as a titer or the highest dilution effective for a certain secondary reaction does not actually indicate the quantity of antibody present. For example, comparisons of titers of antipneumococcal sera and antityphoid sera cannot be made directly because the biological endpoints are different. Although the titer (effective dilution) of one antiserum may be higher than that of an-

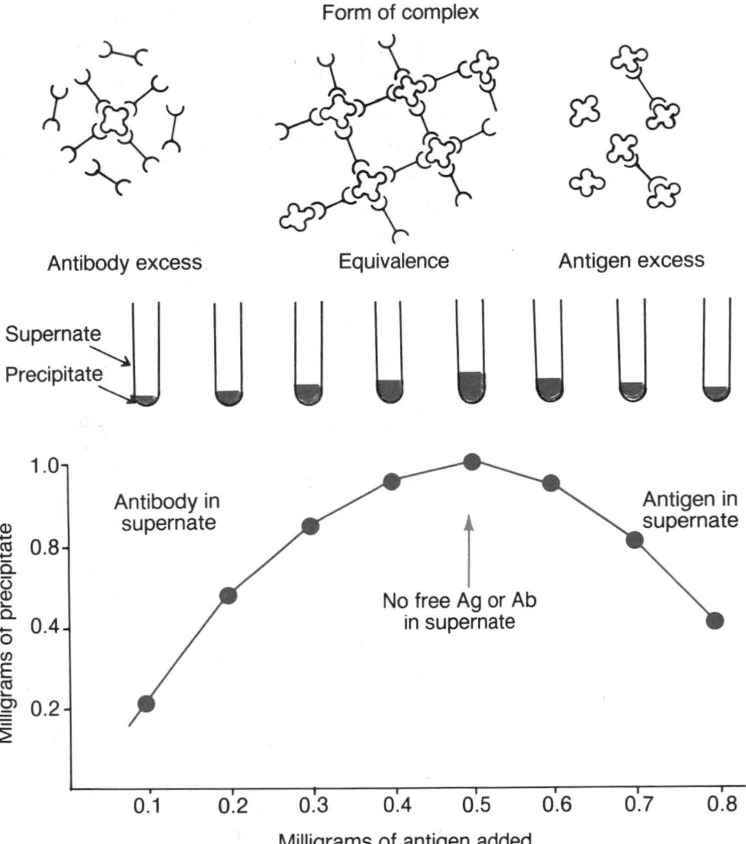

Figure 7-6. The quantitative precipitin reaction. If increasing amounts of antigen are separately added to constant amounts of antiserum, an increase in the amount of precipitate occurs to the maximum point. Further addition of antigen results in a decrease in the amount of total precipitate. This phenomenon is due to formation of antibody–antigen complexes of different compositions. At antibody excess, all the antigenic determinants are covered with antibody and no determinants are available for an antibody to form a bridge between two molecules of antigen. At equivalence, divalent antibodies bind antigenic determinants on different antigen molecules to produce a latticelike structure, which becomes insoluble. At antigen excess, each antibody molecule binds two antigen molecules together to form a lattice. At the point of maximum precipitation, all antibody and antigen should be in the precipitate (equivalence zone). If the antigen is a sugar the amount of antibody can be determined by measuring the amount of protein in the total precipitate formed.

other antiserum, much more antibody may be required to agglutinate or neutralize one kind of microorganism than another. Therefore, a direct comparison of titers in different systems is not possible.

The quantitative precipitin reaction permits measurement of antibody on a weight basis (Fig. 7-6). A series of test tubes each containing the same amount of antiserum is prepared. Increasing amounts of antigen of known quantity are added to this series of test tubes. At the equivalence zone, all of the antibody and all of the antigen added precipitate. The quantity of protein in the precipitate is determined by chemical or spectrophotometric measurement. Since the amount of antigen added is known, this quantity can be subtracted from the value of total precipitate to determine the amount of specific antibody present. The validity of this technique depends upon at least three factors:

1. The antibody–antigen rection must be specific. If a reaction of mixed specificity (more than one antigen and more than one antibody) occurs, it is virtually impossible to reach an equivalence zone as two or more separate antigen–antibody reactions are occurring at the same time.
2. The antiserum being measured must not contain monovalent (nonprecipitating) antibody, as this may not be carried down with precipitate.
3. Other proteins that may affix to antigen–antibody complexes (such as complement) must be eliminated, or an erroneously high value for specific antibody will be obtained because of nonspecific binding of the other proteins.

Nephelometry

Small aggregates of an antibody–antigen complex in a solution create turbidity. This turbidity can be measured by scattering of light passed into the turbid solution. Measurement of the degree of turbidity after addition of a constant amount of antigen to antibody solutions provides a rapid and more sensitive method than the precipitation reaction for quantitation of antigen. High levels of sensitivity are obtained using monochromatic light from a laser. Addition of polyethyleneglycol to the solution increases aggregate size and also increases sensitivity.

Precipitation in Agar

Precipitation reactions resulting from antibody–antigen combinations also occur in agar media. The agar prevents convection currents from disrupting the precipitation pattern. Precipitation-in-agar reactions are extremely valuable for analysis of multiple antigenic components in which each AgAb complex forms a distinct zone of precipitation.

Simple Gel Diffusion

The simple gel diffusion technique evolved directly from the precipitin reaction in solution. If a solution of soluble antigen is layered over antiserum in a small-caliber tube, a line appears at the interface of these solutions as a precipitation reaction occurs. If the antiserum is placed in agar in the tube and a solution of antigen is layered over the antiserum–agar base, a precipitation line appears at the interface. This is known as an *Oudin tube* (Fig. 7-7).

Since the antigen is in solution and the antiserum is distributed evenly in the agar, the location that the precipitation line assumes depends upon six factors: (1) concentration of

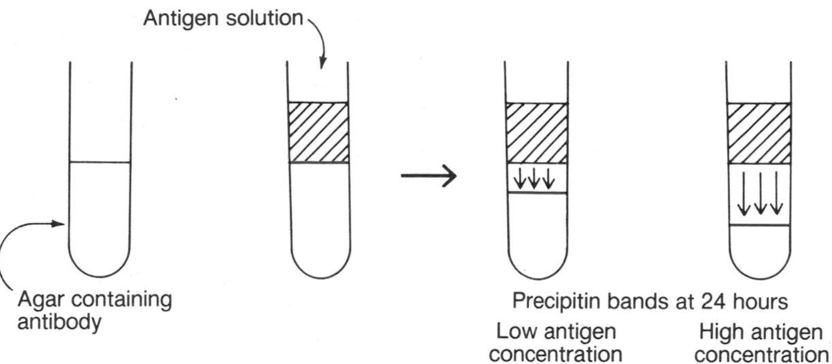

Figure 7-7. Simple gel diffusion, or Oudin tube. If a solution of antigen is placed over agar containing antibody in a tube, a precipitin band will form where the antigen solution meets the antibody. The precipitin band will move into the agar as more antigen from the solution diffuses into the agar. The distance that the precipitin band moves into the agar at any time point is a function of the concentration of the antigen added (higher concentration results in further diffusion into the agar). By comparison of the distance of migration of bands formed by known concentrations of an antigen with the distance of migration of bands produced by solutions containing unknown amounts of the same antigen, an accurate measure of the antigen concentration in the unknown can be made.

antigen, (2) diffusion coefficient of antigen, (3) concentration of antibody, (4) time, (5) temperature, and (6) concentration or density of agar. If the last five variables are held constant, the distance the precipitation line moves into the antiserum–agar layer depends on the concentration of antigen.

Simple gel diffusion may also be carried out on a flat surface (radial diffusion technique). Antiserum is incorporated into agar, which is allowed to gel as a layer on a glass slide. A hole is cut into the agar, and antigen solution is placed into the hole. The antigen will diffuse out into the antibody-containing agar, producing a ring of precipitation. The square of the radius of this precipitation ring depends upon the relative concentration of antigen and antibody. Using a constant dilution of antiserum, antigen concentration may be determined by comparing the diameter of the ring of precipitation produced by a solution of known antigen concentration with that of a ring produced by an unknown solution.

Double Diffusion in Agar

A better technique for analysis of mixtures of antibody–antigen systems is provided by the double diffusion-in-agar (Ouchterlony) technique. When this technique is used, antigen and antisera are separately placed in small wells cut out of a layer of agar on a plate. The antibody and antigen diffuse toward each other. A precipitation band forms where the antibody and antigen interact in the concentrations necessary to meet the requirements of the equivalence zone of the precipitin reaction. If the concentration of the antigen is relatively greater than the concentration of the antibody, the precipitation line appears nearer the antibody well. If the concentrations are equal, the line appears midway between the antibody and the antigen wells. If the antibody concentration is greater than the antigen concentration, the precipitation line appears closer to the antigen well. If multiple antibody–antigen systems are present, a separate line may be observed for each system. The patterns formed by precipitation lines when two or more antigens are compared with one antiserum, or vice versa, may be used to characterize an antigen or antibody preparation (Fig. 7-8).

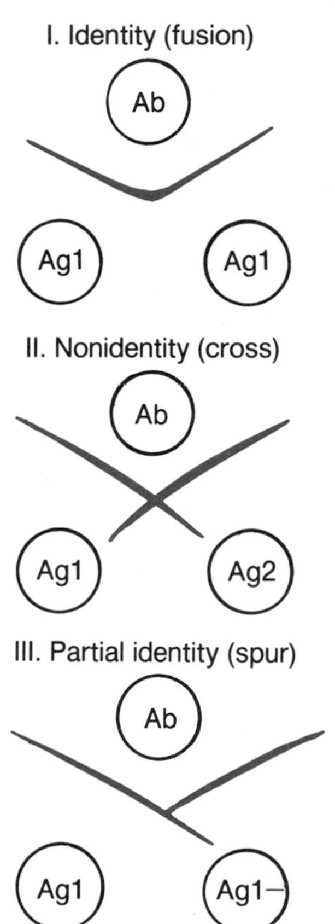

Figure 7-8. Double diffusion in agar reactions. If solution of antigen is placed in one well on the flat layer of agar and the appropriate antiserum placed in an adjacent well, antigen and antibody migrate toward each other, and a precipitation line forms when concentrations of antibody and antigen are at equivalence. If two identical antigen solutions (Ag1) are placed in wells in agar at the base of a triangle, and an appropriate antiserum (Ab) is placed in a well at the apex of the triangle, a precipitation line forms between each antigen well and antiserum well. Since both antigen solutions are the same, separate lines fuse where they meet in the center of a triangle (reaction of identity). If different antigen (Ag1 and Ag2) solutions are placed in base wells, and antiserum-contaning antibodies (Ab) directed against both antigens are placed in an apex well, precipitation lines do not fuse; they cross. The reaction of antibody 1 with antigen 1 essentially does not affect the reaction of antibody 2 with antigen 2, and vice versa, so that the two precipitin lines form independently (reaction of nonidentity). If one antigen solution containing molecules with several antigenic specificities present on the same molecule (Ag1) and a second antigen solution containing molecules with only some of the antigenic specificities of the first antigen (Ag1–) are placed in adjacent wells against antiserum (Ab) which contains antibodies directed toward all specificities present in the first antigen solution, a line of partial identity, or spur formation, is observed. The precipitation line formed between antiserum and antigen with limited antigenic specificities fuses with the line formed by antiserum and antigen containing additional specificities, but this second line extends past the first line, resulting in a spur effect.

If multiple antigen–antibody systems react in agar, it may be difficult to identify and differentiate the number of precipitation bands present. An example is an antiserum prepared in one species (rabbit) by immunization with whole serum proteins of another species (rat). The rabbit antiserum to whole rat serum may produce up to 30 separate precipitation bands when reacted in agar with rat serum. However, it is not possible to differentiate the many different lines by double diffusion in agar. Such a mixture may be analyzed by combining serum protein electrophoresis and immune precipitation in agar.

Immunoelectrophoresis

Many variations combining electrophoresis and immunoprecipitation have been applied to the analysis of mixtures of antigens or antibodies. These include classic immunoelectrophoresis, rocket electrophoresis, two-dimensional electrophoresis, and immune labeling of polyacrylamide gel patterns (Western blot).

Classic Immunoelectrophoresis

The classic combination of electrophoresis in agar followed by reaction with antiserum is illustrated in Figure 7-9. The method is called immunoelectrophoresis.

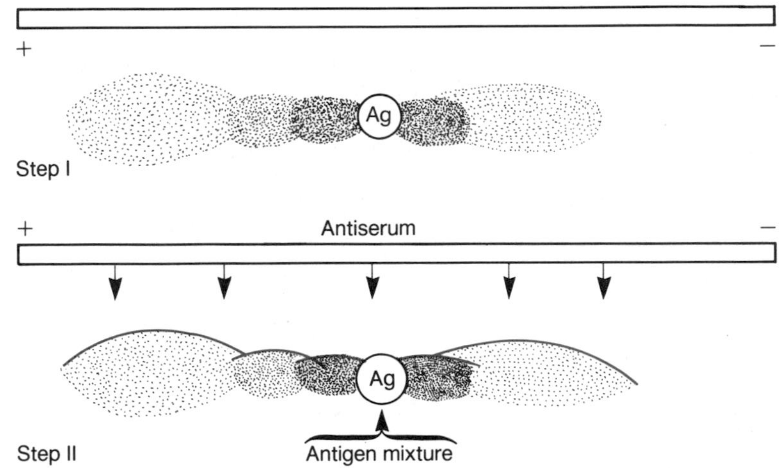

Figure 7-9. Reaction of polyvalent antiserum with a mixture of protein antigens separated by electrophoresis in agar. In step I the mixture of antigens is placed in a small well in a layer of agar on a glass plate or slide. An electric current is applied to the agar. This current acts upon the proteins and results in their migration into the agar. The distance each protein migrates is proportional to the electrostatic charge of the protein. Since proteins in the mixture of antigens differ in charge, separation of proteins due to different migration distances occurs. Location of proteins as they diffuse in agar is represented by shaded areas. In step II following electrophoretic separation, a trough is cut in the agar, a short distance from the well in which the antigen mixture was originally placed. The trough is cut so that its long axis is parallel to electrophoretic separation. Antiserum is then placed in the trough and allowed to diffuse into agar. Antibody to each antigenic protein then separately reacts with that protein in agar, forming precipitation lines where antibody and antigen are in equivalence (solid red lines). Individual antibody-antigen reactions are easier to identify and differentiate because the mixture of antigens has been separated by electrophoresis. Many variations in this basic procedure have been used to provide more exact immunochemical analysis of complex antibody-antigen systems.

Electroimmunodiffusion

A variation of single radial immunodiffusion employing electrophoresis (electroimmunodiffusion) may be used to quantify antigens in dilute fluids. Antiserum is incorporated into the agar layer and an electric current applied across the agar after an antigen solution is placed in a well cut into the agar. The electric field pulls the antigen into the antibody-agar layer. The distance that the antigen-antibody precipitate migrates into the agar layer is proportional to the amount of antigen in the solution.

Rocket Electrophoresis

In this procedure quantitation of antigen may be accomplished by determining the length of an arc of precipitation formed when antigen is electrophoresed into an agar layer containing antibody. This method is not suitable for antigens that migrate to the negative electrode, as the migration must be different from that of the antibody used (Fig. 7-10).

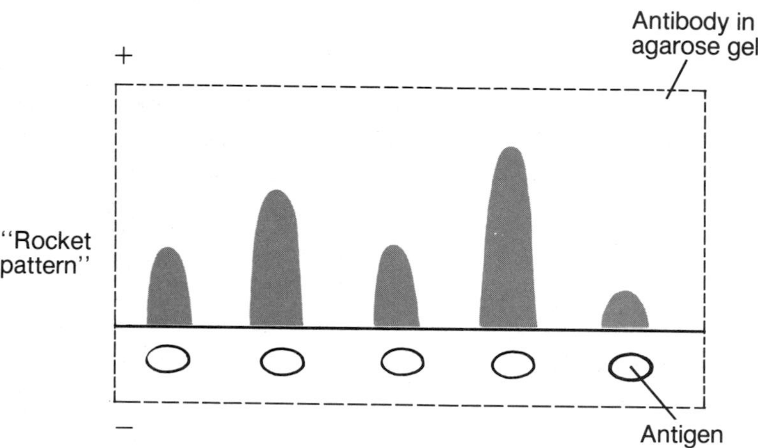

Figure 7-10. Rocket electrophoresis. Antigen that migrates to the positive electrode is pulled into an agar layer containing antibody. The length of the precipitin arc formed is proportional to the concentration of antigen.

Two-Dimensional Electrophoresis

In this variation of rocket electrophoresis an antigen mixture is electrophoresed in agar in one direction; then the antigens are pulled into agar containing antibody by electrophoresis in the perpendicular direction (Fig. 7-11). Using this method several antigens in a mixture may be quantitated.

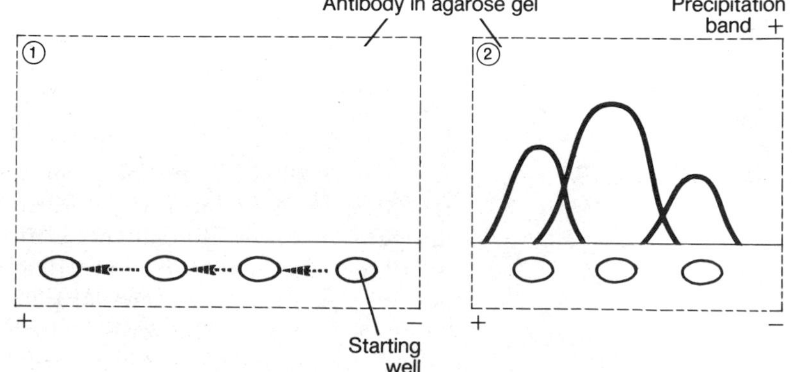

Figure 7-11. Two-dimensional electrophoresis. A mixture of antigens is separated by electrophoresis in agar in one dimension (step I). Then the separated antigens are pulled into a layer of agar containing antibody by electrophoresis in the second dimension (step II).

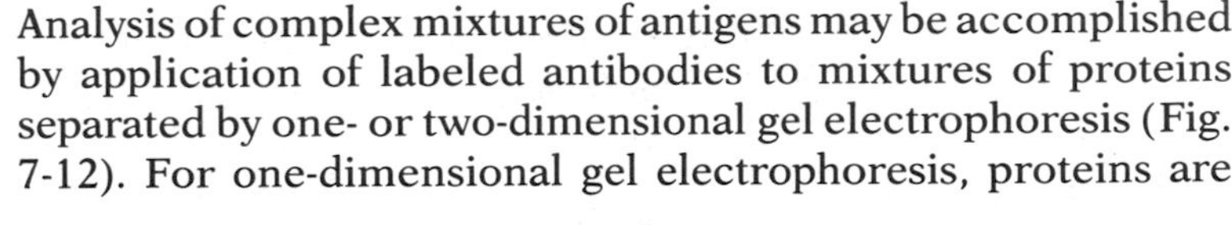

Immunolabeling of Polyacrylamide Gel Patterns (Western Blot or Immunoblot)

Analysis of complex mixtures of antigens may be accomplished by application of labeled antibodies to mixtures of proteins separated by one- or two-dimensional gel electrophoresis (Fig. 7-12). For one-dimensional gel electrophoresis, proteins are placed in a charged field in a polyacrylamide gel slab. The proteins in the mixture will migrate largely on the basis of their molecular weights to form bands in the gel. For two-dimensional gels, the protein mixture is first separated on the basis of charge by isoelectric focusing, then on the basis of molecular weight by polyacrylamide electrophoresis. The gels containing the separated proteins are then electrophoretically transferred to nitrocellulose sheets. These sheets are labeled by specific antibody cither directly using labeled antibody or indirectly where the first antibody is unlabeled and labeling is accomplished by a second labeled antibody, or by any of the labeling procedures described (peroxidase–antiperoxidase, biotin–avidin, labeled protein A). These procedures permit the identification of antigens in complex mixtures of proteins and are

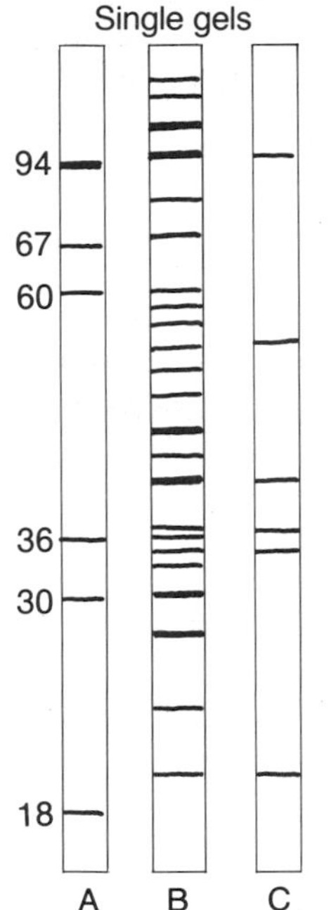

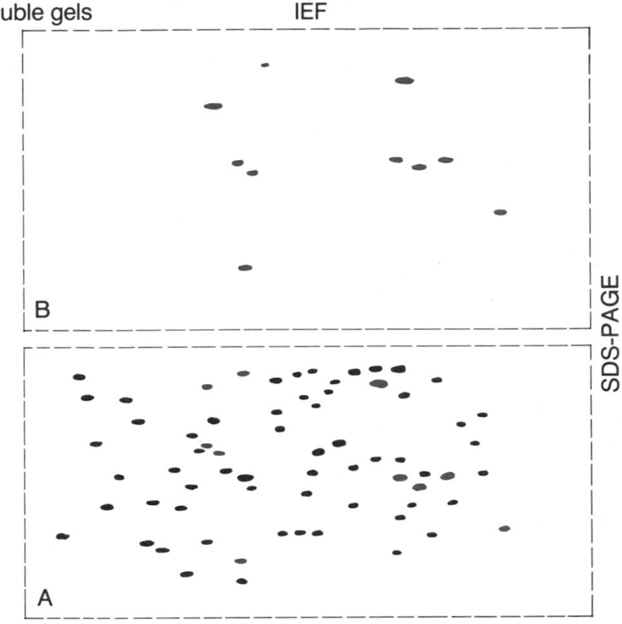

Figure 7-12. Immunolabeling of single- and double-dimension gels. Single gels are sodium dodecyl sulfate–polyacrylamide gels electrophoresis (SDS–PAGE). Lane A is SDS–PAGE of molecular weight markers (MW in thousands); lane B, the presence of all proteins as determined by a protein stain; lane C, labeled by specific antibody. Thus of the 23 proteins identified, 6 are antigens labeled by the antibody. Two-dimensional gels separate the proteins into spots on the basis of isoelectric focusing (IEF) followed by SDS–PAGE. The total proteins are stained in A and immune-labeled in B. Of the 70 proteins identified, 9 are shown to be antigenic.

very useful in analysis of the antigens in bacteria or other infectious agents.

Agglutination

Agglutination of visible antigen particles by antibody occurs by the same mechanism as precipitation of soluble antigen (Fig. 7-13). Simple agglutination results when the antigen is an integral part of the particle, for example, when antibody to erythrocytes, or to bacteria, causes the agglutination of these particles. Passive agglutination results when a soluble antigen is chemically attached to a particle, and antibody is used to agglutinate the coated particle. Materials that have been used for this purpose include latex and bentonite particles and erythrocytes (passive hemagglutination). Addition of the soluble antigen in sufficient amounts to compete for the antibody inhibits the agglutination of the coated particles. Inhibition of passive hemagglutination reactions is an extremely sensitive method for detecting antigen.

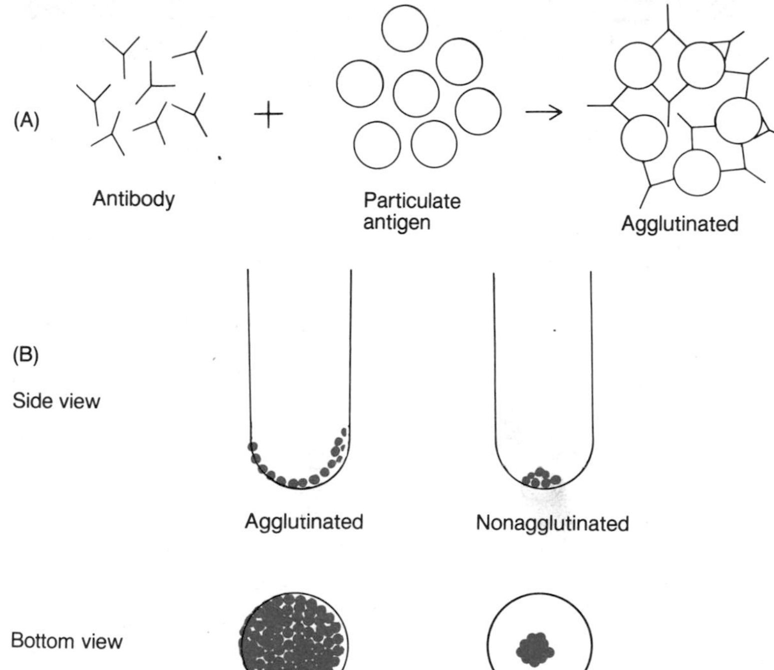

Figure 7-13. Agglutination of antigen by antibody. (A) The reaction of antibody to particulate antigens such as red blood cells results in the cells being bound together by divalent antibodies. (B) If this reaction is carried out in a test tube or tissue culture well, the agglutinated particles do not settle at the bottom as do nonagglutinated particles, but spread out along the bottom and sides of the tube. Such agglutination reactions can be observed by the naked eye if the clumped particles are visible. For example, agglutinated cells are spread out on the bottom of the tube and can be easily distinguished from nonagglutinated cells, which settle into a small compact bottom in round-bottom tubes or wells.

Complement Fixation

The reaction of specific antibody with erythrocytes, bacteria, or other cells in the presence of complement results in the eventual destruction of red cells (hemolysis) or other target cells (e.g., bacteriolysis) (see Chapter 12).

The effect of antibody and antigen on the complement system may be used to measure formation of antibody–antigen complexes. The reaction of antibody and antigen in the presence of complement consumes components of the complement system (complement fixation). If a separate antibody–antigen reaction is allowed to take place in a volume of normal complement-containing serum, the complement activity is depleted by adsorption of active complement components to the antibody–antigen complexes formed. If this mixture is then added to sensitized erythrocytes, lysis does not occur, as the necessary components have been exhausted. This complement fixation reaction provides a sensitive and accurate measurement of antibody or antigen, when one of the reactants is unknown. For complement fixation to occur, a class of antibody (isotype) that can react with complement must be active (complement-fixing antibody); not all immunoglobulins have the capacity to fix complement.

Immunoabsorption

Specific antibody or antigen may be coupled to insoluble carriers, such as cellulose, bentonite, Sepharose, or glass beads, or made insoluble by crosslinking. These solid phase antibody or antigen reagents provide valuable methods for isolation of antigen (by insoluble antibody) or antibody (by insoluble antigen). For instance, a specific antiserum to a given antigen may be utilized to purify that antigen. The gamma globulin fraction of antiserum is coupled to an insoluble carrier, and a solution containing a mixture of antigen and other molecules is added. The specific antigen attaches to the insoluble specific antibody. The contaminating molecules are washed off, and the bound specific antigen is then eluted from the insoluble antibody by lowering the pH of the buffer sufficiently to disrupt the antibody–antigen electrostatic bonds, but not the covalent bond linking the antibody to the insoluble carrier.

Radioimmunoassay

The practical importance of the use of antigen–antibody reactions for the quantification of antigenic material is exemplified by the use of radioimmunoassay for measurement of peptide hormones and other biologically active molecules (Fig. 7-14). Human hormones may have species-specific differences which can elicit specific antiserum in other species. This antiserum may be used to identify and quantify the hormone, even if the hormone represents only a small fraction of the protein in serum. The basic principle is the inhibition of the reaction of a specific antibody and a known amount of antigen by the addition of unknown amounts of antigen. This principle is also used in other secondary antigen–antibody reactions, such as hemagglutination inhibition and precipitation inhibition. However, the use of radiolabeled antigen greatly increases the sensitivity of the test. Radioimmunoassay has been used to measure a large variety of antigenic molecules including hormones, enzymes, and serum proteins.

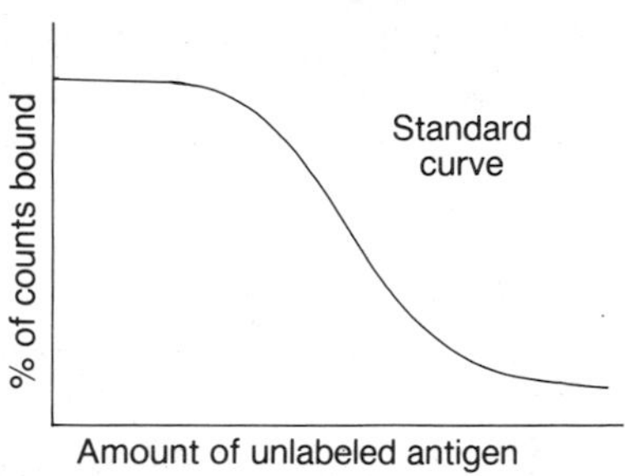

Figure 7-14. Very small amounts of antigen may be measured by the ability of the antigen to compete with radiolabeled antigen binding to antibody in this radioimmunoassay. If a mixture of unlabeled and radiolabeled antigen is added to an antibody solution in slight antigen excess, the amount of labeled antigen bound to antibody is a function of the amount of unlabeled antigen present. On the basis of this competition, a standard curve can be constructed by adding increasing amounts of unlabeled antigen to constant amounts of labeled antigen and antibody. When relatively small amounts of unlabeled antigen are present, all of the radiolabeled antigens are precipitated. As the amount of unlabeled antigen is increased, less radiolabeled antigen is bound to the antibody. When a standard curve using increasing known amounts of unlabeled antigen has been constructed, the amount of antigen in an unknown solution can be determined by comparing the degree of inhibition of binding of labeled antigen by the unknown antigen solution with that produced by known amounts of the same antigen.

Competitive Inhibition Radioimmunoassay

The principle of radioimmunoassay is given in the following reactions:

$$\text{Ab} + {}^{*}\text{Ag} \rightleftharpoons \text{Ab}^{*}\text{Ag}$$
$$\text{Ab} + \text{Ag} + {}^{*}\text{Ag} \rightleftharpoons \text{AbAg} + {}^{*}\text{Ag} + \text{Ab}^{*}\text{Ag}$$

In the first reaction, antibody (Ab) is reacted with a radiolabeled antigen (*Ag) under conditions that result in about 60–70% binding of the antigen. In the second reaction, unlabeled antigen (Ag) is included in the reaction mixture. Because the unlabeled antigen is present, less bound radiolabeled antigen is obtained. By varying the amount of unlabeled antigen present, a quantitative relation can be obtained between the amount of antigen present and the amount of radioactivity in the bound fractions. Once this relationship is determined, a standard curve may be constructed by plotting the percentage of bound label (or, inversely, the percentage in the supernate) against the amount of unlabeled antigen added. The amount of antigen in an unknown mixture can be found by determining the effect of the addition of dilutions of the unknown upon the antibody-labeled antigen system. The amounts of antibody and labeled antigen are kept constant in each determination.

Other properties of an antibody–antigen system may be used to quantify an antigen. Most involve the reaction of varying amounts of antigen or unknown with constant amounts of specific antiserum. As increasing amounts of antigen are added, (1) the amount of unbound antibody decreases; (2) the amount of complex increases; and (3) after equivalence is exceeded, increasing amounts of free antigen are present. The extent of any of these changes, in the presence of a fixed amount of antibody, depends upon the amount of antigen added. This permits variation in the final measurement used to quantify an antigen by immunoassay.

Immunoradiometric Assay

A variation of radioimmunoassay, *immunoradiometric assay,* uses purified radiolabeled antibody instead of labeled antigen. Radiolabeled antibody is added to a solution of antigen. Then, a solid immunoabsorbent antigen is used to separate unbound antibody, leaving the labeled antibody bound to the soluble antigen in the supernatant fluid. The sensitivity of immunoradiometric assays is comparable to that of radioimmunoassays. The choice of assay depends on the feasibility and applicability of an antibody–antigen system to the method.

Enzyme-Linked Immunosorbent Assay

The enzyme-linked immunosorbent assay (ELISA) is similar to the immunoradiometric assay except that the antibody is labeled with an enzyme instead of a radioisotope (Fig. 7-15). For example, unlabeled antibody specific for the antigen in question is allowed to adhere to the bottom of a microplate well, and unbound antibody is washed off. Solution containing an unknown amount of the antigen is added. In the appropriate sensitivity range, the absorbed antibody will be in excess and, therefore, all of the antigen will be bound by antibody. After binding of antigen, a second enzyme-labeled antibody directed against the antigen is added in excess (double-antibody technique). The amount of this second antibody that binds to the antigen depends upon the amount of antigen present. The unbound enzyme-linked antibody is then washed off, and a substrate is added that changes color when acted upon by the enzyme. The intensity of color developed over a certain amount of time depends on the amount of enzyme-linked antibody bound to the antigen in the well. By colorimetric analysis and comparison to known amounts of antigen, a quantitative standard curve is developed. Two of the enzymes commonly used are horseradish peroxidase, which turns a colorless solution of 5-aminosalicylic acid to reddish brown, and alkaline phosphatase, which turns a colorless solution of *p*-nitrophenol to yellow. In practice, the method of running ELISA assays varies. The two most commonly used are the indirect method, similar

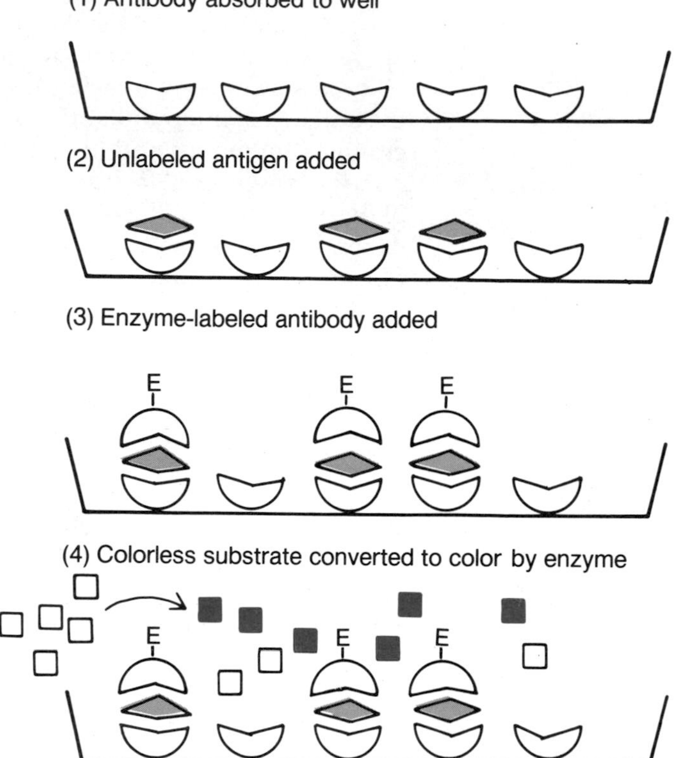

Figure 7-15. Quantification of the enzyme-linked immunosorbent assay (ELISA) depends on the conversion of a colorless substrate to a colored compound by an enzyme coupled to antibody or to antigen. The amount of substrate converted is measured colorimetrically and is dependent upon the amount of enzyme-labeled antibody bound. The amount of antibody bound is in turn dependent upon the amount of antigen bound to unlabeled antibody absorbed to the bottom of the well. The unlabeled antibody absorbed to the well must be added in excess, and the unbound antibody washed off. Then, a standard curve similar to the one shown in Figure 7-14 can be constructed. Variation of the ELISA procedure employing mixtures of antibodies and antigens similar to those shown for immunofluorescence in Figure 7-15 may be used.

to a competitive radioimmunoassay, and the double-antibody method.

Tissue Labeling by Antibody

The location and distribution of antigens in tissues or cells can be accomplished using a variety of techniques that employ markers localized by antigen–antibody reactions.

Immunofluorescence

The most commonly employed dyes for tissue labeling by immunofluorescence are fluorescein (green fluorescence) and rhodamine (red fluorescence). Those compounds may be covalently attached to antibody molecules and emit visible light (fluoresce) when exposed to ultraviolet light of the appropriate wavelength. Fluorescein- or rhodamine-labeled antibody preparations are applied to sections of the unfixed tissue to be examined. The antibody binds to the antigen, if the latter is present in sufficient amounts in the tissue section, forming microprecipitates. If the treated tissue section is washed to remove excess unbound labeled antibody and observed under ultraviolet light, the areas of the tissue section containing the antigen give off visible light that can be observed under the microscope as a red or green fluorescence. Variations of this technique are illustrated in Figure 7-16.

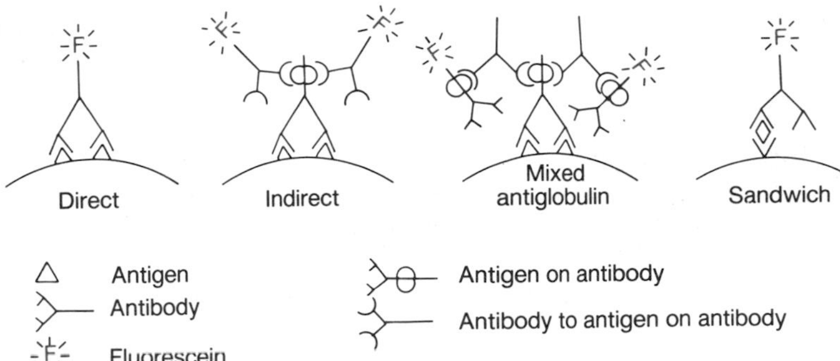

Figure 7-16. Fluorescent antibody techniques. In the direct technique, specific antibody is labeled with fluorescent compound and added to tissue sections. The reaction of specific antibody to antigenic sites in the tissue sections is detected by exposing the section to ultraviolet light and visualizing areas of fluorescence. By means of the indirect technique, unlabeled antibody is reacted with tissue antigen. Fluorescein-labeled antibody to the first antibody is added. The second antibody reacts with the first, which in turn has reacted with tissue antigen. The first antibody added provides more binding sites for second antibody than was provided by tissue antigen, in this way increasing the sensitivity of the technique. In the mixed antiglobulin technique, antigens present on the first antibody are used to react to binding sites of the second antibody. The label can be fluorescent-labeled immunoglobulin of the same species as that of the first antibody. This technique can be particularly useful in labeling surface immunoglobulin molecules. In such a system, the Ig antigens are already present on the cell to be labeled. Anti-immunoglobulin antibody is used to bind labeled Ig to the cell surface Ig. To identify antibody rather than antigen in tissue sections, a "sandwich" technique is used. Antigen is added to tissue and is bound by specific antibody present in the tissue. Specific fluorescein-labeled antibody to antigen is added, which reacts with antigen now fixed to the antibody in the tissue.

Immunofluorescence studies must be carefully controlled to prevent misinterpretation of the staining patterns. (1) Because minute amounts of contaminating antibody to an antigen other than the one of interest may give erroneous results, the specificity of the labeled antibody must be carefully checked by immunochemical controls. (2) The fluorescence produced by the labeled antibody must also be differentiated from nonspecific tissue fluorescence. This can usually be done, because natural tissue fluorescence gives a different color than fluorescein or rhodamine fluorescence. (3) The staining pattern produced by the labeled specific antibody must be clearly different from that which may occur if an adjacent tissue section is treated with labeled nonantibody (normal) immunoglobulins, since the labeled antibody may be nonimmunologically (nonspecifically) bound to the tissue section. (4) The staining pattern should not occur if the tissue section is treated with nonlabeled antibody prior to the addition of the labeled antibody. (5) Specific blocking should also occur if the labeled antiserum is absorbed with authentic nonlabeled antigen prior to the addition of antiserum to the tissue section. Even if these controls are carefully done, the investigator must be careful not to overinterpret the results of immunofluorescence.

Fluorescence Activated Flow Cytometry

Cells that are labeled by a fluoresceinated antibody may be quantitated and separated using a fluorescence-activated cell sorter (FACS) (Fig. 7-17). The FACS delivers single cells in a

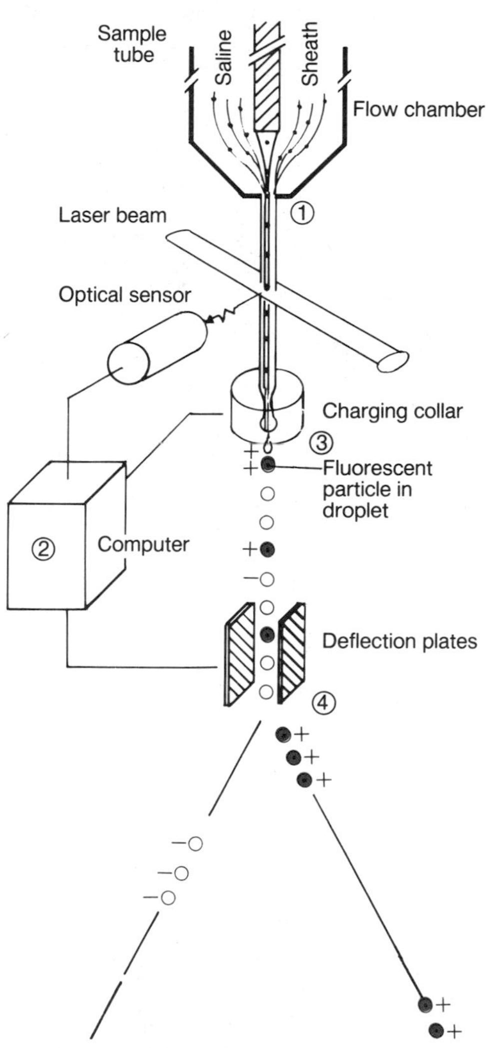

Figure 7-17. Cell separation by sorting. (1) Fluorescently stained cells are forced out of a small nozzle in a liquid jet. (2) Cellular fluorescence, measured immediately below the nozzle, is used to select the cells to be sorted. (3) The jet is broken into droplets. Droplets containing selected cells are electrically charged in a high-voltage field between deflection plates. (4) The charged droplets are electrically deflected into collection tubes.

stream that passes through a laser beam. Light from a laser beam excites the fluorescent dye, which gives a greater or lesser signal depending on the amount of antibody bound. The machine analyzes the distribution of fluorescence in large numbers of cells, giving data as shown in Figure 7-18. Alternatively, the machine can be set up as a cell sorter to separate brightly

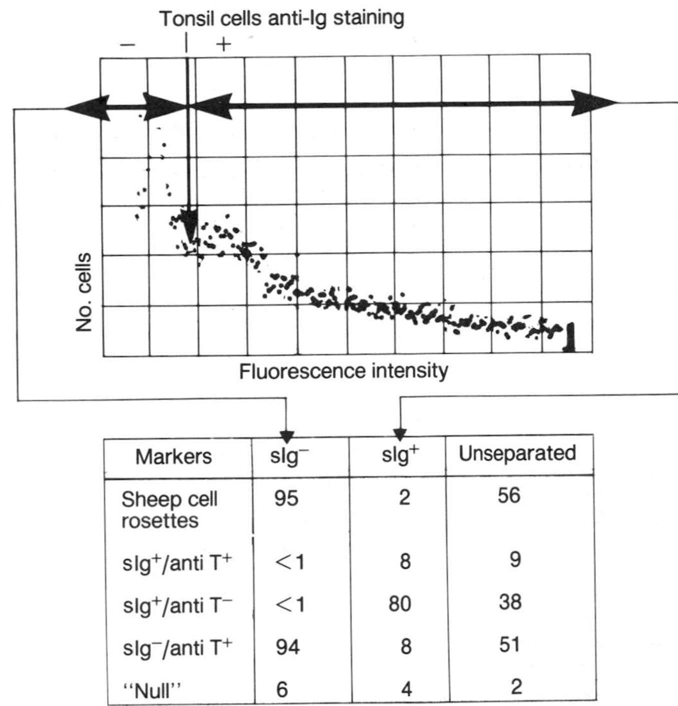

Markers	sIg⁻	sIg⁺	Unseparated
Sheep cell rosettes	95	2	56
sIg⁺/anti T⁺	<1	8	9
sIg⁺/anti T⁻	<1	80	38
sIg⁻/anti T⁺	94	8	51
"Null"	6	4	2

Figure 7-18. Separation of B and T cells with the fluorescence-activated cell sorter. After they are stained with fluorescein-conjugated anti-Ig, the viable cells are analyzed by flow cytofluorometry to give a histogram. The lymphocytes are separated into surface membrane Ig positive ($SmIg^+$) and negative ($SmIg^-$) populations depending on whether the fluorescence intensity is above or below the arbitrary cutoff point. The separated populations may then be reanalyzed for surface Ig and T cell surface markers as shown in the table. Null cells are negative with both anti-Ig and anti-T reagents. (Modified from Roitt I, Essential Immunology, 5th ed. Oxford, Blackwell, 1984, p. 63.)

fluorescent cells from dark ones. This is done by breaking up the stream of negatively charged cells into droplets. The droplets fall between charged plates that direct brightly fluorescence-labeled cells into one stream and unstained cells into another stream, and thusly into separate collection vessels. A recording apparatus measures the intensity of fluorescent staining of each cell as well as the cell size (Fig. 7-18).

Immunoperoxidase

Tissue localization of antigens or antibodies may also be accomplished using enzyme-labeled reagents, such as peroxidase-labeled antibody. Identification of bound antibody is possible through conversion of a colorless soluble substrate to a colored insoluble product by the enzyme. Since different substrates may be activated by the same enzyme, it is possible to localize more than one antigen by the serial addition of peroxidase-labeled antibodies. For instance, double staining of adrenocorticotropin (ACTH) and growth hormone (GH) in the rat anterior pituitary may be accomplished by reaction with rabbit anti-ACTH followed by peroxidase-labeled horse anti-rabbit IgG (double-antibody technique) and incubation with 3,3′-diaminobenzene as substrate. This will produce a known reaction product, which is orange and which will remain fixed on the slide. The slide can then be treated with rabbit anti-GH, peroxidase-labeled horse anti-rabbit IgG, and 4-Cl-1-naphthol. The naphthol substrate will produce a blue reaction product. In this manner, the same section may be examined for localization of ACTH (orange color) and GH (blue color).

Immunoelectron Microscopy

Ultrastructural localization of antigens may be accomplished using essentially the same type of reactions used for immunofluorescence. However, the markers used for electron microscopy are different. These include large or electron-dense molecules such as ferritin, hemocyanin, gold, or virus particles, which are large enough to be visualized by electron microscopy yet can be coupled to antibody or to antigen by chemical means. In addition, peroxidase-labeled antibodies may be used, as the products produced by reaction with the substrates can be seen under the electron microscope. The peroxidase method is more suitable for cytoplasmic localization, the larger particles for cell surface labeling. Even larger particles such as latex beads or larger viruses may be adapted for localization by scanning electron microscopy. Radiolabeled antigens may also be used to detect antigen receptors on cells or in tissues by electron microscopic autoradiography.

The Avidin–Biotin Complex

The extremely high affinity of the glycoprotein avidin for the vitamin biotin provides a system that greatly increases the sensitivity of many immune assays. Avidin has four high-affinity binding sites for biotin ($K_D = 10-15$ moles/liter). Biotin or avidin may be conjugated chemically to antibody, to antigen, or to enzymes or other labeled probes. The variations of labeling permit the use of the avidin–biotin system in immune assay and in immune absorption isolation procedures (Fig. 7-19). Techniques using avidin–biotin labeling are more sensitive and more specific than other enzyme labeling or fluorescent systems. It is estimated that avidin–biotin systems are five times more sensitive than conventional fluorescence for labeling tissue sections.

Microbiological Tests

The effect of bactericidal antibody and complement on certain organisms provides the basis for many microbiological laboratory tests.

Treponema pallidum Immobilization

A specific serologic test for syphilis, *Treponema pallidum* immobilization (TPI), depends upon the presence in an affected individual's serum of antibodies to the causative agent, *T. pallidum*. Motile organisms are mixed with the test serum and normal guinea pig serum (complement source). The mixture is incubated for 16 to 18 hours at 35°C under anaerobic conditions and then examined microscopically. Normally, the *T. pallidum* organisms are motile and are observed to move actively. The action of specific antibody and complement results in loss of this motility.

1. Tissue Localization of Antigen

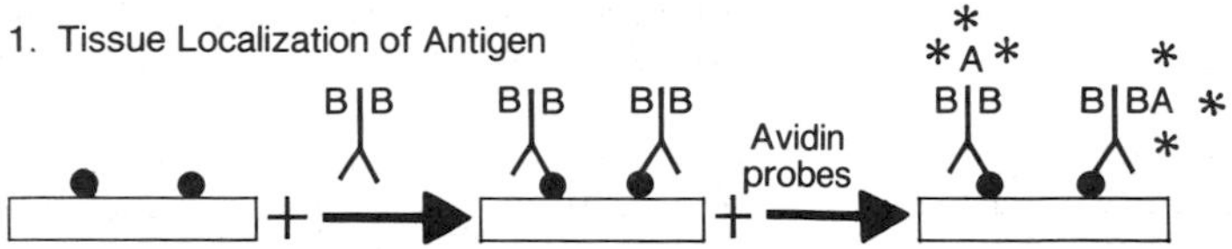

Amount of avidin probe bound depends on antigen in tissue

2. Immune Assay

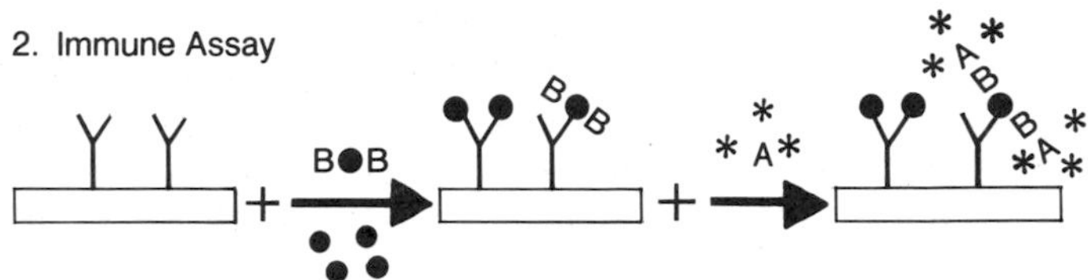

Amount of avidin probe bound related to amount of biotin labeled antigen bounded to antibody; unlabeled antigen competes as in radioimmunoassay

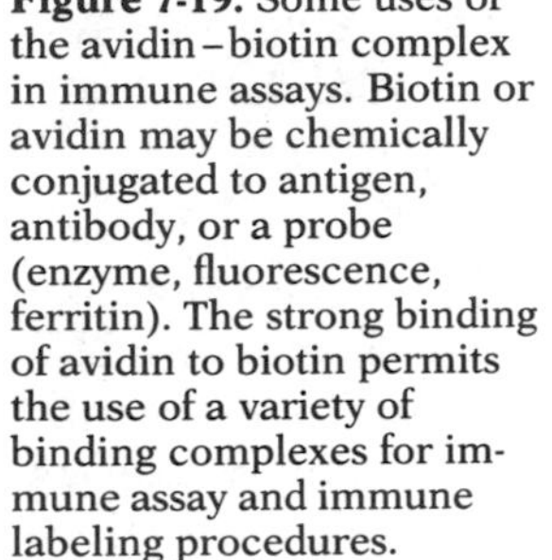

Figure 7-19. Some uses of the avidin–biotin complex in immune assays. Biotin or avidin may be chemically conjugated to antigen, antibody, or a probe (enzyme, fluorescence, ferritin). The strong binding of avidin to biotin permits the use of a variety of binding complexes for immune assay and immune labeling procedures.

3. Ultrastructural Cell Surface Labeling

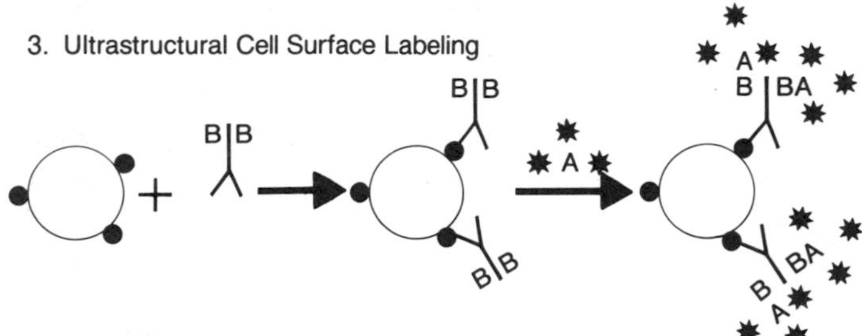

Ferritin detected on cell surface by electron microscopy

4. Immune Absorption

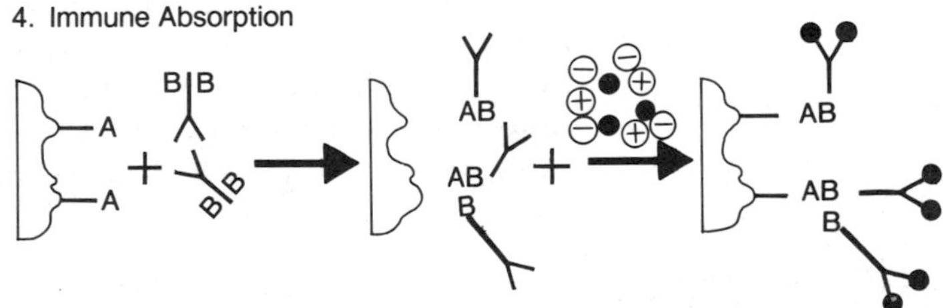

Specific antigen removed from antigen mixture by antibody bound to insoluble matrix

Legend
* Enzyme label ✸ Ferritin ● Antigen B Biotin A Avidin

Opsonization

Opsonization is the reaction of specific antibody and complement with a particle or organism that facilitates or augments phagocytosis of the organism. An opsonic index can be obtained by determining the ratio of activity of a patient's serum to that of normal serum. The activity is determined by the degree of phagocytosis of the test material by microscopic examination of mixtures of serum, complement, and organisms cultured in the presence of macrophages, or by using an O_2

electrode to measure the "O_2 burst" that accompanies phagocytosis.

Neutralization Tests

The activity of antisera to bacteria or viruses may be tested by the ability of such sera to reduce the viability of suspensions of these organisms when cultured in vitro. The effect is usually measured by the activity of dilutions of the antisera or by the rate of neutralization of the target organism by the dilution of the antiserum. The ability to elicit neutralizing antibodies is particularly critical for vaccine development (see Chapter 25). For example, current efforts to produce a vaccine for AIDS may depend on the ability to demonstrate virus-neutralizing antibodies.

Neutralization of the activity of a biologically active molecule or infective organism may also be tested in vivo. A classic example is the toxin neutralization test for anti-diphtheria toxin serum.

Diphtheria Toxin Neutralization. The neutralization potency of an antiserum to diphtheria toxin (antitoxin) is measured by comparison with a standard sample of antitoxin. To test a toxin preparation, increasing amounts of toxin are added to a series of tubes containing 1 unit of a standard antitoxin, and each of the mixtures is injected into a 250-g guinea pig. The amount of toxin that must be mixed with 1 unit of antitoxin to cause death in 4 days is taken as the endpoint and is called the L_+ dose. Conversely, the potency of the unknown antiserum can be determined by mixing increasing dilutions of the antitoxin with one L_+ dose of the toxin and injecting the mixture into guinea pigs. The volume of serum that, when mixed with one L_+ dose of toxin, results in death in 4 days contains 1 unit of antitoxin.

Antigen–Antibody Reactions in Vivo

Antigen–antibody reactions in vivo initiate a number of inflammatory reactions that may be viewed as tertiary effects of antigen–antibody reactions.

Immune Elimination

The presence of antibody in the circulation leads to rapid clearance of antigens injected into the blood (Fig. 7-20). Reaction of antibody with antigen results in formation of aggregated Ig components and activation of complement, which *opsonizes* the complexes and results in clearance of the antigen complexes by the reticuloendothelial system. During the induction phase of antibody formation, antigen will be catabolized at a slow "nonimmune" rate. However, when antibodies are formed, catabolism occurs much more rapidly. During the early phase of immune elimination soluble antigen–antibody complexes in antigen excess are found in the circulation. Solu-

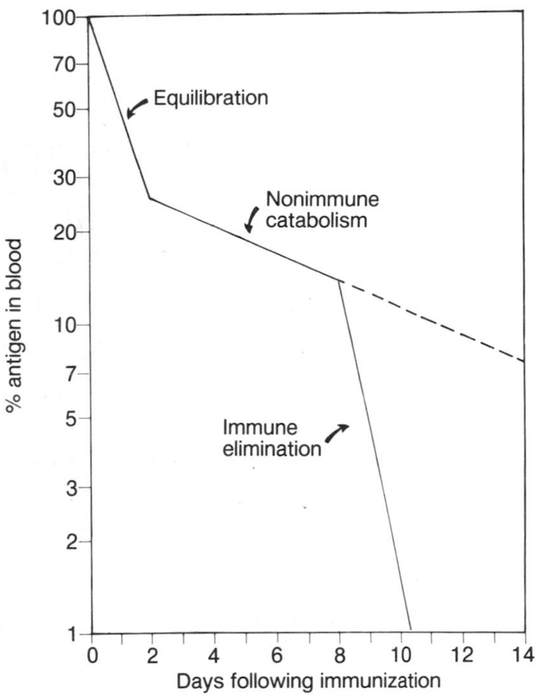

Figure 7-20. Immune elimination. If antibody is present in vivo, antigen is rapidly cleared from the bloodstream. A three-stage elimination of diffusible antigen from the bloodstream of a previously nonimmunized animal has been recognized. Upon intravascular injection of antigen, the blood level of antigen drops rapidly until only about 40% of injected antigen remains in blood. This is due to equilibrium of diffusible antigen between intravascular and extravascular fluids. Following this rapid equilibration, antigen is slowly removed by normal metabolic processes (nonimmune catabolism) until the onset of antibody production between 7 and 10 days after antigen injection. Appearance of antibody results in rapid elimination of antigen (immune elimination) due to formation of antibody–antigen complexes and their removal by the reticuloendothelial system. During the phase of immune elimination, soluble antibody-antigen complex (formed in antigen excess) may be demonstrated in blood. After antigen is completely removed, free antibody appears. If antigen is injected into an animal that already has circulating antibody, antigen is removed in one rapid immune elimination phase.

ble complexes in antigen excess do not contain Fc aggregates, are not opsonized, and may deposit in tissue and be responsible for the lesions of serum sickness.

Antibody–Mediated Inflammatory Reactions

The activity of antibodies in vivo in an actively immunized animal, or an animal that has received antibody by passive transfer of an antiserum prepared in another animal, may result in a reaction involving accessory inflammatory mechanisms. Intravenous injection of antigen into an actively or passively sensitized animal may cause an acute systemic reaction (anaphylaxis). If the antigen is injected into the skin of sensitized animals, erythema (redness) and swelling may be observed. These reactions depend upon tissue inflammatory responses initiated by reactions of antibody or sensitized cells with antigen.

Schick Test

In some cases, antibody can neutralize the inflammatory activity of bacterial toxins, resulting in the absence of a reaction in immune individuals. Historically, in vivo neutralization of diphtheria toxin by antibody was determined by skin testing. A small amount of diphtheria toxin injected intradermally produces a local inflammatory reaction that is maximal at 4 to 5 hours and then fades. In an immunized individual who has antibody to diphtheria toxin, no reaction occurs; the antibody neutralizes the effect of the toxin. This test was pioneered by Bela Schick between 1910 and 1930 and is known as the Schick test. A delayed hypersensitivity reaction to diphtheria toxin may also occur. This is known as a pseudoreaction and can usually be differentiated from the effects of the toxin, as the delayed reaction reaches a maximum at 2 to 3 days and fades by 4 to 5 days.

Dick Test

Some human sera injected into patients with a characteristic scarlet fever rash (scarlatina) can produce a blanching of the rash at the site of injection. Not all human sera can induce this blanching. The effect is due to the presence of specific antibody to the erythrogenic toxin produced by the streptococcal organism responsible. These observations led to the development of the Dick test for antibody to hemolytic streptococcal antigens. Filtrates of cultures of the scarlatinal strains (strains responsible for scarlet fever) of streptococci contain a toxic substance that produces a typical skin reaction in nonimmunized individuals. Individuals with neutralizing antibody do not react to this erythrogenic toxin. The reaction induced by erythrogenic toxin appears as a bright red flush within 6 to 12 hours, is maximum at 24 hours, and fades rapidly. This test measures only resistance to strains of streptococci causing scarlet fever and does not measure protection from or susceptibility to streptococcal throat infection.

Sensitivity of Antigen–Antibody Reactions

The sensitivity of some methods for detection of antibody–antigen reactions is given in Table 7-2. For further information on how to detect and measure both primary and secondary antibody–antigen reactions, the American Society of Microbiology's *Manual of Clinical Immunology* is recommended.

Summary

Antigens react with antibodies to produce antigen–antibody complexes that in turn are responsible for a number of in vitro and in vivo effects. The primary reaction of antigen with antibody involves close approximation of structures on the surface of the antigen (epitopes) with the antibody combining sites

Table 7-2. Sensitivity of Some Methods for Measuring Antibody–Antigen Reactions

Method	Sensitivity (μg antibody N/ml)
Quantitative precipitin	4–10
Simple agar diffusion	5–10
Bacterial agglutination	0.01
Bactericidal	0.0001–0.001
Hemagglutination	0.003–0.006
Hemolysis	0.001–0.03
Complement fixation	0.1
Toxin neutralization	0.01
Passive systemic anaphylaxis (guinea pig)	30
Uterine muscle in vitro	0.01
Passive cutaneous anaphylaxis	0.003
Radioimmunoassay	<0.001

Adapted from Humphrey JH, White RG: Immunology for Students of Medicine, 2nd ed. Oxford, Blackwell, 1963, p201.

(paratopes) so that oppositely charged groups interact and hydrogen bonds and hydrophilic bonds form to join the antigen and the antibody. The strength of these bonds is termed *affinity*. As antibodies have more than one identical paratope and most antigens have many different epitopes, a latticelike complex of antigen and antibody may be formed, which precipitates. This precipitation may be used to quantitate the amount of antibody or antigen in a solution. Other in vitro reactions include agglutination, neutralization, and opsonization. The reaction of antibody with antigen may activate accessory systems such as complement (see Chapter 11) or inactivate biologically active molecules such as bacterial toxins. These effects are the basis for a number of in vitro secondary effects that may be used to measure antibody (or antigen) or to localize antigen cells on tissues. The reaction of antibody with antigens in vivo may activate a number of effector mechanisms. The manifestations of in vivo effects will be presented in more detail in later chapters.

References

Primary Antigen–Antibody Reactions

Benjamin DC, Berzofsky JA, East IJ, et al: The antigenic structure of proteins: a reappraisal. Ann Rev Immunol 2:67, 1984.

Farr RS: A quantitative immunochemical measure of the primary interaction between I*BSA and antibody. J Infect Dis 103:239, 1958.

Kabat EA: The nature of an antigenic determinant. J Immunol 97:1, 1966.

Karush F: Immunological specificity and molecular structure. Adv Immunol 2:1, 1962.

Kitagawa M, Yagi Y, Pressman D: The heterogeneity of combining sites of antibodies as determined by specific immunoabsorbents. J Immunol 95:446, 1965.

Landsteiner K: The Specificity of Serologic Reactions. Springfield, Ill., Thomas, 1936.

Pressman D, Grossberg AL: The Structural Basis of Antibody Specificity. New York, Benjamin, 1968.

Richards FF, Konigsberg WH, Rosenstein RW, et al: On the specificity of antibodies. Biochemical and biophysical evidence indicates the existence of polyfunctional antibody combining regions. Science 187:130, 1975.

Schick AF, Singer SJ: On the formation of covalent linkages between two protein molecules. J Biol Chem 236:2477, 1961.

Monoclonal Antibodies

Cotton RGH: Monoclonal antibodies in the study of structure–functional relationships of proteins. Med Res Rev 5:77, 1985.

Godino J: Monoclonal Antibodies. Principles and Practices. Orlando, Fla., Academic Press, 1983.

Kohler G, Milstein C: Continuous cultures of fused cells secreting antibody of predefined specificity. Nature 256:495, 1976.

Mariuzza R, Strand M: Chemical basis for diversity in antibody specificity analyzed by hapten binding to monoclonal anti-4-hydroxy-3-nitrophenacetyl (NP) immunoglobulins. Mol Immunol 18:847, 1981.

Secondary Antigen–Antibody Reactions

Ackroyd JF: Immunological Methods. Oxford, Blackwell, 1964.

Avrameas S, Ternynck T: The cross-linking of proteins with glutaraldehyde and its use for the preparation of immunoadsorbents. Immunochemistry 6:53–66, 1969.

Bullock G (ed): Techniques in Immunochemistry. Orlando, Fla., Academic Press, Vol 1, 1982; Vol 2, 1983.

Campbell DH, Luescher E, Lerman LS: Immunologic absorbents. I. Isolation of antibody by means of cellulose protein antigen. Proc Nat Acad Sci USA 37:575, 1951.

Crowle AJ: Immunodiffusion. New York, Academic Press, 1961.

Hapke M, Patil K: The establishment of normal limits for serum proteins measured by the rate nephelometer. Hum Pathol 12:1011, 1981.

Heidelberger M: Lectures in Immunochemistry. New York, Academic Press, 1956.

Kabat EA, Mayer MM: Experimental Immunochemistry, 2nd ed. Springfield, Ill., Thomas, 1961.

Lefkowits I, Pernis B: Immunological Methods. Orlando, Fla., Academic Press, Vol 1, 1979; Vol 2, 1980.

Loken MR, Stall AM: Flow cytometry as an analytical and preparative tool in immunology. J Immunol Methods 50:85, 1982.

Mancini G, Carbonara AO, Heremans JF: Immunochemical quantitation of antigens by single radial immunodiffusion. Immunochemistry 2:235, 1965.

Merrill D, Hartley TF, Claman HN: Electroimmunodiffusion (EID): a simple, rapid method for quantitation of immunoglobulins in dilute biological fluids. J Lab Clin Med 69:151, 1967.

Ouchterlony O: Diffusion-in-gel methods for immunological analysis. Prog Allergy 6:30, 1962.

Oudin J: Method of immunochemical analysis by specific precipitation in gel medium. C R Acad Sci (Paris) Ser D 222:115, 1946.

Towbin H, Gordon J: Immunoblotting and dot immunoblotting—current status and outlook. J Immunol Methods 72:313, 1984.

Weetall HH: Preparation and characterization of antigen and antibody adsorbents covalently coupled to an inorganic carrier. J Biochem 117:257–261, 1970.

Weir DM: Antigen–antibody reactions. *In* Cruickshank R (ed): Modern Trends in Immunology. London, Whitefriar, 1963.

Wilchek M, Bocchini V, Becker M, Givol D: A general method for the specific isolation of peptides containing modified residues, using insoluble antibody columns. Biochemistry 10:2828–2834, 1971.

Radioimmunoassay and Enzyme-Linked Immunosorbent Assay

Engvall E, Perlmann P: Enzyme linked immunoabsorbent assay (ELISA). Quantitative assay of immunoglobulin G. Immunochemistry 8:871, 1971.

Rodbard D, Catt KJ: Mathematical theory of radioligand assays: the kinetics of separation of bound from free. J Steroid Biochem 3:255–273, 1972.

Rodbard D, Weiss GH: Mathematical theory of immunoradiometric (labeled antibody) assays. Anal Biochem 52:10–44, 1973.

Schuurs AHWM, Van Weemen BK: Enzyme-immunoassay. Clin Chim Acta 81:1, 1977.

Skelley DS, Brown LP, Besch PK: Radioimmunoassay. Clin Chem 19:146–186, 1973.

Yalow RS: Radioimmunoassay: A probe for the fine structure of biologic systems. Science 200:1236, 1978.

Cell and Tissue Labeling

Avrameas S: Indirect microenzyme techniques for intracellular detection of antigens. Immunochemistry 6:825, 1969.

Coons AH: Histochemistry with labelled antibody. Int Rev Cytol 5:1, 1956.

Hsu SM, Cossman J, Jaffe ES: A comparison of ABC, unlabeled antibody and conjugated immunochemical methods with monoclonal and polyclonal antibodies. An examination of the germinal centers of tonsils. Am J Clin Pathol 80:429, 1983.

Kraenenbuhl JP, Galardy RE, Jamieson JD: Preparation and characterization of an immunoglobulin microscope tracer consisting of a heme-octopeptide coupled to Fab. J Exp Med 139:208, 1974.

Linthicum DS, Sell S: Topography of lymphocyte surface immunoglobulin using scanning immunoelectron microscopy. J Ultrastruct Res 51:55, 1975.

Nakane PK, Pierce GB Jr: Enzyme labeled antibodies for the light and electron microscopic localization of tissue antigens. J Cell Biol 33:307, 1967.

Reisberg MA, Rossen RD, Butler WT: A method for preparing specific fluorescein-conjugated antibody reagents using bentonite immunoadsorbents. J Immunol 105:1151–1161, 1970.

Santer V, Bankhurst AD, Nossal GJV: Ultrastructural distribution of surface immunoglobulin determinants on mouse lymphoid cells. Exp Cell Res 72:377, 1972.

Shnitka TK, Seligman, AM: Ultrastructural localization of enzymes. Annu Rev Biochem 40:375, 1971.

Stein H, Gatter K, Asbahr H, Mason DY: Use of freeze-dried paraffin-embedded sections for immunohistologic staining with monoclonal antibodies. Lab Invest 51:676, 1985.

Microbiological Tests

Dick GF, Dick GH: A skin test for susceptibility to scarlet fever. JAMA 82:265, 1924.

Dick GF, Dick GH: Results with the skin test for susceptibility to scarlet fever. Preventive immunization with scarlet fever toxin. JAMA 84:1477, 1925.

Dochez AR: Etiology of scarlet fever. Medicine 4:251, 1925.

Romer PH: Über den Nachweis sehr kleiner Mengen des Diphtheriegiftes. Z Immunitaetsforsch 3:208, 1909.

Schick B: Die Diphtherietoxin-Hautreaktion des Menschen als Vorprobe der prophylaktischen Diphtherieheilserum-Injection. Munch Med Wochenschr 60:2608, 1913.

Schultz W, Charlton W: Serologische Beobachtungen am Scharlachexanthum. Z Kinderheikd 17:328, 1917.

Schwentker FF, Hodes HL, Kingland LC, Chenoweth BM, Pek JL: Streptococcal infections in a naval training station. Am J Public Health 33:1455, 1943.

Antigen–Antibody Reactions in Vivo

Dixon FJ: The metabolism of antigen and antibody. J Allergy 25:487, 1954.

Talmadge DW, Dixon FJ, Bukantz SC, Dammin GJ: Antigen elimination from the blood as an early manifestation of the immune response. J Immunol 67:243, 1951.

Weigle WO, Dixon FJ: The elimination of heterologous serum proteins and associated antibody response to guinea pigs and rats. J Immunol 79:24, 1957.

Sensitivity of Assays

Gill TJ III: Methods for detecting antibody. Immunochemistry 7:997–1000, 1970.

Minden P, Reid RT, Farr RS: A comparison of some commonly used methods for detecting antibodies to bovine albumin in human serum. J Immunol 96:180, 1966.

8 Cell-Mediated Immunity in Vitro

In the preceding chapter in vitro immune reactions mediated by antibody were described. This chapter covers reactions of immune cells in vitro. *Cell-mediated immunity* refers to the effects of cells of the immune system. As with the reaction of antibodies with antigens in vitro, the reaction of specifically sensitized lymphocytes with antigen may also be measured in vitro. These reactions may also be divided into *primary* and *secondary* reactions. *Primary reactions* refers to direct effects of antigens on sensitized cells, such as binding of antigen or induction of proliferation of the reacting cells. *Secondary reactions* are a result of the effects of immune activated cells on other cells, such as killing of target cells by sensitized lymphocytes, or of the effects of products released from cells (i.e., *lymphokines*). The effect of cell-mediated immunity (CMI) in vivo is exemplified by delayed hypersensitivity and granulomatous reactions. It is not yet possible to duplicate these reactions in vitro. However, in many instances a correlation exists between the effect of cells or cell products as measured by in vitro tests and by in vivo responses. In most instances, T cell populations mediate these effects, but lymphocytes without markers (*null cells*) may also act as effector cells. In addition, accessory cells such as macrophages or polymorphonuclear leukocytes may be recruited (see Chapter 12).

Sensitization of T Cells

The mechanism of sensitization of T cells by antigen has been characterized through in vitro studies. The basic cellular requirements are for immune T lymphocytes and antigen presenting cells to match at the major histocompatibility locus (this subject is presented in detail in Chapters 9 and 10). The antigen-presenting cells are usually macrophages, which are phagocytic, take up the antigen, and also have on their surfaces self antigens that are often used to present soluble protein antigens. The antigen is displayed on the surface of the antigen presenting cell in association with self markers. Then, the T cell receptor binds the antigen and triggers the T cell response.

Primary Cellular Reaction with Antigen

Antigen Binding by Sensitized Cells

T cells that react specifically with antigen as a result of immunization are termed *sensitized cells.* The direct binding of antigen by specifically sensitized cells is measured by using labeled antigens. Radiolabeled antigen, fluorescent or enzyme-labeled antigen, or particulate forms of antigen may be used to demonstrate binding by radioisotopic counting, microscopy, or electron microscopy (Fig. 8-1). Sensitized lymphocytes have cell surface receptors that may bind antigens and activate cell proliferation (blast transformation).

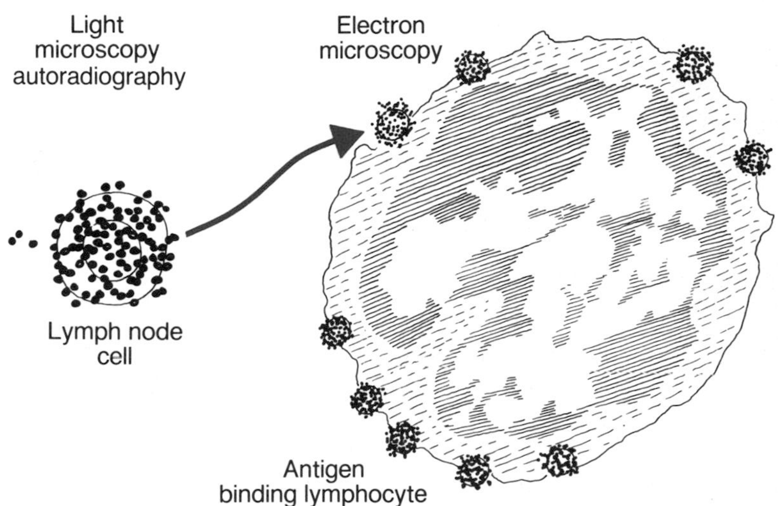

Figure 8-1. Labeling of antigen on surface of lymphocytes. Left: lymph node cell labeled with radiolabeled antigen. (From Diener and Poetkav: Proc Nat Acad Sci USA 69:2366, 1972.) Right: electron microscopic autoradiography of antigen-binding lymphocyte. (From Ada GL: Transplant Rev 5:110, 1970.) In addition, electron-dense antigenic particles, such as whelk hemocyanin, virus, or particles coated with antigen, may be used to label cell surface receptors. Labeling results in a patchy distribution of antigen on the cell surface if carried out at 4°C or in the presence of metabolic inhibitors such as azide. Under physiological conditions the cell surface labeling is lost by modulation (capping, endocytosis, or shedding) of the receptors (see Fig. 8-3). Capping and shedding are energy-dependent processes.

Blast Transformation

Blast transformation measures the proliferation response of sensitized T cells to antigen (Fig. 8-2). The responding cells may have different T cell functions including T_K (killer or cytotoxic), T_D (delayed hypersensitivity), T_H (helper), and T_S (suppressor). The degree of response is measured by visual observation of enlarged "blast" cells or by incorporation of radiolabeled precursors into protein, RNA, or DNA. Because these assays are done in cell culture, the cell numbers can be carefully con-

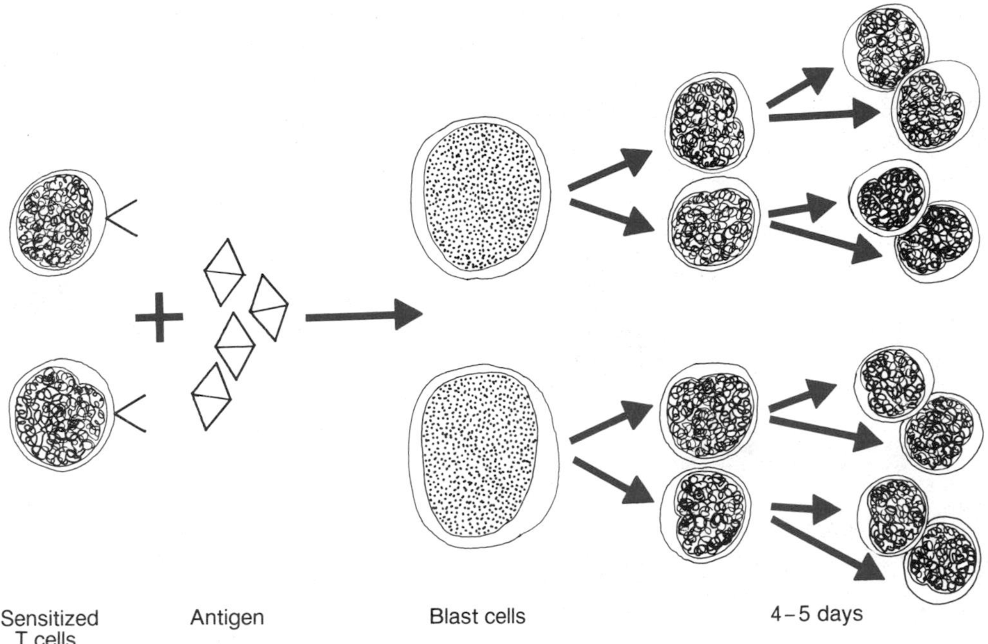

Figure 8-2. Antigen-induced T lymphocyte blast transformation. Antigen added to sensitized T cells in the presence of self-matched antigen-presenting cells stimulates enlargement of cells to "immature blast cells." This enlargement requires RNA and protein synthesis, and is followed by DNA synthesis and mitosis. The response is usually measured by adding one of the four building blocks of DNA as radiolabeled precursors, such as tritiated thymidine, and determining the incorporation of this isotope into new DNA synthesized by the growing cells.

trolled. In such cultures it has been shown that an antigen-processing cell must present the antigen to the responding T cell. The antigen-processing cell displays the antigen on its surface in association with self markers. In addition, T_S cells may inhibit blast transformation of other T cell types, while initially being stimulated to proliferate by antigen.

The early events that occur during activation of blast transformation of T or B cells are very similar to those that are associated with degranulation of mast cells (see Fig. 12-3). Reaction of antigens or mitogens with cell membrane receptors activates phospholipase C in the membrane that cleaves phosphatidylinositol into two second messengers: diacylglycerol and inositol triphosphate. How reaction of mitogen with receptor activates phospholipase C is not known. Diacylglycerol activates protein kinase C, and inositol triphosphate mobilizes Ca^{++} from internal storage sites in the cell into the cytoplasm. Activated protein kinase C in the presence of free Ca^{++} phosphorylates receptor-associated membrane proteins. Subsequent events are not well understood, but may involve increased receptors for, or sensitivity to, activators or growth factors such as interleukins. Mor-

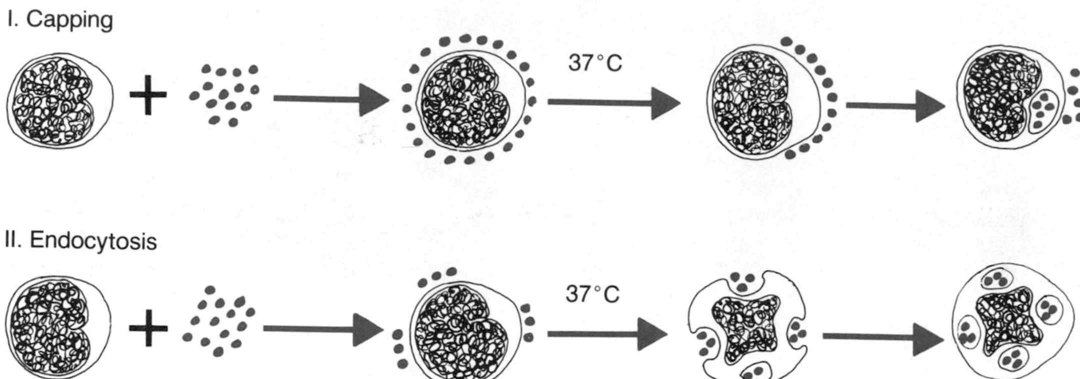

Figure 8-3. Cell surface events associated with lymphocyte activation. Two cell membrane events occur when antigens (or mitogens) react with the cell surface of lymphocytes: (I) diffuse pericellular labeling followed by capping with endocytosis and shedding, or (II) patchy labeling with endocytosis of patches. Both events result in clearing of the cell surface receptor. Activation to proliferation correlates with endocytosis, but not with capping.

phologic studies demonstrate two events at the cell surface: capping and endocytosis (Fig. 8-3). Capping refers to redistribution of the cell surface receptors from over the cell surface to one pole of the lymphocyte. This occurs with many agents that bind to the cell surface and does not necessarily lead to activation of the cell. Endocytosis refers to internalization of the cell surface receptor and bound antigen. This may occur in small patches (clusters of receptors) over the cell surface or in association with capping. Endocytosis does correlate with activation of the lymphocyte to proliferate. The membrane events described above may be required for endocytosis of antigen receptors. The events that follow endocytosis to signal the cell to begin the cell cycle remain unknown. The role of cell–cell interactions and soluble factors in lymphocyte activation and the immune response is discussed in Chapter 10.

The proliferation of immune T cells in culture allows the enrichment of antigen-specific clones: the frequency rises from less than 1 to 10,000 to about 1 in 100. Repeated stimulation in culture can result in pure populations of antigen-specific T cells. These can be diluted to one cell per well and grown in the presence of growth factors to give homogeneous populations of antigen-specific T cells (T cell clones). This form of positive selection in vitro mimics the clonal expansion that occurs in vivo. The ability to call up antigen-specific T cells when they are needed is an essential function of the immune system. T and B cells are committed to producing a single receptor with predetermined specificity prior to antigen stimulation, and a tremendous diversity of antigens must be recognized with a high specificity. Therefore the subset of cells with the desired specificity is quite rare. So antigen-specific cells must be rapidly expanded as they are needed to mount a timely and effective immune response.

Secondary Effects of Antigen Activation of Lymphocytes

Cell-Mediated Cytotoxicity

Five general cell-mediated cytotoxic effector mechanisms have been recognized in vitro (Table 8-1): (1) specifically sensitized effector cytotoxic T cells reacting directly with target cells; (2) specifically sensitized effector lymphocytes (T_D) reacting with antigen and releasing mediators that kill target cells (cytotoxins) or activate other effector cells (macrophages); (3) nonsensitized lymphocytes (null cells) activated by immunoglobulin antibody by Fc binding (antibody-dependent cell-mediated cytotoxicity or ADCC); (4) nonsensitized lymphocytes (natural killer cells, NK) reacting directly with target cells, and (5) activated macrophages. The basis of the reactivity of NK cells is not known. In addition, other cell types such as polymorphonuclear leukocytes or macrophages may function as killer cells via cytophilic antibody. Macrophages may also be activated by nonspecific stimulators such as phorbol esters or polynucleotides. Immune specific delayed hypersensitivity reactions mediated by the first two mechanisms involve T_D (delayed hypersensitivity) or T_K cells. T_K cells are also referred to as cytotoxic T lymphocytes (CTL). T_D activity correlates in vitro with antigen-induced blast transformation.

Table 8-1. Mechanisms of Lymphoid Cell-Mediated Immunity

T_K cells (CTL)	Sensitized to target cell — direct killing
T_D cells	Sensitized to target cell — lymphokine release, indirect killing (accessory cells)
Null cells + specific antibody	Antibody-dependent cell-mediated cytotoxicity (ADCC)
NK cells	Natural killing
Activated macrophages	Phagocytosis and digestion

Cytotoxic T lymphocyte activity is measured as the ability of T cell populations to kill target cells in vitro. Intracellular components of target cells may be labeled by addition of isotopes such as ^{51}Cr and cytolysis determined by the release of label from the target cell (Fig. 8-4). The cytotoxic effect of a population of T cells is expressed as the percentage of specific killing at a given effector-to-target-cell ratio (E/T ratio). This does not necessarily relate directly to the number of killer cells present. Different CTL may express different lytic capacity. In addition, one CTL may lyse more than one target cell. Thus, in measuring cytolysis by release of intracellular components, the

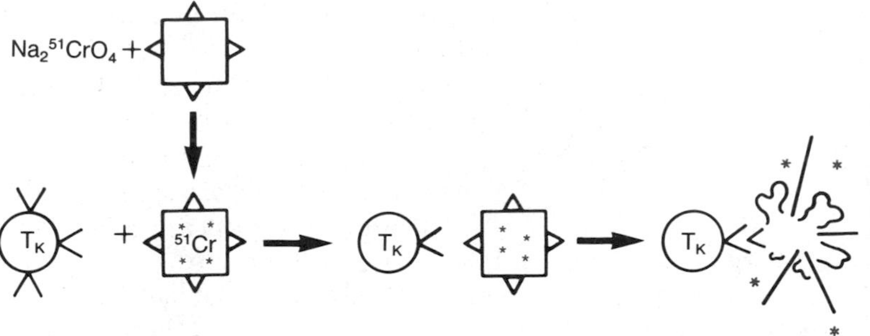

Figure 8-4. ^{51}Cr release assay for lymphocyte-mediated cytotoxicity. The release of intracellular components by the action of killer cells is determined. Target cells are labeled by incubation with $Na_2{}^{51}CrO_4$. Killer cells are then added to the labeled target cells. After incubation, the amount of intracellular and extracellular label remaining is determined by counting the radioactivity in the supernate and/or centrifuged cells. The percentage of specific lysis is calculated from the formula

$$\frac{\text{experimental } {}^{51}\text{Cr release} - \text{spontaneous release}}{\text{maximal release} - \text{spontaneous release},} \times 100$$

where the experimental release is that from the target cells treated with killer cells, the spontaneous release is that from untreated target cells, and the maximal release is that observed by lysing the target cells by freezing and thawing or by solubilizing them in detergent.

relative degree of activity of two populations of killer cells can be estimated by the E/T ratio of each that gives the same percentage of specific release. The T cell population that has greater cytotoxic activity will give 50% release at a lower E/T ratio.

The specificity of killing can be assayed by cold target inhibition of specific ^{51}Cr release (Fig. 8-5). Cytotoxic T lympho-

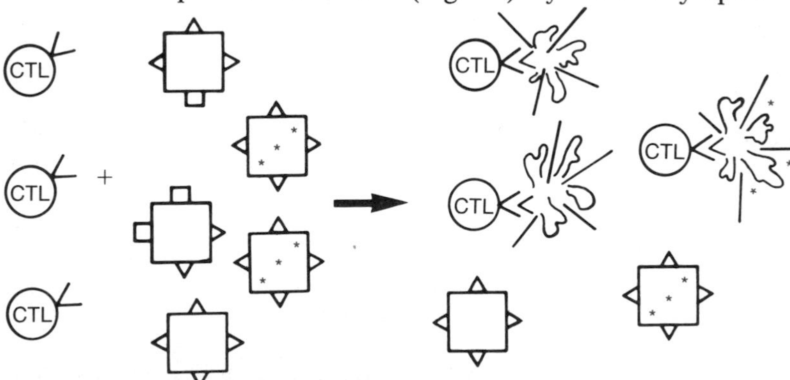

Figure 8-5. Cold target inhibition assay. Unlabeled target cells may be used to compete with labeled target cells in a lymphocyte-mediated cytotoxicity assay. The killer cells are added to a mixture of labeled and unlabeled target cells. If the unlabeled target cells contain some of the same antigenic specificities as the labeled target cells to which the CTL are reactive, the amount of ^{51}Cr released from the labeled target cells in a given period of time will be decreased. Quantitation of this inhibition of the CTL-mediated lysis may be used to determine antigenic relationships among different target cell populations and the specificity of reactivity of different CTL in a mixed population. In the example shown, only half as much radiolabel is released as would have occurred if no unlabeled target cells were present, because the CTL act on a mixture of labeled and unlabeled target cells.

cytes (T_K) are added to a mixture of unlabeled target cells and labeled target cells. The unlabeled target cells compete for the specific CTL and decrease the amount of label released from the labeled target cells. In a manner similar to a radioimmunoassay, the degree of antigenic cross-reactivity may be estimated by the amount of cold target inhibition obtained. In this manner, shared antigens recognized by CTL cells in different tissues may be identified.

Killing of target cells by specifically sensitized lymphocytes is an immune-specific effector function of the cellular arm of the immune response. Immunization with cells expressing foreign antigens on the cell surface results in expansion of populations of T_K (or cytotoxic T) lymphocytes with specific receptors for the antigen. CTL activity is specific for antigens on the target cells, does not require antiserum or complement to be effective, and is active against foreign MHC class I antigens (graft rejections), viral antigens expressed on cell surfaces, or tumor antigens. Upon second contact with antigen in vivo this population of cells is available to kill cells expressing the antigen (memory).

Agents that inhibit direct lymphocyte-mediated cytolysis have been used to study the mechanism of direct killing of target cells by specifically sensitized T_K lymphocytes. The activity of the killer cell during killing may be divided into three phases: (1) initial recognition of target cell antigens by sensitized CTL; (2) CTL activation and lethal attack; and (3) target cell lysis (Fig. 8-6). Following killing of a target cell, a CTL may go on and kill other target cells. A direct transfer of killer cell products to target cells is thought to produce a membrane defect in the target cell similar to that produced by the membrane-attack complex of complement (see Chapter 12), which results in a lethal hole in the target cell membrane. Intimate contact between killer T cells and target cells is required for cell killing.

Monolayer Plaques

The interaction of sensitized lymphocytes and target cells may be studied morphologically by observing the effect of sensitized lymphocytes on target cells growing in monolayers. Plaques or holes occur in the monolayer when sensitized lymphocytes are added. Sensitized lymphocytes surround the target cells and eventually cause their detachment from the monolayer. Figure 8-7 depicts the destruction of monolayer target cells. As long as the target cells remain attached to the monolayer, they appear to be viable; however, upon separation from the monolayer, the target cell undergoes morphologic alterations indicative of cell death. These alterations include vacuolization and disintegration of the cytoplasm and condensation of nucleus and cytoplasm. Although close contact between the sensitized lymphocytes and target cells occurs, the exact mechanism of target cell death remains unclear.

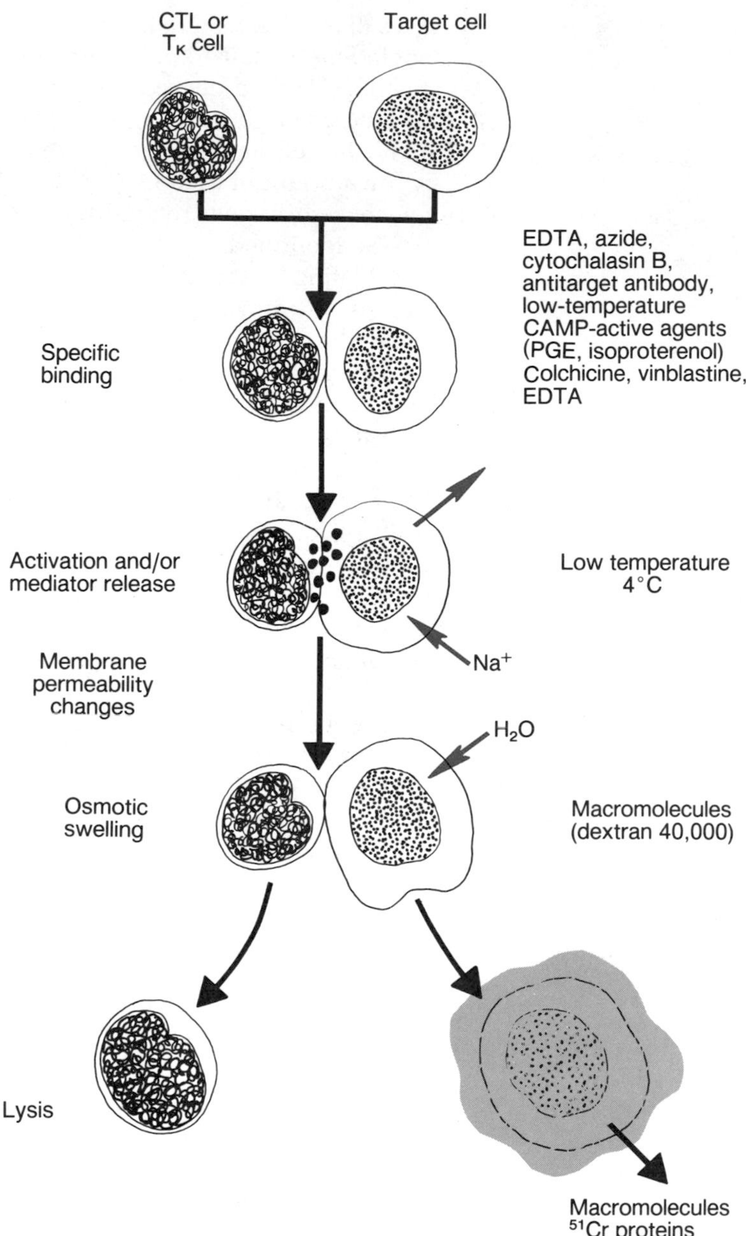

Figure 8-6. Stages of CTL (T_K)-mediated target cell lysis. Reaction of specifically sensitized T_K cell with target cell is followed by sequential changes culminating in lysis of the target cell. The T_K cell can then detach and attack another target cell. The use of inhibitors suggests that binding occurs via an antigen receptor and is an energy-requiring process involving membrane modulation. Following binding, energy-requiring activation of T_K cells may occur in some situations, as indicated by the effect of metabolic inhibitors. However, membrane permeability changes in the target cell occur within minutes of killer cell binding. Further lysis proceeds without an energy requirement. Activated T_K cells have granules containing lysosomal enzymes, which may be released after contact with the target cell. The terminal stages of lysis involve continued osmotic uptake of H_2O into the cell due to the increase in membrane permeability. (Modified from Henney CS: J Reticuloendothel Soc 17:4, 1975.)

An identical type of interaction between lymphocytes and target cells may occur in vivo in tissue reactions mediated by lymphocytes. Figure 8-8 shows the pathologic changes occurring during the development of experimental allergic thyroiditis. As in the target cell monolayer system, lymphocytes pass between the thyroid-follicle-lining cells, causing them to separate from each other and from the basement membrane, eventually destroying the thyroid cells. The basement membrane appears intact during the development of the lesion. Infiltra-

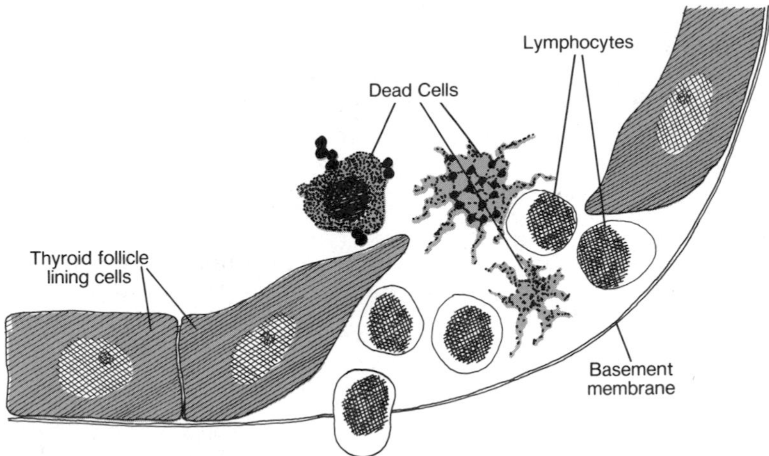

Figure 8-7. Reaction of sensitized lymphocytes with target cells in vitro. T lymphocytes from a sensitized donor infiltrate and surround monolayer target cells, seemingly without effect on viability or morphologic appearance of target cells. As a result of this infiltration, monolayer cells become separated from each other and from culture surface. Monolayer cells that retain contact with the monolayer remain viable, but when they are separated from other monolayer cells, morphologic changes consistent with cell death occur. These alterations do not occur in tissue culture cells that become separated from the monolayer in the presence of normal lymphocytes. Fluids and washings taken from monolayers treated with sensitized lymphocytes cannot be used to initiate new cultures, whereas fluids or washings of cultures treated with normal lymphocytes can. DC, dead or dying cells separated from monolayers; L, lymphocytes; MTC, monolayer target cells. (Modified from Biberfield P, Holm G, Perlmann P: Exp Cell Res 52:672, 1968. Copyright © Academic Press.)

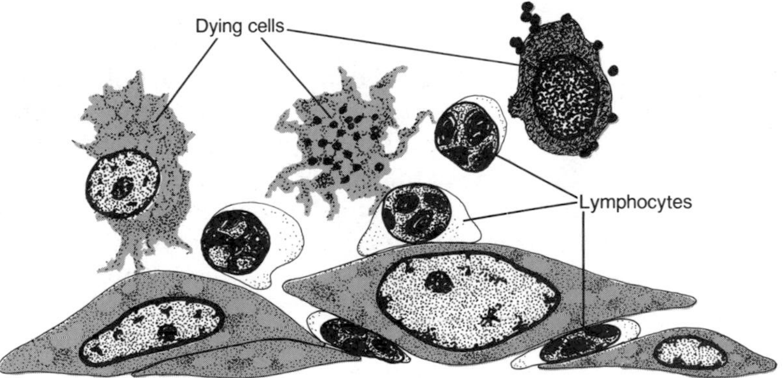

Figure 8-8. Reaction of sensitized lymphocytes with target cells in vivo (morphologic changes in experimental allergic thyroiditis). Changes similar to those illustrated in Figure 8-7 for reaction of sensitized lymphocytes with tissue culture monolayers occur with thyroid-follicle-lining cells in allergic thyroiditis. Mononuclear cells appear first in perivenular areas and then invade stroma of thyroid. Invasion of follicles follows. Lymphocytes appear to pass through the basement membrane of the thyroid follicle, separating thyroid-follicle-lining cells from basement membrane and from other follicular cells. Death of lining cells occurs when these cells are isolated from basement membrane and from other follicular cells. DC, dead or dying cells; L, lymphocytes; TFC, thyroid-follicle-lining cells. (Modified from Flax MH: Lab Invest 12:199, 1963. Copyright © 1963, International Academy of Pathology.)

tion of mononuclear cells, with separation, isolation, and destruction of target cells, may be observed in contact dermatitis, classic graft rejection, and many autoallergic diseases believed to be mediated by specifically sensitized cells (e.g., destruction of thyroid-follicle-lining cells in experimental allergic thyroiditis and destruction of germinal epithelium in experimental allergic orchitis).

T_D Lymphocytes

T_D lymphocytes initiate delayed hypersensitivity inflammatory reactions in vivo. The activity of these cells may also be measured in vitro (Fig. 8-9). Sensitized T_D cells are activated to

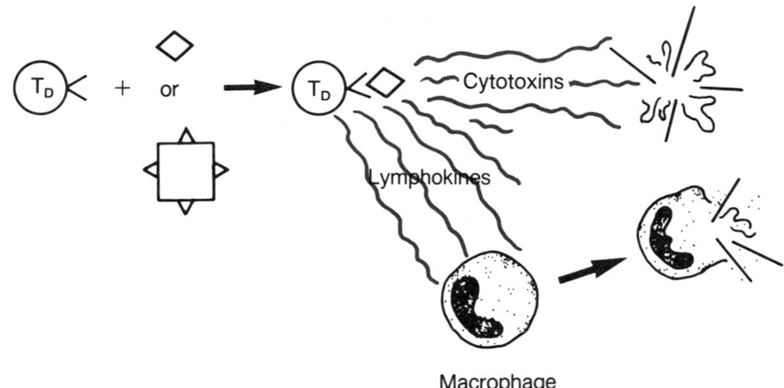

Figure 8-9. T_D cell-mediated immunity. T_D cells are activated by reaction with antigen, either soluble or cell surface, to release lymphocytic mediators (lymphokines). These mediators attract and activate accessory cells, in particular macrophages, which destroy the target cell.

proliferate in the presence of antigen and to produce and release a variety of lymphocyte mediators termed *lymphokines*. Proliferation may be directly measured as blast transformation (see above). Lymphokine production may be measured by determining a variety of effects on other cells, some of which may be measured in vitro. The role of lymphocytes and lymphokines in inflammation is presented in Chapter 12. Lymphokines may activate macrophages to produce damage to cells not bearing the specific antigen recognized by the T_D effector cell ("innocent bystander" effect). Thus reactions of T_D cells with antigen on one cell may ultimately cause damage to an antigenically unrelated cell if a severe inflammatory response is generated. Experimentally, measurement of the activity of lymphokines may often be used to detect T_D cell-mediated immunity. However, some of the techniques used are not readily applicable for widespread use. Another in vitro technique used to measure the effects of antigen on T_D cells is leukocyte (macrophage) migration inhibition.

Migration Inhibition

Migration inhibition measures the effect of mediators from sensitized lymphocytes (lymphokines) on migration of peritoneal exudate macrophages in the presence or absence of antigen. Extracts of antigen-treated lymphocytes may also be assayed for migration inhibition factor (MIF). Quantitation is achieved by measuring the area of migration of antigen- or MIF-treated cells on an agar layer, comparing the area to that of nontreated cells, and calculating the percentage of migration inhibition (Fig. 8-10). This assay has been used extensively in experimental and clinical studies.

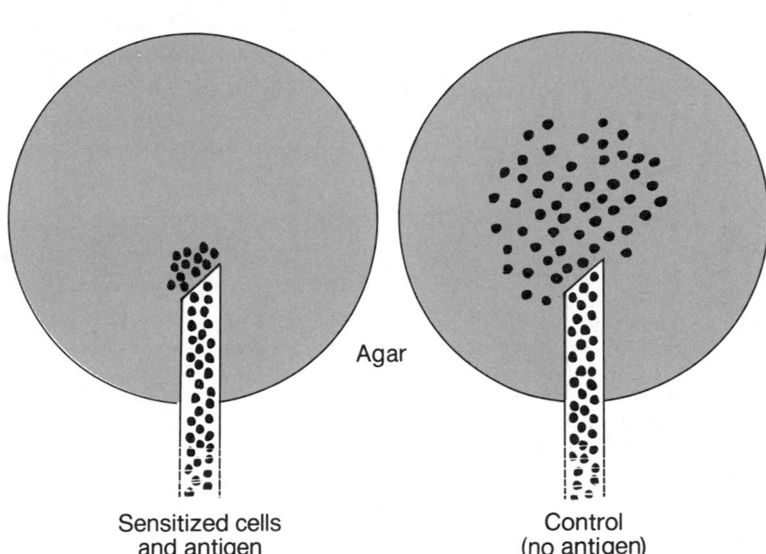

Figure 8-10. Macrophage migration inhibition. To measure the migration of macrophages a population of cells is collected in a capillary pipette. The pipette is placed on an agar layer. After incubation in vitro the cells migrate over the agar (control). However, if sensitized lymphocytes and antigen or migration inhibition factor (MIF) are present, the macrophages do not migrate out of the capillary pipette.

Lymphokine-Activated Cells

Normal unsensitized T lymphocytes may be activated to become killers following non-antigen-specific stimulation with a variety of mitogens (Fig. 8-11). This activation may be caused by

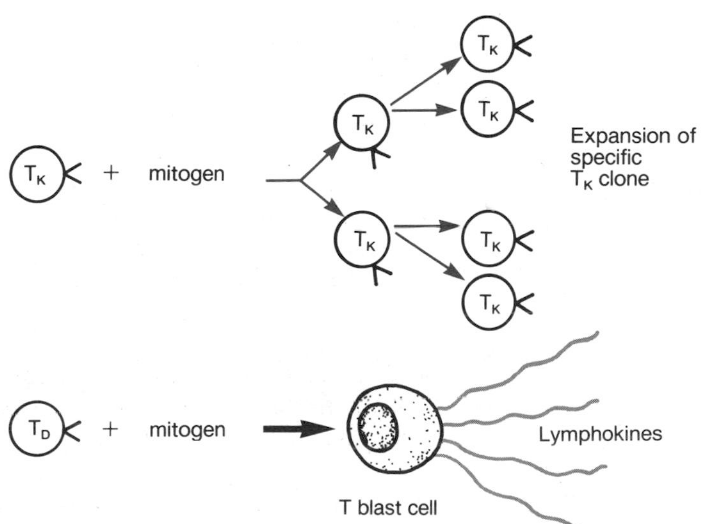

Figure 8-11. Mitogen-activated cell-mediated immunity. Mitogens activate T cell killing either by expanding the numbers of T_K cells by proliferation or by nonspecifically inducing the production of lymphokines by T_D cells.

the increased numbers of T killer cells generated by mitogen stimulation or the generation of cytotoxic or macrophage-activating lymphokines (see above). Whereas some evidence exists that mitogens may act at least in part by agglutinating activated killer cells to target cells, this is not the case with concanavalin A (ConA)-activated killer cells. ConA presumably acts by stimulating preexisting T_K cell populations to expand and thus express their genetically determined immune specificity to foreign target cells. The in vivo significance of mitogen-induced cytotoxicity remains uncertain. However, this phenomenon does indicate the inherent killing spectrum of activated T cells and suggests that nonspecific activation produces killer cells that might act on foreign cells or organisms.

In a somewhat similar fashion one lymphocyte mediator, interleukin 2, has been shown capable of expanding and activating a new class of cytolytic cells, lymphokine-activated killer cells (LAK). These cells can be shown to be potent killers of fresh tumor cells in vitro and in vivo. Unlike that caused by CTL, chromium release caused by LAK in vitro is not antigen specific, more than one type of tumor may be lysed, and killing is not self restricted. However, on the basis of cell surface markers, IL2 works on a precursor cell that differentiates into the activated killer, LAK. These cells , when given back to donor mice along with high doses of IL2, have been shown to proliferate in vivo and to kill tumor cells actively. They are totally dependent on exogenous IL2 and disappear when the interleukin is not given. However, LAK therapy at the present time is associated with considerable toxicity to the lungs, generalized edema apparently of nonspecific localization, and release of various lymphokines. The basis of the tumor-specific killing is unknown at this time. Recent reports of clinical efficacy in treating melanomas and certain carcinomas need to be verified.

Sensitization of Killer Cells in Vitro

CTL may be induced in vitro. Cell populations containing nonsensitized CTL are mixed with stimulator cells and incubated for 4 to 7 days (Fig. 8-12). During this time the specifically reactive cells proliferate and develop the specific capacity to kill the target cells. Cells that respond in mixed lymphocyte reactions with stimulator cells of foreign histocompatibility type develop cytotoxic activity to specific histocompatibility antigens. Fibroblast cultures have been used for this purpose. Using fibroblast monolayers, it is possible to sensitize lymphocytes to foreign histocompatibility antigens. Tumor cell monolayers may be used to sensitize to tumor specific transplantation antigen. Virus-infected target cells may be used to induce CTL specific for viral antigens. Self antigens may be

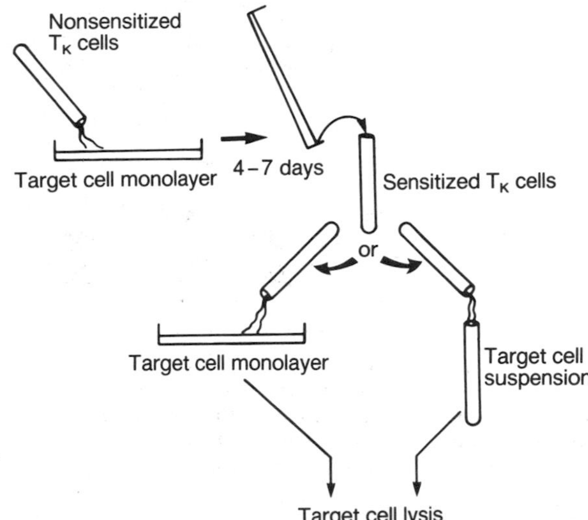

Figure 8-12. Sensitization of CTL in vitro. Nonsensitized populations of CTL may be sensitized in vitro by incubation with target cells. After 4 to 7 days, the CTL removed specifically lyse target cells containing antigens to which they were exposed in vitro. This is due to a specific expansion of CTL (proliferation).

recognized by culturing lymphocytes on autologous fibroblast cultures, thus inducing autoallergy in vitro. Macrophages are required for optimal sensitization of T cells in vitro, but macrophages do not usually take part in the killer cell effector stage of the reaction.

In vitro secondary sensitization or boosting may also be used to demonstrate antigenic cross-reactivity between different target cell populations. In vitro boosting is accomplished in the same manner as in vitro priming, except that the lymphoid cells are obtained from donor animals that have been immunized to a given target cell line. If a marked increase in killing is evidenced after in vitro exposure to a second target cell line as compared with the effect of exposure of lymphoid cells from unimmunized donors to that cell line, then an antigenic relationship between the cell line used for in vivo priming and that used for in vitro boosting has been demonstrated.

Antibody-Dependent Cell-Mediated Cytotoxicity

Target cells may be lysed by effector cells that are not themselves specifically sensitized, but bind onto the target cell by antibodies on the target cell surface (Fig. 8-13). The cells active as effectors in antibody-dependent cell-mediated cytotoxicity (ADCC) bear cell surface receptors for the Fc domains of aggregated immunoglobulin that is usually of the IgG class. ADCC effector populations include polymorphonuclear leukocytes and macrophages as well as lymphocytes. Killing requires effector target cell interaction that is accomplished by the antibody attaching to the target cell by its antigen-binding site and to the effector cell by its Fc piece. The in vivo significance of ADCC is also not clear, but such a mechanism could act to augment antibody-mediated effector mechanisms and can be shown to kill larval stage parasites in vitro.

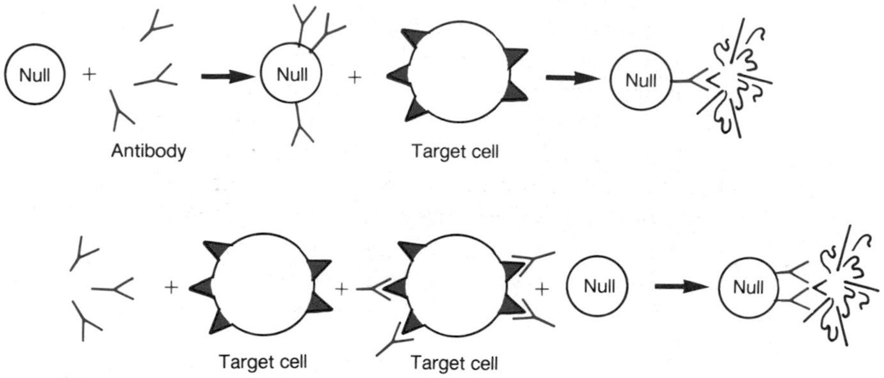

Figure 8-13. Antibody-dependent cell-mediated cytotoxicity (ADCC) is due to the attachment of effector cells to aggregated antibody on target cells. This bestows on previously nonimmune reactive cells the capacity to react specifically with antigens on cells and kill them. Other cells such as polymorphonuclear leukocytes and macrophages may also function as effector cells through passively absorbed antibody.

Natural Killer Cells

Some lymphocytes with neither T nor B cell markers are able to cause death of certain target cells without specific antibody-mediated direction. These cells are called *NK (natural killer)* cells. Natural killer cell activity is also measured by a cytotoxic assay (Fig. 8-14). It is directed against a variety of target cell lines and may be inhibited by carbohydrates, suggesting that NK cell receptors react to carbohydrate antigens. NK activity exists without stimulation but may be enhanced by interferon.

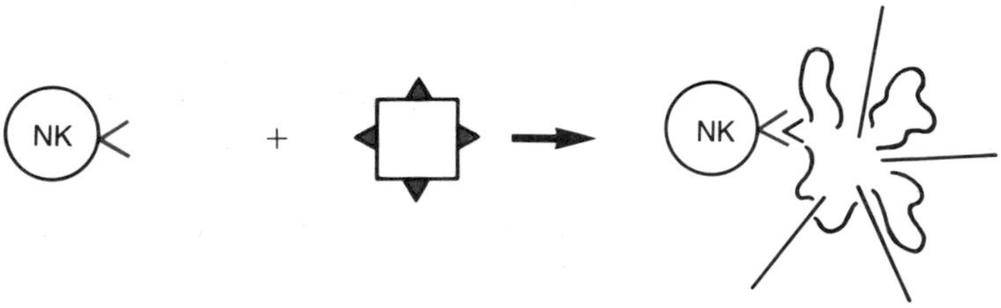

Figure 8-14. Natural killer cells. Nonimmune persons have cells that are able to kill target cells. The nature of the antigen receptor for such cells is unknown, although the effect appears to be target cell antigen specific.

Activated Macrophages

The macrophage has an important accessory role for CMI (Fig. 8-15). In delayed hypersensitivity reactions in vivo it is usually

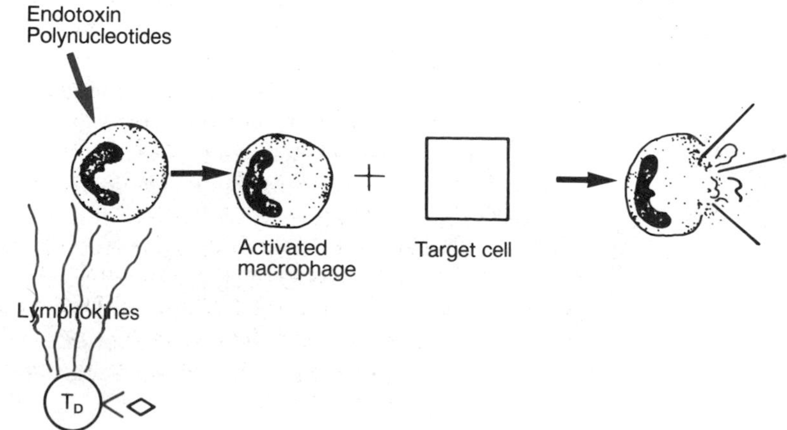

Figure 8-15. Activated macrophages. Macrophages may be activated nonspecifically by endotoxin or polynucleotides or by lymphokines released by T_D cells reacting with specific antigens. Activated macrophages will kill target cells nonspecifically.

the macrophage that actually performs the lytic or destructive step. Thus, T_D cells kill indirectly by producing lymphokines that activate macrophages to become killers. Macrophages also may become *armed* by attachment of *cytophilic antibody* and function as immune specific killers. In addition, macrophages may be activated by a variety of agents (biological response modifiers) to become more efficient killers, presumably by increasing the amount of lysosomal enzymes and cellular metabolism. Increased in vitro activity of the macrophage may reflect an enhanced state of resistance to infectious agents in vivo. (See Chapter 12.)

Summary

Cell-mediated immunity refers to the measurement of reactions mediated by immune lymphocytes. Primary reactions are the direct effect of antigen on sensitized cells; secondary reactions are the result of immune-activated lymphocytes on other cells. Direct effects include antigen binding and activation of sensitized cells to proliferate. Secondary effects include T_K (killer) or T cytotoxic cell (CTL) activity, mitogen-induced killing or lymphokine production, antibody-dependent cell-mediated cytotoxicity, natural killer cell activity, and killing by activated macrophages. The mechanisms responsible for most cellular reactions in vivo are T_K (CTL) and T_D. T_K activity is measured by the effect of specificially sensitized T_K cells on target cells in vitro (cytotoxicity); T_D activity is measured by proliferation or lymphokine production after antigen stimulation.

References

General

Bloom BR, David JR: In Vitro Methods in Cell Mediated and Tumor Immunology. New York, Academic Press, 1976.

Cohen S: The role of cell-mediated immunity in the induction of inflammatory responses. Am J Pathol 88:502, 1977.

Antigen Binding

Ada GL: Antigen binding cells in tolerance and immunity. Transplant Rev 5:105, 1970.

Ada GL, Ev PL: Lymphocyte receptors and antigen receptors on B and T cells. *In* Sela M (ed): The Antigens, vol 3. Academic Press, New York, 1975, p 190.

Basten A, Miller JFAP, Warner NL, Dye J: Specific infection of thymus-derived (T) and non-thymus derived (B) lymphocytes by ^{135}I labeled antigen. Nature 231:104, 1971.

Cone RE, Gershon RK, Askenase PW: Nylon adherent antigen-specific rosette-forming T cells. J Exp Med 146:1390, 1977.

Greaves MF, Moller E: Studies on antigen binding cells. I. The origin of reactive cells. Cell Immunol 1:372, 1970.

Noar D, Sulitzeanu D: Binding of radiolabeled bovine serum albumin to mouse spleen cells. Nature 214:687, 1967.

Sell S, Asofsky R: Lymphocytes and immunoglobulins. Prog Allergy 86:95, 1968.

T Cell Activation and Blast Transformation

Dutton RW, Bulman RW: The significance of the protein carrier in the stimulation of DNA synthesis by hapten–protein conjugates in the secondary response. Immunology 7:54, 1964.

Hirschhorn K, Back F, Kolodny RL, Firschein IL, Hashem N: Immune response and mitoses of human peripheral blood lymphocytes in vitro. Science 142:1185, 1963.

Kirchner H, Blaese RM: Pokeweed mitogen-, concanavalin A-, and phytohemagglutinin-induced development of cytotoxic effector lymphocytes. An evaluation of the mechanisms of T cell-mediated cytotoxicity. J Exp Med 138:812, 1973.

Ling NR: Lymphocyte Stimulation. Amsterdam, North-Holland, 1968.

Marshall WH, Valentine FT, Lawrence HS: Cellular immunity in vitro: clonal proliferation of antigen stimulated lymphocytes. J Exp Med 128:327, 1969.

Moller G (ed): Interleukins and lymphocyte activation. Immunol Rev 63, 1982.

Nedrud J, Touton M, Clark WR: The requirement for DNA synthesis and gene expression in the generation of cytotoxicity in vitro. J Exp Med 142:960, 1975.

Oppenheim JJ, Rosenstreich DL: Mitogens in Immunobiology. Academic Press, New York, 1976.

Pearmain G, Lycette RR, Fitzgerald PH: Tuberculin-induced mitosis in peripheral blood leukocytes. Lancet 1:637, 1963.

Robbins AH: Tissue culture studies of the human lymphocyte. Science 146:1648, 1964.

Valentine IT: The transformation and proliferation of lymphocytes in vitro. *In* Revillard JP (ed): Cell Mediated Immunity: In Vitro Correlates. Baltimore, University Park Press, 1971, p6.

T_D Activities in Vitro

Aarden LA, et al: Letter to the Editor. Revised nomenclature for antigen nonspecific T cell proliferation and helper factors. Mol Immunol 17:641, 1980.

Bennett B, Bloom BR: Reactions in vivo and in vitro produced by a soluble substance associated with delayed-type hypersensitivity. Proc Nat Acad Sci USA 59:756, 1968.

Bloom BR, Bennett B: Mechanism of a reaction in vitro associated with delayed hypersensitivity. Science 153:80, 1966.

Bloom BR, Jimenez L: Migration inhibitor factor and the cellular basis of delayed hypersensitivity reactions. Am J Pathol 60:453, 1970.

Carpenter RR: In vitro studies of cellular hypersensitivity. I. Specific inhibition of migration of cells from adjuvant-immunized animals by purified protein derivative and other protein antigens. J Immunol 91:803, 1963.

David JR: Delayed hypersensitivity in vitro: its mediation by cell free substances formed by lymphoid cell–antigen interaction. Proc Nat Acad Sci USA 56:72, 1966.

David JR, Al-Askari S, Lawrence HS, Thomas L: Delayed hypersensitivity in vitro. I. The specificity of inhibition of cell migrations by antigen. J Immunol 93:264, 1964.

George M, Vaughan JH: In vitro cell migration as a model for delayed hypersensitivity. Proc Soc Exp Biol Med 111:514, 1962.

Green JA, Cooperband SR, Kibrick S: Immune specific induction of interferon production in cultures of human blood lymphocytes. Science 164:1415, 1969.

Heise ER, Hans S, Wiser RS: In vitro studies on the mechanism of macrophage migration inhibition in tuberculin sensitivity. J Immunol 101:1004, 1968.

Lawrence HS, Landy M (eds): Mediators of Cellular Immunity. New York, Academic Press, 1969.

Likhite V, Sehon A: Migration inhibition and cell-mediated immunity: a review. Rev Can Biol 30:135, 1971.

Pekarek J, Krecj J: Survey of the methodologic approaches to studying delayed hypersensitivity in vitro. J Immunol Methods 6:1, 1974.

Salvin SB, Nishio J: In vitro cell reactions in delayed hypersensitivity. J Immunol 103:138, 1969.

Wagner H, Rollinghoff M, Nossal GJV: T-cell-mediated immune responses induced in vitro: a probe for allograft and tumor immunity. Transplant Rev 17:3, 1973.

Waksman BH: Studies on cellular lysis in tuberculin sensitivity. Annu Rev Tuberc 68:746, 1953.

Waksman BH, Namba Y: On soluble mediators of immunologic regulation. Cell Immunol 21:161, 1976.

Ward PA, Remold HG, David JR: Leukotactic factor produced by sensitized lymphocytes. Science 163:1079, 1969.

Wunderlich JR, Canty TG: Cell mediated immunity induced in vitro. Nature 228:62, 1970.

Cytotoxic Lymphocytes

Berke G, Amos GB: Mechanism of lymphocyte-mediated cytolysis: the LMC cycle and its role in transplantation immunity. Transplant Rev 17:71, 1973.

Biberfield P, Holm G, Perlmann P: Morphologic observations on lymphocyte peripolesis and cytotoxic action in vitro. Exp Cell Res 52:672, 1968.

Brunner KT, Mauel J, Rudolf H, Chapuis B: Studies of allograft immunity in mice. I. Induction, development and in vitro assay of cellular immunity. Immunology 18:501, 1970.

Canty TG, Wunderlich JR: Quantitative in vitro assay of cytotoxic cellular immunity. J Nat Cancer Inst 45:761, 1970.

Chism SE, Burton RC, Grail DL, Bell PM, Warner NL: In vitro induction of tumor specific immunity. VI. Analysis of specificity of immune response by cellular competitive inhibition. Limitations and advantages of the technique. J Immunol Methods 16:254, 1977.

Flax MH: Experimental allergic thyroiditis in the guinea pig. II. Morphologic studies on the development of the disease. Lab Invest 12:199, 1971.

Goldstein P, Smith ET: Mechanism of T-cell-mediated cytolysis: the lethal hit stage. Contemp Top Immunol 7:273, 1977.

Granger GA: Mechanisms of lymphocyte-induced cell and tissue destruction in vitro. Am J Pathol 59:469, 1970.

Hayry P, Defendi V: Mixed lymphocyte cultures produce effector cells: model of in vitro allograft rejection. Science 168:133, 1970.

Hellstrom I, Hellstrom KE, Sjogren HO, Warner G: Demonstration of cell-mediated immunity to human neoplasms of various histologic types. Int J Cancer 7:1, 1971.

Hellstrom KE, Hellstrom I: Lymphocyte-mediated cytotoxicity and blocking activity to tumor antigens. Adv Immunol 18:209, 1974.

Henkart PA: Mechanism of lymphocyte mediated cytotoxicity. Annu Rev Immunol 3:31, 1985.

Henney CS: On the mechanism of T-cell mediated cytolysis. Transplant Rev 17:37, 1973.

Henney CS: T cell mediated cytolysis: an overview of some current issues. Contemp Top Immunol 7:245, 1977.

Hodes RJ, Handwerger BS, Terry WD: Synergy between subpopulations of mouse spleen cells in the in vitro germination of cell-mediated cytotoxicity. J Exp Med 140:1646, 1974.

Lohmann-Matthew ML, Fisher H: T cell cytotoxicity and amplification of the cytotoxic reaction by macrophages. Transplant Rev 17:150, 1973.

Martz E: Mechanisms of specific tumor cell lysis by alloimmune T lymphocytes: resolution and characterization of discrete steps in the cellular interaction. Contemp Top Immunol 7:301, 1977.

Moller G (ed): Mechanism of action of cytotoxic T cells. Immunol Rev 72:1983.

Nabholz M, MacDonald HR: Cytotoxic T lymphocytes. Annu Rev Immunol 11:273, 1983.

Perlmann P, Holm G: Cytotoxic effects of lymphoid cells in vitro. Adv Immunol 11:117, 1970.

Perlmann P, Perlmann H, Wigzell H: Lymphocyte-mediated cytoxicity in vitro. Induction and inhibition by humoral antibody and nature of effector cells. Transplant Rev 13:91, 1972.

Plata F, Cerottini J-C, Brunner KT: Primary and secondary in vitro generation of cytolytic T lymphocytes in the murine sarcoma virus system. Eur J Immunol 5:227, 1975.

Podack ER, Koningsburg PJ: Cytotoxic T cell granules. J Exp Med 160:695, 1984.

Rosenau W, Moon HD: Lysis of homologous cells by sensitized lymphocytes in tissue culture. J Nat Cancer Inst 27:471, 1961.

Ruddle NH: Lymphotoxic redux. Immunol Today 6:156, 1985.

Takasugi M, Klein E: A microassay for cell-mediated immunity. Transplantation 9:219, 1970.

Taylor HE, Culling CFA: Cytopathic effect in vitro of sensitized homologous and heterologous spleen cells on fibroblasts. Lab Invest 12:884–894, 1963.

Williams TW, Granger GA: Lymphocyte in vitro cytotoxicity: mechanism of lymphotoxic-induced target cell destruction. J Immunol 102:911, 1969.

Wilson DB: Quantitative studies on the behavior of sensitized lymphocytes in vitro. I. Relationship of the degree of destruction of homologous target cells to the number of lymphocytes and to the time of contact in culture and consideration of the effect of isoimmune serum. J Exp Med 122:143, 1975.

Winn HJ: Immune mechanisms in homotransplantation. II. Quantitative assay of the immunologic activity of lymphoid cells stimulated by tumor homografts. J Immunol 86:228, 1961.

Antibody-Dependent Cell-Mediated Cytotoxicity

Balch CM, Ades EW, Loken MR, Shope SL: Human "null" cells mediating antibody-dependent cellular cytotoxicity express T lymphocyte differentiation antigens. J Immunol 124:1845, 1980.

Herlin D, Herlin M, Steplewski Z, Koprowski H: Monoclonal antibodies in cell-mediated cytotoxicity against human melanoma and colorectal carcinoma. Eur J Immunol 9:657, 1979.

Kay AD, Bonnard CD, West WH, Herberman RB: A functional compression of human Fc receptor-bearing lymphocytes active in natural cytotoxicity and antibody dependent cellular cytotoxicity. J Immunol 118:2058, 1977.

Parrillo JE, Fauci AS: Apparent direct cellular cytotoxicity mediated via cellular antibody. Multiple Fc receptor bearing effector cell populations mediating cytophilic antibody induced cytotoxicity. Immunology 33:839, 1977.

Payne CM, Linde A, Kibler R, et al: Surface features of human natural killer cells and antibody dependent cytotoxic cells. J Cell Sci 77:27, 1985.

Perlmann P, Holm G: Cytotoxic effects of lymphoid cells in vitro. Adv Immunol 11:117, 1969.

Perlmann P, Perlmann H, Biberfeld P: Specifically cytotoxic lymphocytes produced by preincubation with antibody complexed target cells. J Immunol 108:558, 1972.

Perlmann P, Perlmann H, Muller-Eberhard HJ, Manni JA: Cytotoxic effects of leukocytes triggered by complement bound to target cells. Science 163:937, 1969.

Takasugi J, Koide Y, Takasugi M: Reconstitution of natural cell-mediated cytotoxicity with specific antibodies. Eur J Immunol 7:887, 1977.

Van Boxel JA, Paul WE, Green I, Frank M: Antibody-dependent lymphoid cell-mediated cytotoxicity: role of complement. J Immunol 112:398, 1974.

Natural Killer Cells

Granger GA, Kolb WB: Lymphocyte in vitro cytotoxicity: mechanisms of immune and nonimmune small lymphocyte-mediated target L cell destruction. J Immunol 101:111, 1968.

Herberman RB (ed): NK Cells and Other Natural Effector Cells. Orlando, Fla., Academic Press, 1982.

Herberman RB, Nunn ME, Lavrin DH: Natural cytotoxic reactivity of mouse lymphoid cells against syngeneic and allogeneic tumors. Int J Cancer 16:216, 1975.

Herberman RN, Reynolds CW, Ortaldo J: Mechanisms of cytotoxicity by natural killer cells. Annu Rev Immunol 4:651, 1986.

Moller G (ed): Natural Killer Cells. Immunol Rev 44, 1979.

Ortaldo JR, Herberman RB: Heterogeneity of natural killer cells. Annu Rev Immunol 2:359, 1985.

Takasugi M, Koide Y, Akira D, Ramseyer A: Specificities in natural cell mediated cytotoxicity by the cross-competitive assay. Int J Cancer 19:291, 1977.

Takasugi M, Mickey MR, Terasaki PI: Reactivity of lymphocytes from normal persons on cultured tumor cells. Cancer Res 33:2898, 1973.

Macrophage Activation

Adams DO, Hamilton TA: The cell biology of macrophage activation. Annu Rev Immunol 2:283, 1984.

Gotoff SP, Vizral IF, Malecki TJ: Macrophage aggregation in vitro. Transplantation 10:443, 1970.

Hibbs JB, Remington JS, Stewart CC: Modulation of immunity and host resistance by microorganisms. Pharmacol Ther 8:37, 1980.

Keller R: Mechanisms by which activated normal macrophages destroy syngeneic rat tumor cells in vitro. Immunology 27:285, 1974.

Mackaness GB: Resistance to intracellular infection. J Infect Dis 123:439, 1971.

Mackaness GB, Blanden RV: Cellular immunity. Drug Allergy 11:89, 1967.

Mooney J, Waksman BH: Activation of normal rabbit macrophage monolayers by supernatants of antigen stimulated macrophages. J Immunol 105:1138, 1970.

Nathan CF, Karnovsky ML, David JR: Alterations of macrophage functions by mediators from lymphocytes. J Exp Med 133:1356, 1971.

Nelson DS (ed): Immunology of the Macrophage. New York, Academic Press, 1976.

Raffel S: Types of acquired immunity to infectious diseases. Annu Rev Microbiol 3:221, 1949.

9 The Major Histocompatibility Complex and the Immunoglobulin Gene Superfamily

The major histocompatibility complex (MHC) is a series of genes that code for protein molecules responsible for cell–cell recognition. The MHC of mammalian species contains three groups of genes: class I, class II, and class III. Class I and class II genes code for cell surface recognition molecules, and class III codes for some complement components (the complement system is presented in Chapter 12). Class I and II region products control recognition of self and nonself; T cells not only recognize antigens but also have receptors that recognize the MHC products of other cell types from the same individual as self, and the products of cells from other individuals as nonself (foreign). All nucleated cells express class I MHC antigens on their surface. Class II antigens are expressed on some cells (B cells, macrophages) but not on others (most parenchymal cells do not express class II MHC). Class II markers may appear on some activated cells, that is, activated T cells, or may be induced to higher levels in some class II marker–expressing cells, that is, macrophages under the influence of interferon. The MHC is part of the immunoglobulin supergene family, which also codes for the recognition molecules of T and B cells for antigens.

Self–Nonself Recognition

The ability of cells to recognize other cells as self or from another genetically different individual (nonself) is an important property in maintaining the integrity of tissue and organ structure. As discussed in Chapter 1, primitive organisms have the ability to distinguish cells of the same species from cells of different species through cell surface glycoprotein molecules. During mammalian embryogenesis, developing tissues must have means of interacting with some cell types and avoiding interaction with other cell types. The major histocompatibility system also prevents an individual from being invaded by cells from another individual. For example, transplants from one individual generally cannot survive in another individual, because of histocompatibility differences. Histocompatibility differences between the mother and fetus during gestation may provide a mechanism preventing the mother from being invaded by fetal tissues and the fetus from being invaded by maternal cells.

Major histocompatibility complex products also play a major regulatory role in the immune response. Histocompatibility similarities are required for cellular cooperation in induction of the immune response and provide a mechanism to ensure that T cells and B cells of a given individual can recognize each other for cooperation, yet bear immunoglobin supergene receptors that recognize foreign structures at the same time (see Chaper 10). Class I products determine to a large extent the specificity of graft rejection, whereas class II region products control cell interactions during induction of immunity.

Although we do not know why 80 different variations of class I MHC antigens are carried in the human population (see below), such diversity might prove advantageous in avoiding a catastrophic viral infection that might destroy the entire population. Instead, the diversity of tissue types could ensure that no single infectious agent could evade the immunity of all individuals with widely different tissue types. Class I MHC antigens are commonly recognized by cytolytic T cells specific for virally infected cells. Even if one tissue type were associated with a poor immune response to the infection, only a small percentage of the population would be lost, and the infection could be contained by the immunity of the rest of the population.

Genetics of Tissue Transplantation

The ability of the immune system to recognize tissue from a different individual of the same species as foreign is determined by tissue antigens controlled largely by MHC class I products. If solid tissue, such as a donor kidney, from one individual of a species is transplanated to a second, genetically different individual of the same species, a characteristic reaction termed *allograft* (homograft) rejection is observed. If transplantation occurs from one part of the body to another in the same individual *(autograft)* or between two genetically identical individuals *(synograft* or *isograft)*, for example between monozygotic twins or between individual animals of an inbred strain, this reaction does not take place. If transplantation is made between individuals of different species *(xenograft)*, a more brisk and intense rejection may result.

The genetic control of transplantation antigens as demonstrated by the behavior of skin grafts among inbred strains of

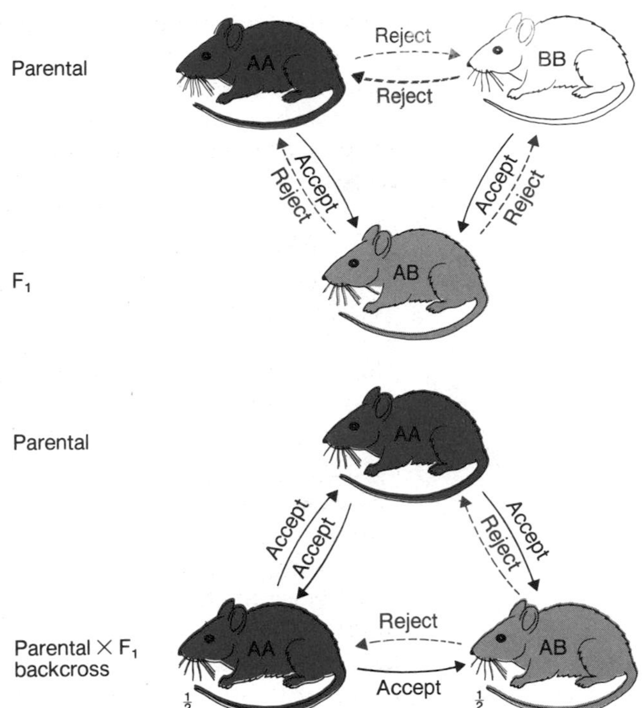

Figure 9-1. Genetics of transplantation. The behavior of skin grafts between two inbred mouse strains differing at a major histocompatibility locus (H-2) and the behavior of grafts to and from various hybrids and backcrosses to one of the parental strains are illustrated. Arrows indicate a graft from a given donor to a given recipient. Rejection occurs when the donor contains a specificity not present in the recipient. Capital letters indicate specificities present in inbred parental strains and designated progeny. Dotted lines indicate rejection of graft; solid lines, acceptance.

mice and their hybrid offspring is illustrated in Figure 9-1. MHC genes controlling transplantation antigens are usually inherited according to codominant Mendelian rules. Grafts between the homozygous parental strains are rapidly rejected. Since the F_1 contains both specificities of each parental strain, F_1 hybrids will accept grafts from each parental strain. However, grafts from F_1 mice will be rejected by each parental strain, as the F_1 carries the MHC products of the other parental strain. The results of a parental – F_1 backcross (mating of F_1 mice to one of the parental strains) are indicated at the bottom of Figure 9-1. Half these offspring will be identical to the parental strain and half to the F_1, and thus transplants to and from these mice will behave accordingly. Through the thorough study of the behavior of grafts among different strains of mice and their offspring and the correlation of this with the serologically identifiable lymphocyte antigens, the transplantation genetics and histocompatibility loci of the mouse have been identified.

Genetic Control of the Immune Response

The ability to produce an immune response is controlled by class II region gene products. The function of MHC gene products in induction of antibody formation has been delineated by studies in genetic low responder mice. Mice of the same strain or MHC type will show the same magnitude of response (high, intermediate, or low) to selected T-dependent antigens. Low responder mice generally produce very low levels of antibodies to some antigens and do not convert from an IgM (low primary response) to an IgG response after stimulation by antigen. However, low responder animals of a given MHC class II–controlled antigen can produce normal amounts of antibody if the antigen is complexed to an immunogenic carrier. Therefore, low responder animals have B cells that can recognize and produce antibody to the antigen. This implies that the B cells of low responders are functionally intact, but lack T cell help. Low responder strains also have low T cell proliferative responses to antigens, supporting the conclusion that genetic unresponsiveness is due to a specific defect in T cells. Class II region genes are linked to, but are different from, the class I genes responsible for tissue graft rejection.

The function of MHC genes in T and B cell interactions was determined by passive transfer experiments. If cells from different MHC thymus donors are transferred to nude mice (congenitally athymic, T cell deficient), the recipient nude mouse is able to respond to T-dependent antigens only when the MHC types of the thymus cell donor and the B cells in the recipient nude mouse are the same (Fig. 9-2). The B cells of the

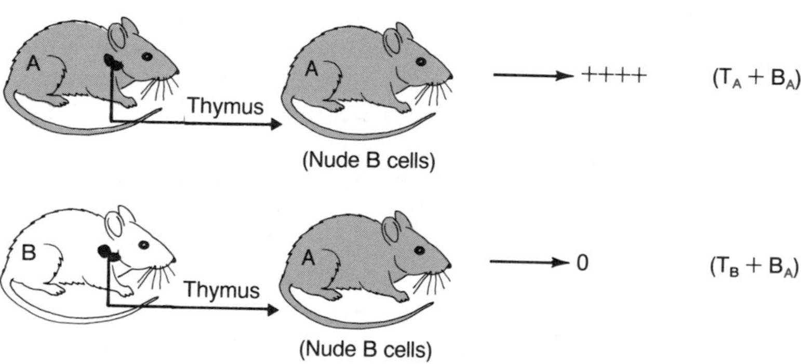

Figure 9-2. MHC restriction of T cell–B cell cooperation. In this experimental model, the capacity of nude mice, which lack T cell functions, to become immunized to a T-dependent antigen is restored by thymus cells from major histocompatibility complex (MHC)-identical donors, but not by thymus cells from MHC-different donors. If strain A thymus cells are transferred to another strain A nude mouse, an immune response may be induced; if strain B thymus cells, which differ in the MHC, are transferred to a strain A recipient, no response can be generated. Thus, in order for T and B cells to cooperate during induction of antibody production, they must share some MHC-controlled structures.

recipient must match the MHC of the thymus donor to be helped by the T cells. If they do not match, the B cell cannot respond to T cell help. Similarly, in irradiated F_1 recipients of mixtures of mature parental cells, a T-dependent antigen stimulates a response in the F_1 recipients only when the transferred parental T and B cells have the same MHC type (Fig. 9-3).

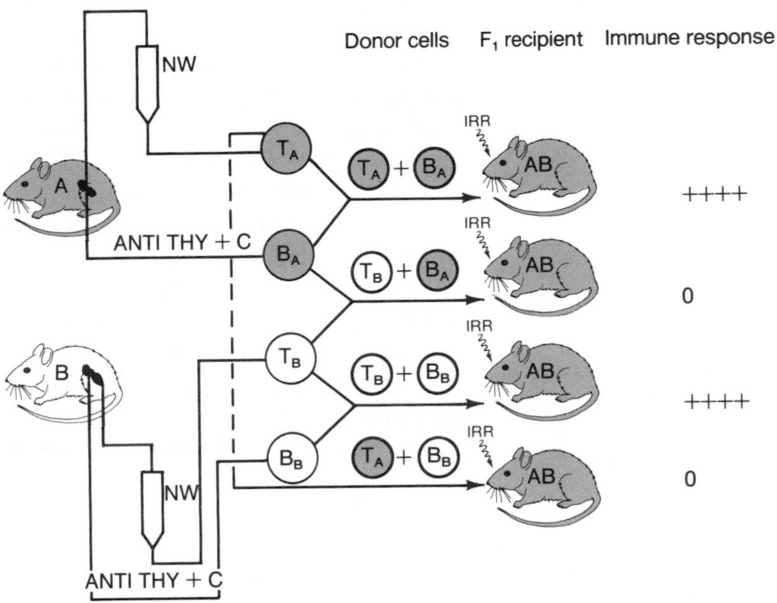

Figure 9-3. MHC control of antibody production in F_1 mice reconstituted with mixtures of parental T and B cells. The ability of F_1 (A + B) irradiated recipients to respond to T-dependent antigens is determined by MHC matching of donor T and B cells. Parental T cells are obtained by passage over nylon wool columns that retain B cells. Parental B cells are isolated by treatment with anti-T cell serum and complement (B cells survive, T cells are killed). Only when irradiated F_1 recipients are reconstituted with T and B cells of the same parental MHC type are the F_1 recipients able to mount an immune response.

Macrophage Restriction

Evidence for a macrophage–T cell MHC restriction comes from studies using inbred guinea pigs of strains 2 and 13 (Fig. 9-4). The system of analysis involves antigen-induced T cell

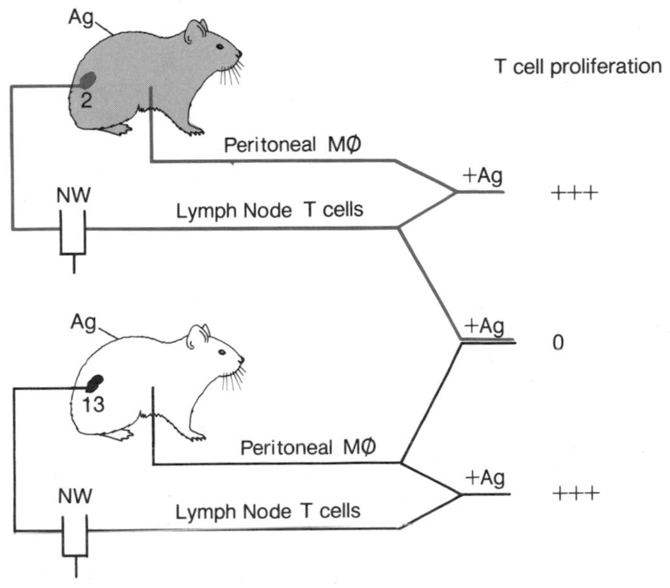

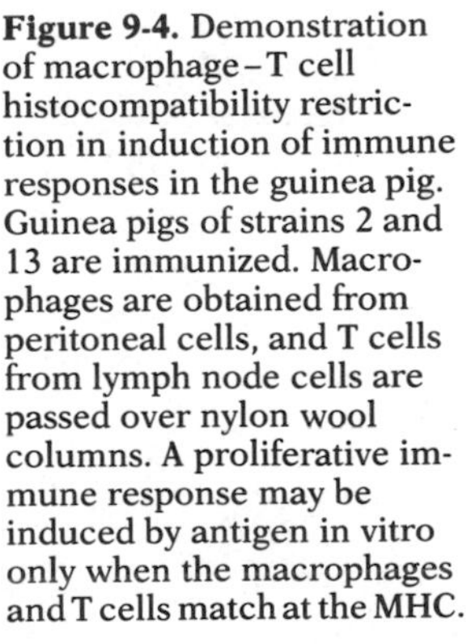
Figure 9-4. Demonstration of macrophage–T cell histocompatibility restriction in induction of immune responses in the guinea pig. Guinea pigs of strains 2 and 13 are immunized. Macrophages are obtained from peritoneal cells, and T cells from lymph node cells are passed over nylon wool columns. A proliferative immune response may be induced by antigen in vitro only when the macrophages and T cells match at the MHC.

proliferation (blast transformation). In order for antigen to induce transformation of T cells, histocompatible macrophages must be present. Mixtures of peritoneal exudate macrophages (glass adherent) and lymph node T cells (fractionated over nylon wool columns) from the same strain after immunization with antigen respond to antigen in vitro by blast transformation, whereas mixtures of macrophages and T cells from different strains do not. The compatible macrophages can be pulsed with antigen, washed, and then added to T cells. From this, a good response can be obtained. The conclusion is that the macrophage processes antigen and must be histocompatible with T cells to present the antigen to them. Macrophages must express a class II (MHC) product, and the class II product may actually function as an antigen-binding structure of macrophages that is recognized in turn by T cells that react with both antigen and the class II molecule (see below).

A simplified representation of the most likely relationship of macrophage–T helper–B cell collaboration and MHC restriction is shown in Figure 9-5. In this model, the macrophage

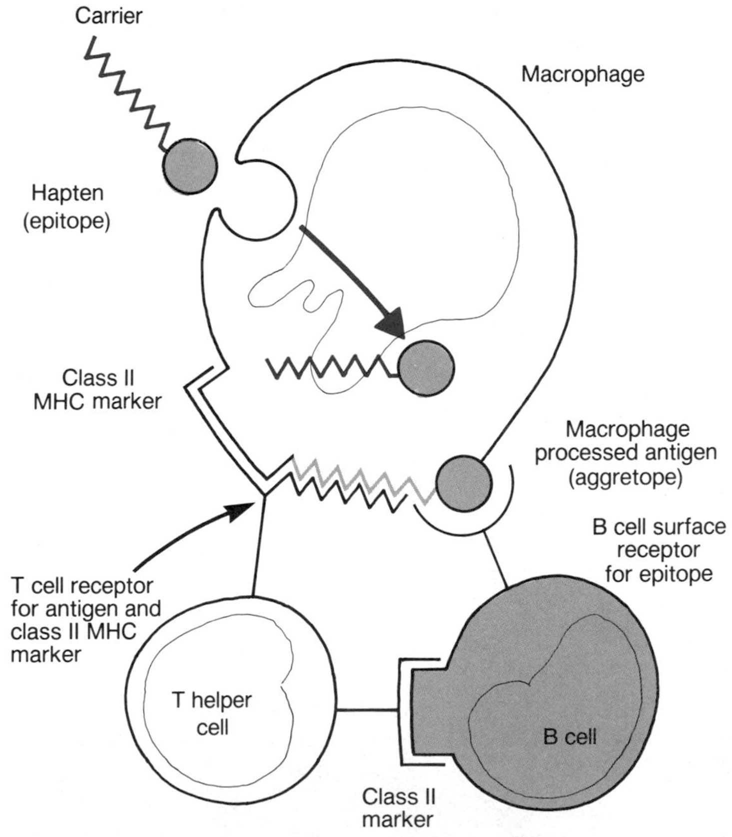

Figure 9-5. Class II region–determined recognition interaction of T cells, B cells, and macrophages during induction of antibody formation. Class II restriction requires that the T helper cell be able to recognize class II markers on macrophages. The same T cell receptor reacts with antigen and class II MHC marker on the macrophage during T cell activation and on the B cell when providing T helper function. Dual specificity (antigen and MHC marker) comes from the same pair of T cell receptor α and β chains (see Chapter 10).

and the B cell bear class II determinants and the T helper cell has receptors for these. In addition, the T cell has a receptor for antigens on the carrier, and the B cell a receptor for hapten determinants. The macrophages process antigen after phagocytosis and partial digestion by lysosomal proteases into peptide fragments 10–20 amino acids long and then present the antigenic fragments to T cells in association with class II MHC determinants. The T helper cell must be able to recognize carrier and class II markers on both the macrophage and the B cell. When each of these requirements is fulfilled, the B cell will be stimulated to proliferate, which greatly increases the number of cells capable of synthesizing specific antibody. These then differentiate into plasma cells, which secrete large amounts of antibody. The nature of the stimulating signals is presented below. A similar model employing class II receptors on T suppressor cells and class II MHC markers on macrophages and B cells may be operative in induction of T suppressor activity, which turns off antibody production (see Chapter 10).

The requirement for class II region recognition for induction of antibody responses may serve to focus T helper effects on appropriate cells, such as macrophages and B cells. During induction of immunity, T helper cells would not be useful reacting with other cell types such as heart and kidney. The presence of class II antigens on macrophages and B cells assures that T helpers will act on these cells. In addition, since T helper cells react with class II markers in the context of antigen, specific T helper cells are activated in the presence of antigen and the specific cells required for an antibody response.

The principles of self recognition by immune competent cells must be taken into consideration in attempts to reconstitute humans with immune deficiency diseases. Thus in bone marrow or thymus transplantation, the donor cells must share some histocompatibility antigen specificities with the recipient. If not, the appropriate cellular reactions required to generate an effective immune response may not be able to take place.

Structure of the Major Histocompatibility Gene Complex

In recent years extensive studies of the mouse and human have led to a much better understanding of the genetic control of immune reactions and the major histocompability complex. Since much more is known about the MHC of the mouse than that of the human, the characteristics of the mouse MHC are described in detail and compared with those of the human MHC. The MHC has been localized to the H-2 gene complex in mouse chromosome 17 and the HLA complex in human chromosome 6.

The Mouse MHC (H-2)

The pioneering work of Little, Gorer, Snell, and others who used serological methods and congenic mice has led to the current understanding of this chromosomal region in the mouse. The structure of the MHC region has been determined largely by analysis of congenic mice. Snell produced congenic mice by repeated backcrossing of selected progeny with the parental strain to the point that the genetic background of the inbred mice was identical to that of the parent except for MHC traits. As a first step (see Fig. 9-1), inbred mice of strain A and strain B are mated to produce an $(A \times B)F_1$. The first backcross of the F_1 with parent A can be expected to produce half of the progeny with MHC phenotype (A × B). These were selected for B-type MHC based on rejection of their skin grafted onto the A parent strain. The selected mice are again mated with parent A and tested by skin grafting. This process of backcrosses and selection is repeated 20 times. During all those generations, the random assortment of chromosomes will dilute out all of the unselected chromosomes coming from the B parent. In addition, crossing over between pairs of chromosome 17 will result in a segment of chromosome 17 copying the selected trait (B phenotype at the MHC), whereas the rest of chromosome 17 will come from the A strain.

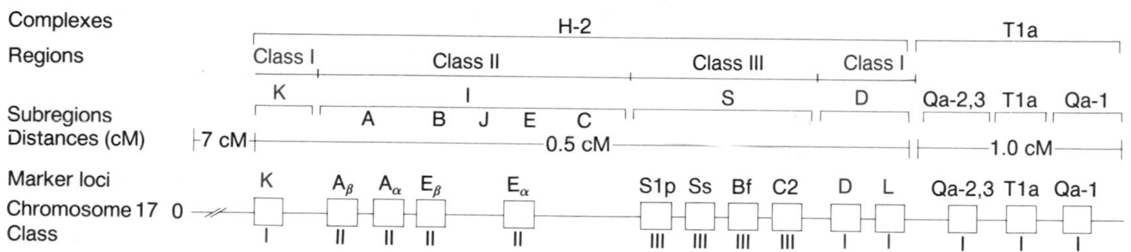

Figure 9-6. Fine-structure map of the mouse major histocompatibility complex. The mouse major histocompatibility (H-2) complex is located on chromosome 17 and contains genetic regions that control a variety of immune reactions. The H-2K and H-2D regions control the expression of tissue antigens that are recognized by immune allograft rejection. The I region controls various immune responses. The classic depiction of the I region is shown, although only genes for the A and E regions have been confirmed by gene cloning. The S1 region controls the serum concentration of components of complement. Qa1 and Qa2,3 control some erythrocytic alloantigens, and Tla the thymus-leukemia (TL) antigens. One centimorgan (CM) is equivalent to a 1% recombination frequency per generation.

Class I Genes (H-2K and H-2D)

Although the map of the mouse MHC complex is changing rapidly because of new information being collected, it may be schematically recorded as shown in Figure 9-6. The major histocompatibility antigens responsible for graft rejection (allogeneic or within-species transplantation antigens) are controlled by the class I genetic regions, H-2K and H-2D. Class I regions code for cell surface antigens that serve as targets for antibody- or cell-mediated immune reactions. H-2K and H-2D specificities also play a major role in recognition of an individual's own tissue cells. During viral infections the viral antigens expressed on infected cells are recognized by cytotoxic T cells in association with class I MHC markers. The infected cells are recognized as "altered self" and lysed by T effector lymphocytes.

Class II Genes (the "I Region")

Using congenic mice, it was found that matching of class I genes was neither necessary nor sufficient for T cell–B cell cooperation; matching for a subregion of the class II region (the "I region") was required for a mixture of T and B cells to respond to immunization with T-dependent antigens. The I region (immune response region) codes for recognition structures that control interactions of macrophages, T cells, and B cells or the respective factors produced by these cells (see Chapter 10 for details). The I region has been divided into at least five subregions, A, B, J, E, and C, which are delineated in recombinant strains of mice and by genetic crossovers that have occurred within the MHC region and result in different patterns of immune responses to a variety of antigens. However, it seems likely that only the I-A and I-E subregions actually produce gene products that function as class II MHC markers.

The A subregion of class II controls the extent of antibody formation to a variety of T-dependent antigens, including various synthetic amino acid polymers such as poly(Tyr, Glu, Ala, Lys) as well as some larger protein molecules such as ovalbumin and lysozyme. The E region controls the levels of antibody production to an additional series of natural proteins such as pigeon cytochrome *c* and synthetic polypeptides such as poly(Glu, Lys, Phe). The E region shows genetic complementation in effect by collaboration with the A region as follows: two genetic low responder strains with different A and E regions may produce F_1's that are high responders. This seemingly paradoxical result is explained by the A region of one parental strain and the E region of the other parental strain complementing each other by each producing one of the subunits of the I-E molecule. Together these subunits form a functional I-E molecule so that a high immune response may be generated. The I region class II genes code for cell surface products, Aα, Aβ, Eα, and Eβ, that are present mainly on B cells and macrophages (see below). Some are, however, also present on T cells. These molecules determine the compatibility of lymphoid cell interactions in induction of immune responses.

Class III Genes

The class III genes, located in the S region, encode for components of the complement system. S/p and Ss encode for different forms of C_4, C_2 for C_2, and Bf for factor B (see Chapter 12).

The Human MHC (HLA)

The human MHC is called HLA, because the serologically defined markers were first found on lymphocytes (human lymphocyte antigens). Understanding of the role of the HLA

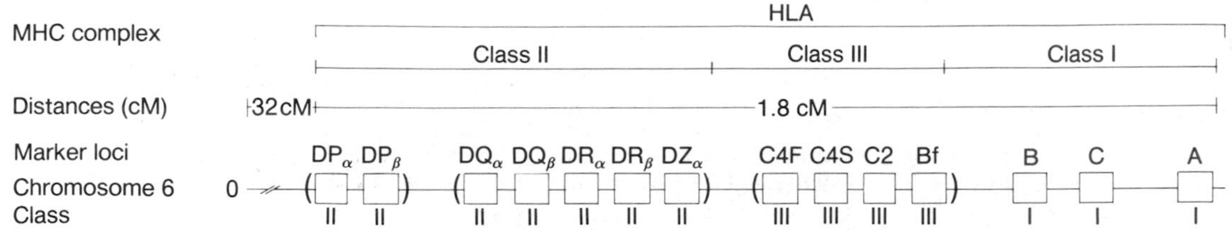

Figure 9-7. Proposed map of the human major histocompatibility (HLA) gene complex. The genes for HLA antigenic specificity are located on the sixth human chromosome in the relative order shown. There is room in this complex for many other genes. Each gene contains information for one specificity in each series.

complex in human immune responses is still incomplete. A map of the HLA complex is shown in Figure 9-7. The HLA gene complex is located on chromosome 6. Three class I genes code for transplantation antigens A, B, and C; the class II genes are DP, DQ, DR, and DZ, and the class III products are complement components C_2, C_4, and Bf. The organization of the human MHC differs from that of the mouse, but the function and the products appear analogous. In the human MHC the class I, II, and III gene regions are uninterrupted, whereas in the mouse MHC the class I gene (K) is separated from the other class I gene (D) by class II and III genes. Class I genes code for antigenic determinants present on all nucleated cells and are detected serologically (SD-defined determinants). Class II genes code for determinants recognized by mixed lymphocyte reactions (lymphocyte-defined or LD determinants). The class II gene products are now also detected serologically. Class II antigens are found primarily on B cells and macrophages, including tissue macrophages such as Kupffer cells of the liver, glial cells in the brain, and Langerhans cells in the epidermis.

The production of linked MHC specificities has given rise to the term *haplotype,* that is, specificities controlled by linked loci (see Fig. 9-15). Also present on the human chromosome 6 are genes for some red blood cell antigens. The role of class I genes in controlling human immune responses is less well understood than in the mouse. There is suggestive evidence that the antibody titers to diphtheria and measles may be MHC linked. The association of certain diseases, such as alkylosing spondylitis and uveitis, with the HLA-B27 specificity and the practical application of the relationship of HLA antigens to graft rejection are presented below.

MHC Products and the Cell Surface

Class I

Class I MHC gene products are glycoproteins of approximate MW 45,000 that are noncovalently bound to a MW 12,000, 96-amino-acid peptide termed β_2-microglobulin. The orientation of the MHC class I molecule and β_2-microglobulin in the cell membrane is illustrated in Figure 9-8. The class I compo-

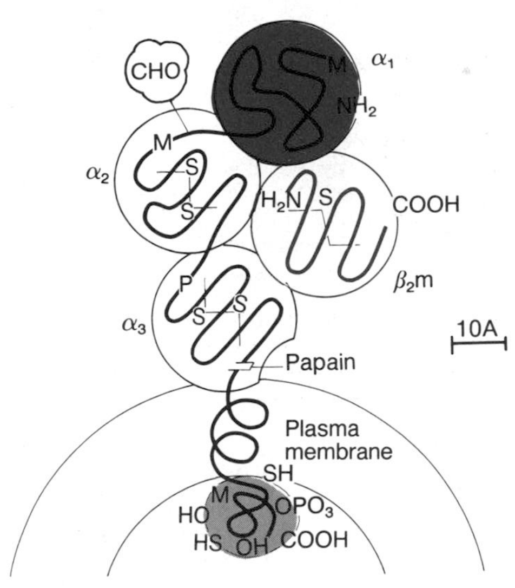

Figure 9-8. Structure of transplantation (class I) antigen. The heavy chain consists of 340 amino acids with three extracellular domains of approximately 90 residues each, a transmembrane segment of 40 amino acids, and an intracellular peptide of 30 residues. Two of the outer domains (α_2 and α_3) have intrachain disulfide bonds (forming 60-residue loops with considerable homology with Ig). Allotypic specificites are located in the α_1 and α_2 domains; α_3 is relatively invariant. β_2-Microglobulin is folded into the α_3 domain and is also invariant. The location of a variable domain at the carboxy end of the molecule with three or four invariant domains at the amino terminal is similar to the immunoglobulin heavy chain and suggests an origin from a common ancestral gene.

nent is referred to as the heavy chain and the β_2-microglobulin as the light chain. The heavy chain structure is organized with three exposed domains, α_1, α_2, and α_3, which extend from the cell surface and are attached to a hydrophobic transmembrane domain and a short cytoplasmic "anchor" segment within the cell. Each of the external domains contains about 90 amino acids, the transmembrane domain about 40 amino acids, and the cytoplasmic domain 30 amino acids. The light chain (β_2-microglobulin) is about the same size as one of the α external domains of the heavy chain. Each domain is immunoglobulin-like, consisting of 90 amino acids in a folded β pleated sheet structure held together by a disulfide bond at the ends, giving a plane-like surface that can be used to build a macromolecule. The β_2 chain folds with the α_3 domain of the heavy chain, and the α_1 and α_2 domains also pair.

The β_2-microglobulin gene is located on a chromosome different from that containing the MHC. Its structure is essentially invariant, whereas that of the heavy chains varies extensively from one individual to another because of differences in amino acid sequences of the external domains. The polymorphism of the heavy chain is contributed primarily by the α_1 domain and to a lesser degree by the α_2 domain. The homology between the MHC gene products and the immunoglobulins raises the possibility that the genes have a common evolutionary origin (see below).

Class I genes are organized into eight coding regions (exons) separated by seven intervening sequences (introns). The different coding regions each code for different structural domains, including the external domains (Fig. 9-9) and the

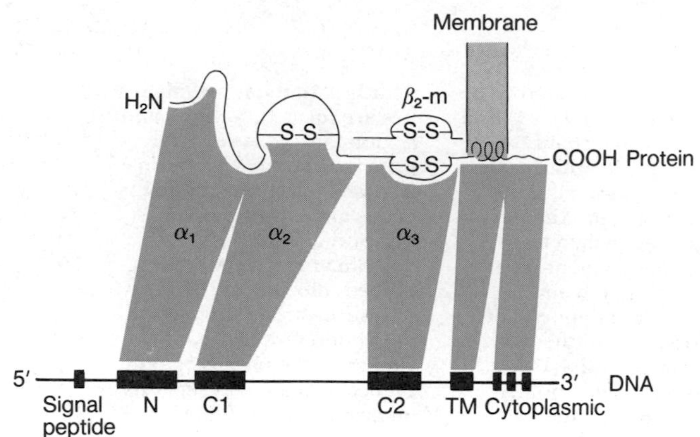

Figure 9-9. Schematic representation of class I genes and their product. Class I MHC determinants are controlled by α_1 (N) and α_2 (C1) domains. The α_3 (C2) domain associates with β_2-microglobulin and can be exchanged between different H-2 alleles or genes without affecting epitopes recognized by alloreactive or H-2 restricted CTL. (Modified from Forman et al.: Immunol Rev 81:203, 1984.)

transmembrane domain. Three small exons code for the cytoplasmic domain. The enormous degree of variation in the sequences of the class I molecules allows between 8 and 49 different versions (alleles) of each genetic locus. Expression of the class I genes is codominant. Each individual F_1 mouse expresses K$A\beta$, K$B\beta$, D$A\beta$, and D$B\beta$ on all cells. The total number of combinations is the product of the number of alleles of these three loci, and is increased further by having two MHC genes at each locus (one on each sixth chromosome). Thus it is not surprising that matching between two unrelated individuals for a tissue graft is an extremely rare occurrence.

Other class I genes are also located within the MHC region of mice. Most of these are in the Qa and Tla regions; the functions of the Qa and Tla gene products are not clearly defined as yet. The product of the D or the HLA-A, B, C genes becomes inserted in the cell membrane where the extracellular domains are recognized as transplantation antigen.

Class II

The products of the class II genes are less well characterized. In the mouse the class II gene product (Ia) consists of two polypeptide chains (α and β, Fig. 9-10). The α chain has a molecular

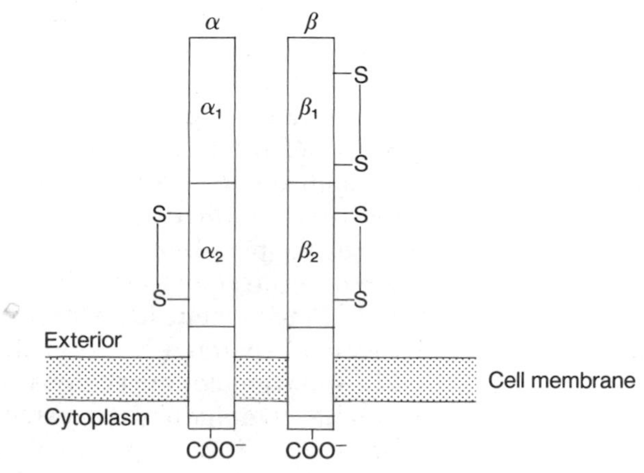

Figure 9-10. A model of the class II MHC molecule. The α and β chains are divided into two external domains (α_1 and α_2 or β_1 and β_2), a transmembrane domain, and a cytoplasmic domain. The cysteine residues that participate in disulfide bridge formation are indicated by S, and the glycosylation sites on the external domains are indicated by CHO.

weight of 33,000, and the β chain 29,000. A third chain of MW 33,000 is invariant and is associated with the $\alpha\beta$ heterodimer before it is expressed on the cell surface. It may have an important role in transport of the heterodimer to the cell surface. Each class II polypeptide contains two external domains of 90 amino acids, a transmembrane domain of about 30 amino acids, and a cytoplasmic domain of 10–15 amino acids.

A genetic map of the class II region of the mouse is shown in Figure 9-11. The Aα, Aβ and Eβ genes are in the I-A subregion,

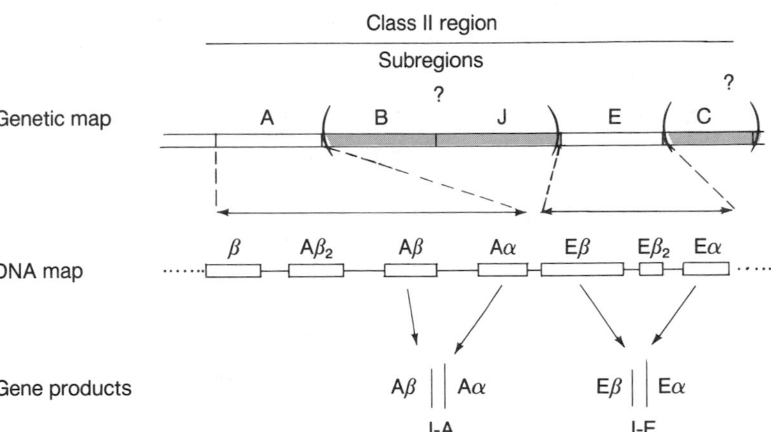

Figure 9-11. Genetic map of the class II region of the mouse based on recombination, with a DNA map based on molecular biology.

and the Eα gene is in the I-E region. These are codominantly expressed. β and Aβ2 are pseudogenes that are not expressed. Products of the B, J, and C regions have not been clearly identified. Based on functional studies, it has been postulated that a suppressor factor, I-J, is produced by genes in the J region, but there does not appear to be room on the chromosome for such a gene on the basis of recombinant DNA mapping of the class II region. Most recombinations within this region have occurred at a "hot spot" in or near the E gene. Since genetic distance is based on recombination frequency, this "hot spot" may have exaggerated the apparent distance between the I-A and I-E loci. DNA mapping shows them to be much closer, leaving little or no space for postulated B and J regions.

The gene products of the different alleles of the same locus on each chromosome can combine to form a new I-A marker. Thus in an (H-2^a × H-2^b)F_1 heterozygous mouse, the Aα chain of the "a" haplotype combines with either the Aβ chain of the "a" type or the Aβ chain of the "b" type. In the latter case, the $A^a\alpha$–$A^b\beta$ molecule is a hybrid determinant that can be recognized by some T cells in the F_1 mouse. This is yet another mechanism for increasing the diversity of class II markers recognized by T cells.

A map of the human class II region is shown in Figure 9-12. Much less is known about the human class II region than about that of the mouse. Mouse I-A and I-E molecules are homologous to the

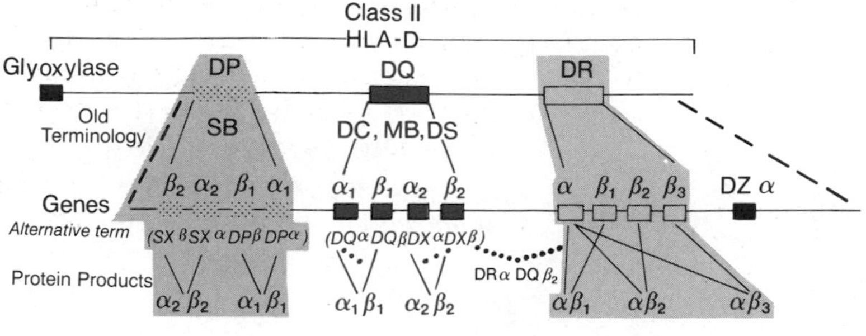

Figure 9-12. A schematic map of the human class II region. The numbers in front of α or β, such as 2α or 1α, identify different genes. The DQ region contains two α genes and two β genes that could provide the DQ region gene product. In the DR region there is one nonpolymorphic α gene and three β genes. The DP region contains two α and two β genes and the DZ region contains an α gene, but little else is known about this subregion. (See Immunology Today, March 1985, for additional information.)

human DQ and DR molecules; analogs to the DP and DZ products have not been identified in the mouse. If one can assume two α and two β chains per subregion for the four class II allelic subregion genes in the human, then up to four different products can be expressed for each class II subregion, or 16 different class II products per cell in a heterozygous individual. This provides great variability in the markers that lymphoid cells can use to identify self from nonself.

Class III

Class III gene products are complement components C2 and C4 of the classical pathway and factor B of the alternate pathway (see Chapter 12). These components are functionally related in that they are each involved in activation of the third component of complement (C3). The significance of their linkage with the MHC is not known.

Figure 9-13. Similarities in structure of lymphoid cell surface receptors: Thy 1, MHC class I, MHC class II, IgM, and T cell receptor. Receptors contain extracellular, transmembrane, and cytoplasmic domains. Thy 1 is a common T cell differentiation antigen of the mouse that is roughly analogous to CD3 in the human.

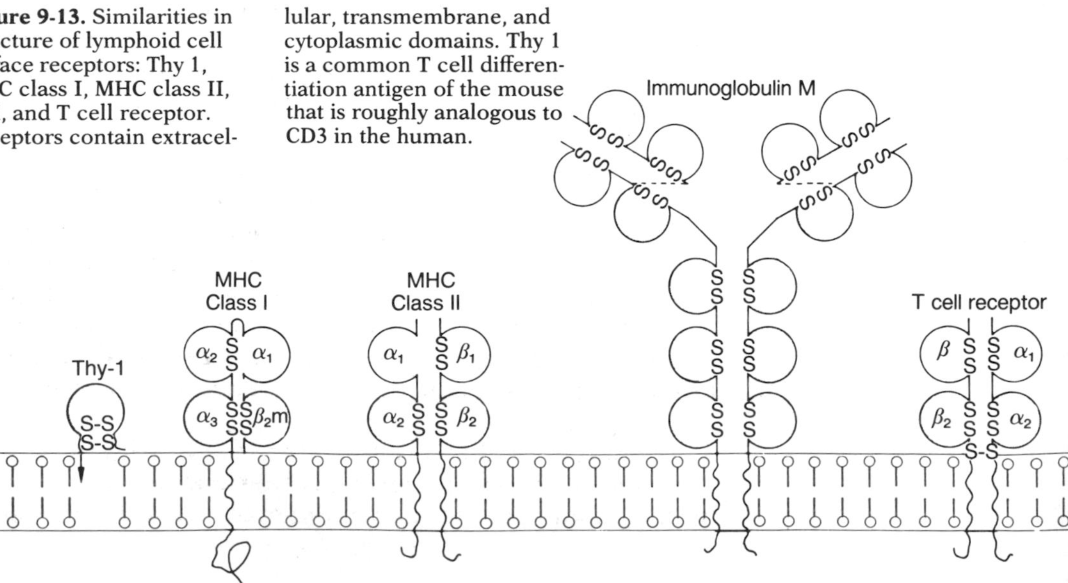

Comparison of Cell Surface Molecules of Lymphocytes

A comparison of the structure of lymphocyte cell surface receptors is illustrated in Figure 9-13. Similarities in structure and sequence homologies among the polypeptide chains in various domains suggest a common evolutionary origin of these molecules (Fig. 9-14).

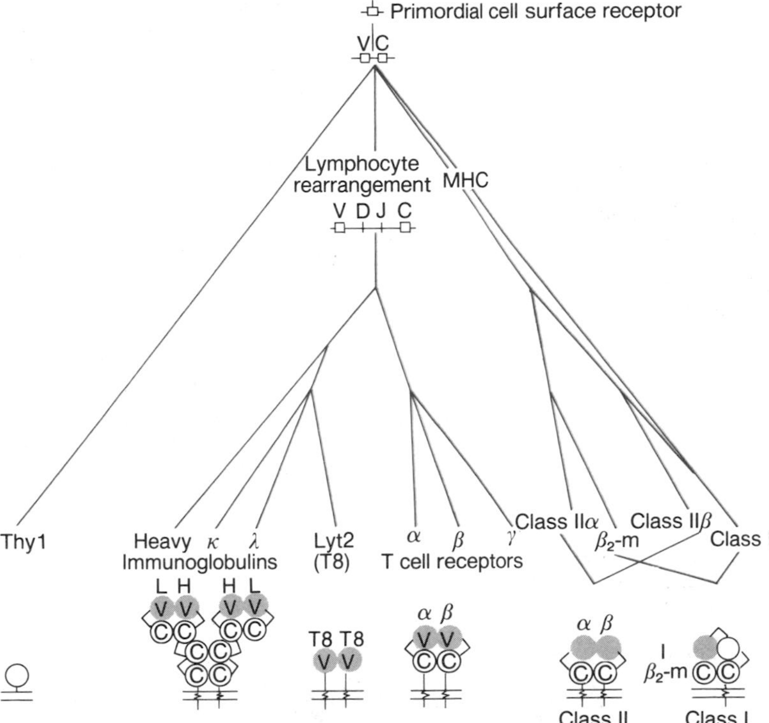

Figure 9-14. A schematic representation of the evolution of the immunoglobulin gene superfamily. V and C denote V- and C-like homology units, respectively. The open circles for the MHC molecules do not exhibit significant sequence similarity with the immunoglobulin homology units, although they are of similar length. The Thy 1 homology unit does exhibit sequence similarity, although it is not easily classified as V or C and may have diverged prior to the V–C divergence. The horizontally paired homology units represent probable domain structures apart from those hypothesized for the CD8 molecule. (Modified from Hood L, Kronenberg M, Hunkapiller T: T cell antigen receptor and the immunoglobulin supergene family. Cell 40:225–229, 1985.)

The MHC and Tissue Transplantation

Historically, the major importance of the identification of the products of the MHC involved their role in human tissue transplantation. Transplants between identical twins are not rejected, whereas rejection occurs where there are differences at the MHC. Tissue grafts from one genetically different individual to another (allografts) require suppression of the immune response if the graft is to survive.

Donor–Recipient Matching in Human Transplantation

Although immunosupression has prolonged human graft survivial, the results are frequently not satisfactory. Better tissue matching of recipient and donor combined with less vigorous immunosuppression might be the most advantageous approach. Extensive serological testing is now done in attempts to match donor and recipient histocompatibility antigens, but the results have not been as productive as expected. Complementary DNA probes for human MHC genes will provide better tissue-typing results.

Histocompatibility antigens are those cellular determinants specific for each individual of a species that are responsible for immune rejection when attempts are made to transfer or transplant cellular material from one individual of the same species to another. Identical twins are the only known human individuals who share all histocompatibility antigens. Perhaps the most familiar example of histocompatibility antigens is the ABO blood group system. The A and B antigens are found not only on erythrocytes but also on other tissue cells. Therefore, no attempt to transfer solid organs from one individual to another should be made across a known AB blood group difference. However, other histocompatibility antigens are obviously important, because matching of the ABO or other erythrocyte antigen systems between donor and recipient is not enough to provide a compatible relation.

During the 1960s many attempts were made to develop tests for histocompatibility antigens and matching tests for potential donors and recipients. Tests that have been used to select organ donors include the mixed lymphocyte culture reaction (MLR) and the analysis and matching of histocompatibility antigens by serologic tests. The in vitro systems are not only useful for matching donors and recipients of grafts but provide a means of evaluating immunologic recognition and its significance.

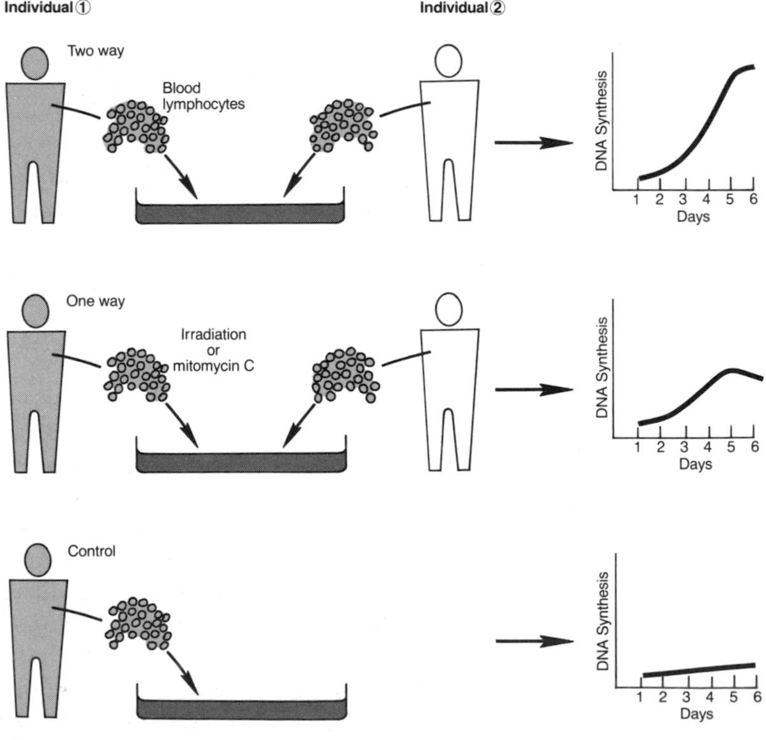

Figure 9-15. Mixed lymphocyte reaction (MLR). The degree of stimulation in an MLR correlates to the degree of histocompatibility difference between the lymphocyte donors. This is a two-way test (a cross-match test), because the lymphocytes of each donor interact with each other. The test can be made one-way by preventing the response of one set of lymphocytes, the organ donor's, by treatment with radiation or an antimetabolite such as mitomycin C. This gives an estimate of the rejection response of a potential recipient (living cells) against the cells of a potential organ donor (the treated cells). Stimulation is measured by an increase in DNA synthesis, occurring 5–7 days after interaction in culture, that is not seen when the cells of only one individual are cultured (control). The ability to store lymphocytes in vitro in liquid nitrogen freezers permits tissue typing even when a given donor is no longer living.

Mixed Lymphocyte Reactions

The mixed lymphocyte reaction (MLR) test is based on the observation that cultures of mixtures of lymphocytes from two genetically different individuals produce transformed immature blast cells that synthesize DNA (Fig. 9-15).

Although it was first suspected that MLR reactions depended upon the class I A, B, and C antigens defined by humoral antibodies (see below), it is now known that the extent of a mixed lymphocyte reaction is dependent not upon class I differences but upon the class II gene products. The cell that responds in the MLR is a T cell. The stimulator cell containing the antigen to which the responding T cell reacts is a macrophage or B cell. The class II antigens detected serologically are present on macrophages and B cells, but not on T cells. Class I specificities may stimulate mixed lymphocyte reactions weakly or increase class II–induced reactions, but for practical purposes MLR is considered to be the result of class II differences. A second aspect of the MLR is the generation of cytotoxic T lymphocytes (CTL) that react specifically with the class I region markers of the stimulator cells. These cells are generated from a subset of precursor T cells different from the cells that proliferate in the MLR. The killing is directed to class I MHC markers (see Chapter 10). Thus the MLR proliferation response depends upon class II products; the cytotoxicity response upon class I products (Fig. 9-16).

Serologically Defined Histocompatibility Antigens

In addition to the antigens detected by the MLR, there are serologically defined cell membrane components that are recognized during allograft rejection and are directly related to the rejection reaction. The identification of these histocompatibility antigens in the laboratory depends upon the serologic (antibody-mediated) recognition of MHC products on lymphocytes. Most tissue antigens appear to be shared by lymphocytes and solid tissue. The identification of a given antigen on a lymphocyte can be determined by the ability of an antiserum to react with the antigen, activating complement and causing the death of the lymphocytes.

Antihistocompatibility antisera that reacted with lymphocytes were recognized as long as 50 years ago, but the significance of such antibodies with respect to histocompatibility was not apparent until more recently. Antibodies in human sera to human lymphocytes are found in patients with certain diseases, in multiparous women, and in patients receiving multiple blood transfusions. In retrospect these latter situations were found to be caused by genetically controlled differences in MHC specificities among human individuals (allotypy). In the 1950s, the reaction patterns of such antisera with lymphocytes from a number of different individuals were revealed. For instance, some antisera reacted with lymphocytes from essentially the same donors in a panel (e.g., 20 of 50 donors), whereas

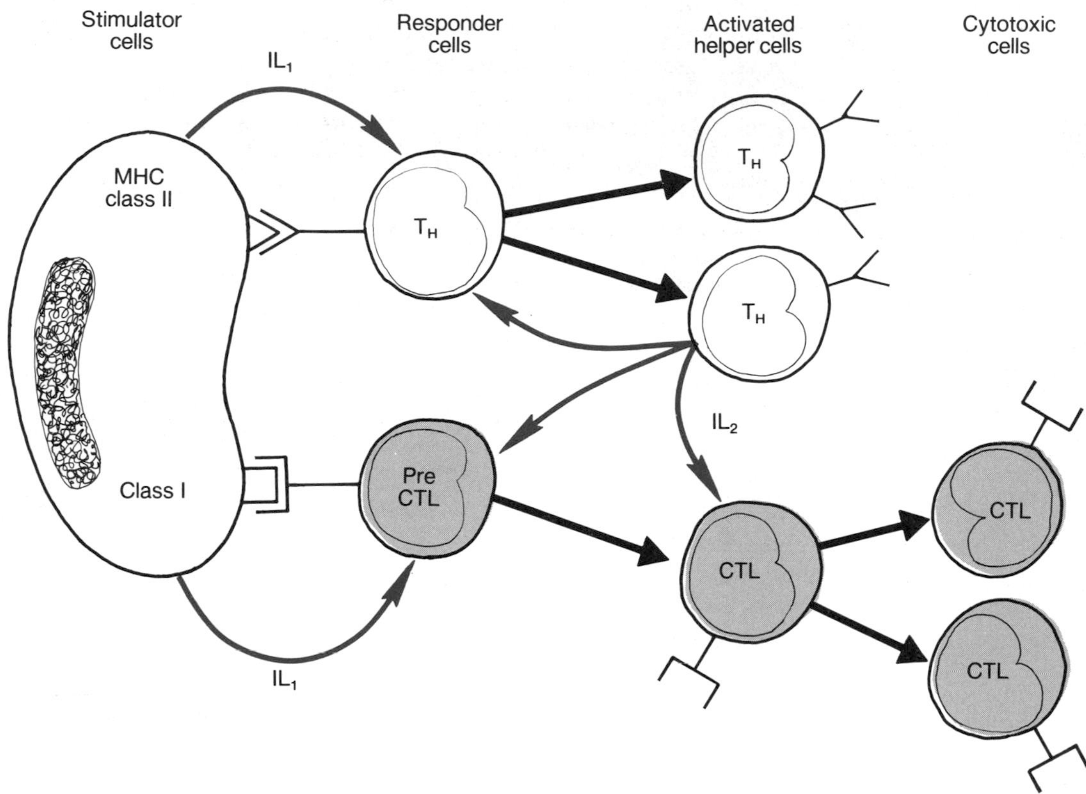

Figure 9-16. Interaction of T helper/inducer T cells and precursors of CTL during generation of CTL responsible for graft rejection. T_H cells are stimulated by reaction with class II MHC products to proliferate and produce IL2. IL2 acts on CTL precursors activated by reaction with class I MHC product to support proliferation and differentiation of CTL.

other antisera reacted with lymphocytes of different donors. The reaction patterns observed were extremely complicated and, it seemed, unresolvable. However, in the early 1960s Van Rood introduced computer analysis of the reaction patterns, a method that was soon adopted by others. This resulted in resolution of the reaction patterns of many different antisera. In the mid-1960s, a number of individuals who had been testing such antisera held a series of conferences at which many of the problems involving detection techniques and reaction patterns were compared. The result was an example of the contribution that can be made to scientific understanding by unselfish cooperation of different investigators.

Genetics of Human Histocompatibility Antigens

It is now generally accepted that human histocompatibility antigens, comprising over 50 different specificities, are controlled by the MHC. The serologic identification of MHC gene products using conventional sera from multiparous women, as well as monoclonal antibodies, has resulted in the identification of 23 A, 49 B, 8 C, 19 DW, 16 DR, 3 DQ, and 6 DP specificities (Table 9-1). Historically, typing has involved mainly A, B, and D antigens. An example of the inheritance of HLA-A, -B, and -D types is shown in Figure 9-17.

Table 9-1. Complete Listing of Recognized HLA Specificities

A	B		C	D	DR	DQ	DP
A1	B5	Bw47	Cw1	Dw1	DR1	DQw1	DPw1
A2	B7	Bw48	Cw2	Dw2	DR2	DQw2	DPw2
A3	B8	B49(21)	Cw3	Dw3	DR3	DQw3	DPw3
A9	B12	Bw50(21)	Cw4	Dw4	DR4		DPw4
A10	B13	B51(5)	Cw5	Dw5	DR5		DPw5
A11	B14	Bw52(5)	Cw6	Dw6	DRw6		DPw6
Aw19	B15	Bw53	Cw7	Dw7	DR7		
A23(9)	B16	Bw54(w22)	Cw8	Dw8	DRw8		
A24(9)	B17	Bw55(w22)		Dw9	DRw9		
A25(10)	B18	Bw56(w22)		Dw10	DRw10		
A26(10)	B21	Bw57(17)		Dw11(w7)	DRw11(5)		
A28	Bw4	Bw58(17)		Dw12	DRw12(5)		
A29(w19)	Bw6	Bw59		Dw13	DRw13(w6)		
A30(w19)	Bw22	Bw60(40)		Dw14	DRw14(w6)		
A31(w19)	B27	Bw61(40)		Dw15			
A32(w19)	B35	Bw62(15)		Dw16	DRw52		
Aw33(w19)	B37	Bw63(15)		Dw17(w7)	DRw53		
Aw34(10)	B38(16)	Bw64(14)		Dw18(w6)			
Aw36	B39(16)	Bw65(14)		Dw19(w6)			
Aw43	B40	Bw67					
Aw66(10)	Bw41	Bw70					
Aw68(28)	B44(12)	Bw71(w70)					
Aw69(28)	B45(12)	Bw72(w70)					
	B45(12)	Bw73					
	Bw46						

Antigens followed by a number in parentheses are recognized as splits of the antigen in parentheses; for example, A23 is a split of A9.

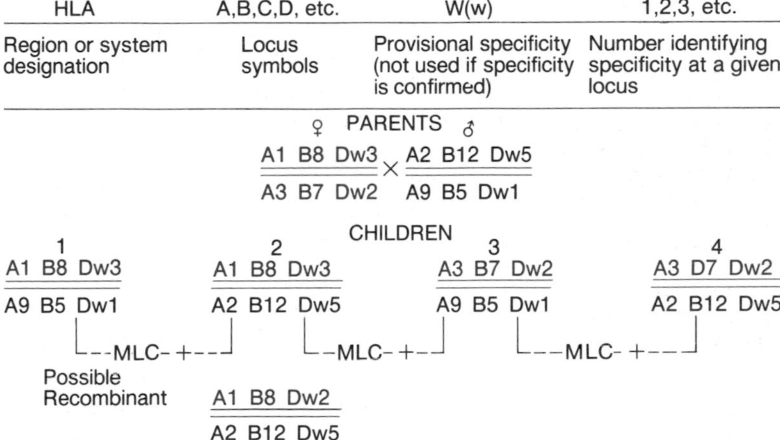

Figure 9-17. Inheritance of HLA-A, -B, and -D types. Genetically linked HLA-A, -B, and -D types are inherited as a unit on one chromosome (haplotype). The haplotype is written on one line (A1 B8 Dw3). From a given pair of parents only four haplotype combinations are possible. Thus in a family of five or more siblings, at least one pair must have identical HLA types unless a recombination of chromosomes has occurred. The recombination listed has a crossover between B and D. The identification of crossover frequencies permits a relative localization of HLA regions in the HLA supergene. MLC indicates a positive mixed lymphocyte culture reaction because of HLA-D difference. (Modified from Bodmer WF, et al.: Proc R Soc Lond [Biol] 202:93, 1978.)

The distribution of MHC genes within a family dictates that only four combinations of HLA antigens occur among siblings unless recombination occurs. Each parent has two MHC haplotypes, each made up of four HLA antigens. If the haplotypes are designated AB for one parent and CD for the other parent, the four possible haplotype combinations in their children are AC, AD, BC, and BD. Thus, in a family of five children of the same parents, two of the children will have an identical match for all HLA markers. The likelihood of crossing over between two parental chromosomes given a recombinant haplotype (part from each parental haplotype) is about 1% and is a function of the distance along the chromosome occupied by the MHC region. Such an individual would have no chance of finding an MHC matched sibling.

HLA Testing and Graft Survival

It was once thought that the HLA antigens could provide a means of identifying individuals who had similar or identical tissue antigens and who would not reject tissue grafts. Using skin grafts, it was observed that grafts between identical twins would survive indefinitely; grafts between unrelated HLA-nonidentical individuals are usually rejected within about 10 days. Grafts between HLA-matched unrelated individuals lasted only slightly longer than those between HLA-nonidentical unrelated individuals, whereas grafts between HLA-identical siblings survived 20 to 40 days. Clearly more than HLA antigen matching is required to select a histocompatible donor. At least two other factors must be considered: other HLA loci and minor histocompatibility loci (non-HLA antigens).

The existence of HLA antigens in other loci is possible. The presence of additional HLA loci adds an additional variable to the problem of tissue matching (see above). Since standard tissue typing can take into account only detectable specificities, matches presently classified as identical indicate identity only at the known HLA loci, so that nonidentity at another locus might explain some of the lack of correlation of matching to graft survival.

Transplantation studies in mice have resulted in the concept of strong and weak histocompatibility antigens. At least 11 histocompatibility systems have been identified in the mouse. The MHC system is termed the *strong* histocompatibility system because organ grafts between individual mice differing in antigenic specificities controlled by the MHC evoke strong rejection reactions. If organ donor and recipient are matched for the MHC but differ in one of the other systems, rejection is not as rapid or as severe. Therefore, these histocompatibility antigen systems are called *weak*. It is apparent that weak histocompatibility systems are also present in humans, but they remain to be defined. The evidence regarding weak histocompatibility antigens indicates that differences in these systems can be more readily overcome by immunosuppressive therapy than can differences in strong histocompatibility antigens.

The clinical experience in regard to HLA matching and renal and other tissue graft survival has been disappointing. Some representative data are presented in Figure 9-18. The

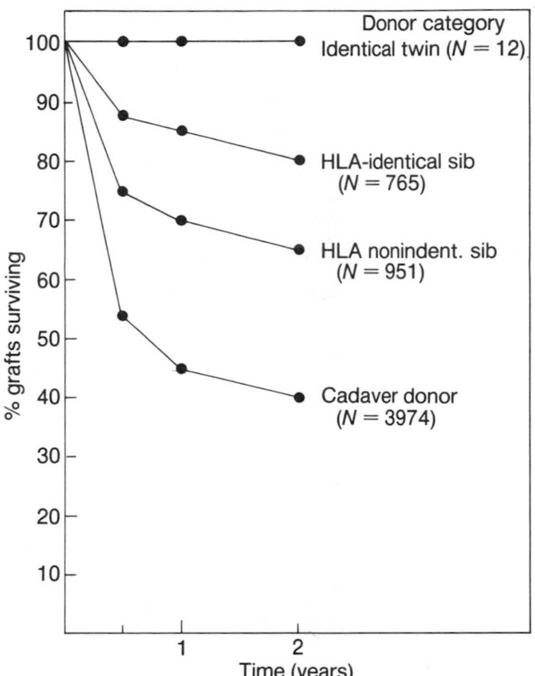

Figure 9-18. Survival times of kidney allografts among people of different genetic relationships, ranging from identical twins to unrelated individuals (cadaver donors). (From Hildemann WH: Tissue Antigens 22:1–6, 1983.)

survival of grafts reflects the histocompatibility differences (MHC and others) as well as other factors (complicating diseases, infection, etc.). The difference in survival of renal grafts between identical twins and HLA-identical siblings probably reflects non-MHC differences and indicates that non-MHC differences contribute to 15% of transplant failures. The difference between HLA-identical siblings and HLA-nonidentical siblings at 1 year suggests that MHC differences also contribute 15% to transplant failure.

Additive effects of MHC plus non-MHC alloantigens probably account in large part for the 60% failure rate in unmatched cadaver donors. At this time there appears to be little correlation between HLA-A and -B matching and graft survival. There does appear to be some correlation between HLA-DR matching and renal graft survival in North America, but not in Europe. Thus HLA typing has had decreasing influence on transplantation programs, whereas controlled immunosuppression has received greater emphasis.

Human MHC and Disease Associations

Certain HLA phenotypes are found associated with some human diseases. Of particular interest are immune-related diseases (Table 9-2), such as ankylosing spondylitis, Reiter's disease, and acute anterior uveitis, which are strongly associated with HLA-B27. The HLA-B27 specificity may be linked to an immune response (IR)–type gene that influences the response to an infectious agent or degree of inflammation in rheumatoid diseases. Reiter's disease consists of an infectious urethritis followed by arthritis, uveitis, and chronic skin lesions indistinguishable from psoriasis. The incidence of urethritis is not influenced by HLA-B27, but the incidence of the subsequent arthritis and skin lesions is. In addition, a small number of individuals may develop arthritis following intestinal infection with *Yersinia enterocolitica*. Again, the incidence of infection is not related to HLA type, but the incidence of arthritis is much higher in individuals with HLA-B27. In these diseases the finding of a B27 marker may aid diagnosis. Although the data are not as convincing, HLA-B8 and HLA-Bw15 are associated with systemic lupus erythematosus, and HLA-B13 with pemphigus. Thus, there may be an inherited tendency to produce an immunopathologic response to infections or inflammatory stimuli in certain individuals. The finding that the inheritance of some of these tendencies is linked to HLA specificities could assist in identification of new infectious agents or pathogenic mechanisms associated with rheumatoid disease.

In one instance a specific molecular defect has been described for a class I association. Individuals with congenital

Table 9-2. HLA and Disease Associations

Disease	Number of Studies	HLA SD Antigen	Frequency in Patients (%)	Frequency in Controls (%)	Average Relative Risk
Ankylosing spondylitis	5	B27	90	7	141.0
Reiter's disease	3	B27	76	6	46.6
Acute anterior uveitis	2	B27	55	8	16.7
	6	B13	18	4	5.0
Psoriasis	6	Bw17	29	8	5.0
	4	Bw16	15	5	2.9
Graves' disease	1	B8	47	21	3.3
Celiac disease	6	B8	78	24	10.4
Dermatitis herpetiformis	3	B8	62	27	4.5
Myasthenia gravis	5	B8	52	24	4.6
Systemic lupus erythematosus	2	Bw15	33	8	5.1
Multiple sclerosis	4	A3	36	25	1.7
		B7	36	25	1.5
Acute lymphatic leukemia	7	A2	63	37	1.7
	8	Bw35	25	16	1.6
Hodgkin's disease	7	A1	39	32	1.3
	7	B8	26	22	1.3
Chronic hepatitis	1	B8	68	18	9.5
Ragweed hay fever, Ra5 sensitivity	1	B7	50	19	4.0

adrenal hyperplasia have a deletion of the 21-hydroxylase gene that also deletes a portion of the class III region associated with C4 as well as a part of the neighboring HLA-B class I subregion. This deletion converts the HLA-B13 gene into the rare HLA-Bw47 that is always associated with the disease.

Summary

The major histocompatibility complex (MHC) is a series of linked genes on chromosome 6 of humans and chromosome 17 of the mouse. Class I region genes control the expression of tissue antigens responsible for graft rejection; class II region genes code for the lymphoid cell surface markers that are required for self recognition between cells and cooperation in the induction of the immune response; and class III region genes code for some of the components of complement. Histocompatibility antigens are complex cell surface structures that are recognized as foreign by one individual of a species when exposed to tissue of another individual of that species (allografts). Immune response antigens are controlled by the class II genes and determine the ability of T lymphocytes of a given individual to recognize and cooperate with macrophages and B cells of the same class II type in the response to foreign antigen. Understanding the human MHC is important for tissue matching prior to organ grafting and for determining the genetic susceptibility to certain diseases.

References

Self–Nonself Recognition

Burnet FM: The Clonal Selection Theory of Acquired Immunity. London, Cambridge University Press, 1959.

Burnet FM: The Integrity of the Body: A Discussion of Modern Immunological Ideas. Cambridge, Harvard University Press, 1962.

Burnet FM: Multiple polymorphism in relation to histocompatibility antigens. Nature 245:359, 1973.

Cohen IR, Welerle H: Regulation of autosensitization. The immune activation and specific inhibition of self recognizing thymus derived lymphocytes. J Exp Med 137:224, 1973.

Dorf ME (ed): The Role of the Major Histocompatibility Complex in Immunobiology. New York, Garland/STM Press, 1985.

Gotze D (ed): The Major Histocompatibility System in Man and Animals. New York, Springer-Verlag, 1977.

Jerne NK: The somatic generation of immune recognition. Eur J Immunol 1:1, 1971.

Hoffman GW: A theory of regulation and self–nonself discrimination. Eur J Immunol 5:638, 1975.

Klein E: Parental variants. Transplant Proc 3:1167, 1971.

Klein J: Biology of the Mouse Histocompatibility-2 Complex. New York, Springer-Verlag, 1975.

Ohno S: The original function of MHC antigens as the general plasma membrane anchorage site organogenesis-directing proteins. Immunol Rev 33:59, 1977.

Reigmann J, Miller RG: Polymorphism and gene function. Rev Comp Immunol 7:403, 1983.

Thorsby E: Biological function of HLA. Tissue Antigens 11:321, 1978.

Zinkernagel RM: Thymus and lymphohemopoietic cells: their role in T cell maturation, in selection of T cell H_2 restriction-specificity and H_2 linked Ir gene control. Immunol Rev 42:224, 1978.

Zinkernagel RM: Major transplantation antigens in host response to infection. Hosp Pract 13:83, 1978.

Genetics of Tissue Transplantation

Amos DB: Genetic aspects of human HL-A transplantation antigens. Fed Proc 29:2018, 1970.

Bach FH (ed): Immunobiology of Transplantation. New York, Grune & Stratton, 1974.

Bodmer WF, Jones EA, Barnstable CJ, Bodmer JG: Genetics of HLA: the major human histocompatibility system. Proc R Soc Lond [Biol] 202:93, 1978.

Howard JG, Michie JG: Transplantation immunology. *In* Cruickshank R (ed): Modern Trends in Immunology. London, Whitefriars, 1963.

Klein J (ed): The Biology of the Mouse Histocompability 2 Complex. New York, Springer-Verlag, 1975.

Klein J, Figueroa F, Nagy Z: Genetics of the major histocompatibility complex: the final act. Annu Rev Immunol 1:119, 1983.

Merrill JP: Human tissue transplantation. Adv Immunol 7:276, 1967.

Moller G (ed): Genetic and Biological Aspects of Histocompatibility Antigens. Transplant Rev 15, 1973.

Snell GD: Histocompatibility genes of the mouse. II. Production and analysis of isogenic resistant lines. J Nat Cancer Inst 21:843, 877, 1958.

Snell GD, Stimpfiing JH: Genetics of tissue transplantation. *In* Green EL (ed): Biology of the Laboratory Mouse, 2nd ed. New York, McGraw–Hill, 1966.

Staats J: Standardized nomenclature for inbred strains of mice: sixth listing. Cancer Res 36:4333, 1976.

Genetic Control of Immune Reactions

Bechtol KB, Freed JB, Herzenberg LA, McDevitt HO: Genetic control of the antibody response to poly-L-(Tyr, Glu)–poly-D, L-Ala–poly-L-Lys in $C_3H \leftrightarrow$ CWB tetraparental mice. J Exp Med 140:1660, 1974.

Benacerraf B: Role of MHC gene products in immune regulation. Science 212:1229, 1981.

Benacerraf B, McDevitt HO: The histocompatibility linked immune response gene. Science 175:273, 1972.

Bevin MJ, Hunig T: T cells respond preferentially to antigens that are similar to self. Proc Nat Acad Sci USA 78:1843, 1981.

Bluestein HG, Green I, Benacerraf B: Specific immune response genes of the guinea pig. I. Dominant genetic control of immune responsiveness to copolymers of L-glutamic acid and L-alanine and L-glutamic acid and L-tyrosine. J Exp Med 134:458, 1971.

Gasser DL, Silbers WK: Genetic determinants of immunologic responsiveness. Adv Immunol 18:1, 1974.

Green I, Paul WE, Benacerraf B: A study of the passive transfer of delayed hypersensitivity to DNP-poly-L-lysine and DNP-GL in responder and nonresponder guinea pigs. J Exp Med 126:959, 1967.

Haverkorn MJ, Hofmann B, Masurel N, Van Rood JJ: HLA linked genetic control of immune response in man. Transplant Rev 22: 120, 1975.

Heber-Katz E, Wilson D: Collaboration of allogeneic T and B lympholymphocytes in the primary antibody response to sheep erythrocytes in vitro. J Exp Med 142:928, 1976.

Kantor FS, Ojeda A, Benacerraf B: Studies on artificial antigens. I. Antigenicity of DNP-poly-lysine and DNP-copolymer of lysine and glutamic acid in guinea pigs. J Exp Med 117:55, 1963.

Kappler JW, Marrack PC: Helper T cells recognize antigen and macrophage components simultaneously. Nature 262:797, 1976.

Katz DH, Benacerraf B (eds): The Role of Products of the Histocompatibility Gene Complex in Immune Responses. New York, Academic Press, 1976.

Kindred B, Shreffler DC: H-2 dependence of cooperation between T and B cells in vivo. J Immunol 109:940, 1972.

McDevitt HO (ed): Ir Genes and Ia Antigens. New York, Academic Press, 1978.

McDevitt HO, Benacerraf B: Genetic control of specific immune responses. Adv Immunol 11:31, 1969.

Moller G (ed): Conditions for T cell activation. Immunol Rev 35, 1977.

Moller G (ed): Ir genes and T lymphocytes. Immunol Rev 38:1, 1978.

Rosenthal AS, Shevach EM: Functions of macrophages in antigen recognition by guinea pig T lymphocytes. I. Requirement for histocompatibility macrophages and lymphocytes. J Exp Med 138:1194–1212, 1974.

Sasportes M, Fradelizi D, Nunez-Roldan A, Wollman E, Giannopoulos Z, Dausset J: Analysis of stimulating products involved in primary and secondary allogeneic proliferation in man: I, II, and III. Immunogenetics 6:29, 43, 55, 1978.

Schwartz RH: T-lymphocyte recognition of antigen in association with gene products of the major histocompatibility complex. Annu Rev Immunol 3:237, 1985.

Shreffler DC, David CS: The H-2 major histocompatibility complex and the I immune response region: genetic variation, function and organization. Adv Immunol 20:125, 1975.

Thomas DW, Yamashita U, Shevach EM: The role of Ia antigens in T cell activation. Immunol Rev 35:97, 1977.

Unanue ER: The regulatory role of macrophages in antigenic stimulation. Adv Immunol 15:95, 1972.

Von Boehmer H, Hudson L, Sprent J: Collaboration of histoincompatible T and B lymphocytes using cells from tetraparental bone marrow chimeras. J Exp Med 142:989, 1975.

MHC T Cell Killing Restriction

Berke G, Amos GB: Mechanism of lymphocyte-mediated cytolysis: the LMC cycle and its role in transplantation immunity. Transplant Rev 17:71, 1973.

Germain R, Dorf M, Benacerraf B: Inhibition of T lymphocyte mediated tumor-specific lysis by alloantisera directed against the H_2 serologic specificities. J Exp Med 142:1023, 1975.

Klein J: Genetics of cell mediated lymphocytotoxicity in the mouse. Semin Immunopathol 1:31, 1978.

Matzinger P, Bevan MJ: Induction of H-2–restricted cytotoxic T cells: in vivo induction has the appearance of being unrestricted. Cell Immunol 33:92–100, 1977.

Moller G (ed): MHC restriction of anti-viral immunity. Immunol Rev 58, 1981.

Moller G (ed): Mechanism of action of cytotoxic T cells. Immunol Rev 72, 1983.

Shearer GM, Schmitt-Verhulst A-M: Major histocompatibility complex restricted cell-mediated immunity. Adv Immunol 25:55, 1977.

Zinkernagel R: Virus specific T-cell–mediated cytotoxicity across the H-2 barrier to virus altered alloantigen. Nature 261:139, 1976.

Zinkernagel RM, Althage A, Cooper S, Callahan G, Klein J: In irradiation chimeras, K or D region of the chimeric host, not of the donor lymphocytes, determines immune responsiveness of antiviral cytotoxic T cell. J Exp Med 148:805, 1978.

Zinkernagel RM, Callahan GN, Althaga A, Cooper S, Klein DA, Klein J: On the thymus in the differentiation of "H-2 self-recognition" by T cells: evidence for dual recognition. J Exp Med 147:882, 1978.

Zinkernagel RM, Doherty PC: H_2 compatibility requirement for T-cell–mediated lysis of target cells infected with lymphocytic choriomeningitis virus. J Exp Med 141:1427, 1975.

MHC Genes

Amos DB: The evolution of the supergene: observation on the major histocompatibility complex. *In* Zalesk MB, Abeyounis CJ, Kano K (eds), Immunobiology of the Major Histocompatibility Complex. Basel, Karger, 1981.

Clark SS, Forman J: Allogeneic and association recognition determinants of H-2 molecules. Transplant Proc 15:2090, 1983.

Germain RN, Malissen B: Analysis of the expression and function of class-II major histocompatibility complex molecules by DNA mediated transfer. Annu Rev Immunol 4:28, 1986.

Gonwa T, Peterlin BM, Stobo JD: Human Ir genes: structure and function. Adv Immunol 34:71, 1983.

Hansen TH, et al.: The immunogenetics of the mouse major histocompatibility gene complex. Annu Rev Genet 18:99, 1984.

Hood L, Steinmetz M, Malissen B: Genes of the major histocompatibility complex of the mouse. Annu Rev Immunol 1:529, 1983.

Klein J, Figueroa F, Nagy Z: Genetics of the major histocompatibility complex: the final act. Annu Rev Immunol 1:119, 1983.

Lew AM, et al.: Class I genes and molecules: an update. Immunology 57:3, 1986.

Mengle-Gaw L, McDevitt HO: Genetics and expression of mouse Ia antigens. Annu Rev Immunol 3:363, 1985.

Nathenson SG, et al: Murine major histocompatibility complex class-I mutants: molecular analysis and structure–function implications. Annu Rev Immunol 4:471, 1986.

Steinmetz M, Hood L: Genes of the major histocompatibility complex in mouse and man. Science 222:727, 1983.

MHC Products

Algranati ID, Milstein C, Ziegler A: Studies on biosynthesis, assembly and expression of human major transplantation antigens. Eur J Biochem 103:197, 1980.

Crumpton MJ, Snary D, Walsh FS, Barnstable CJ, Goodfellow PN, Jones EA, Bodmer WF: Molecular structure of the gene products of the human HLA system: isolation and characterization of HLA-A, -B, -C and Ia antigen. Proc R Soc Lond [Biol] 202:159, 1978.

Ferrone S, Allison JP, Pellegrino MA: Human DR (Ia-like) antigens: biological and molecular profile. Contemp Top Mol Immunol 7:239, 1978.

Frelinger JA, Shreffler DC: The major histocompatibility complexes. *In* Benacerraf B (ed): Immunogenetics and Immunodeficiency. Baltimore, University Park Press, 1975, p81.

Grey HM, Kubo RT, Colon SM, Poulik MD, Cresswell P, Springer T, Turner M, Strominger JL: The small subunit of HL-A antigens is β_2 macroglobulin. J Exp Med 138:1608, 1973.

Henriksen O, Appella E, Smith DF, Tanigaki N, Pressman D: Comparative chemical analysis of the alloantigenic fragment of HL-A antigens. J Biol Chem 251:4214, 1976.

Hood L, Kronenberg M, Hunkapiller T: T cell antigen receptors and the immunoglobulin supergene family. Cell 40:225, 1985.

Kaufman JF, et al: The class II murine major histocompatibility complex. Cell 36:1, 1984.

Moller G (ed): MHC and MLS Determinants. Immunol Rev 60, 1981.

Moller G (ed): Structure and Function of HLA-DR. Immunol Rev 66, 1982.

Nathenson SG: Biochemical properties of histocompatibility antigens. Annu Rev Genet 4:69, 1970.

Nathenson SG, et al.: Murine major histocompatibility complex class I mutants: molecular analysis and structure function relationship. Annu Rev Immunol 4:47, 1986.

Norcross MA, Kanehisa M: The predicted structure of the Ia β1 domains: a hypothesis for the structural basis of major histocompatibility complex–restricted T-cell recognition of antigens. Scand J Immunol 21:511, 1985.

Pctcrson PA, Rask L, Lindblom JB: Highly purified papain-solubilized HL-A antigens contain β-2-microglobulin. Proc Nat Acad Sci USA 71:35, 1974.

Reisfeld RA: Isolation and serological evaluation of HL-A antigens solubilized from cultured human lymphoid cells. *In* Korn ED (ed): Methods in Membrane Biology. New York, Plenum, 1974, p143.

Reisfeld RA, Pellegrino MA, Ferrone S, Kahan BD: Chemical and molecular nature of HL-A antigens. Transplant Proc 5:447, 1973.

Strominger JL, Ferguson W, Fuks A, Giphart M, Kaufman J, Mann D, Orr H, Parham P, Robb R, Terhorst C: Isolation and structure of HLA antigens. Birth Defects 14:235, 1978.

Walford RL, Waters H, Smith GS: Human transplantation antigens. Fed Proc 29:2011, 1970.

Walker LE, Reisfeld RA: Human histocompatibility antigens: isolation and chemical characterization. J Immunol Methods 49:R25, 1982.

MHC and Organ Transplantation

Albert ED, Baver MP, Mayr WR (eds): Histocompatibility Testing 1984. New York, Springer-Verlag, 1984.

Albert E, Gotze D: The major histocompatibility system in man. *In* Gotze E (ed): Histocompatibility Antigens. Berlin, Springer-Verlag, 1978, p7.

Albrechtsen D, Bratlie A, Nousianinen H, Solheim BG, Winther N, Thorsby E: Serological typing of HLA-D: predictive value in mixed lymphocyte cultures (MLC). Immunogenetics 6:91, 1978.

Amos DB: Genetic and antigenetic aspects of human histocompatibility system. Adv Immunol 10:251, 1969.

Amos DB, Kostyu DD: HLA–a central immunological agency of man. Adv Hum Genet 10:137, 1980.

Bach FH: Transplantation: pairing of donor and recipient. Science 168:1170, 1970.

Bodmer J, Bodmer W: Histocompatibility 1984. Immunol Today 5:251, 1984.

Bodmer WF (ed): The HLA system. Br Med Bull 34, 1978.

Bodmer WF, Bodmer J, Batchelor R, Festenstein H, Morris P: Joint Report from the Seventh International Histocompatibility Workshop in Histocompatibility Testing 1977. Copenhagen, Munksgaard, 1978.

Cheigh JB, Chami J, Stenzl KH, Riggio RR, Saal S, Mouradian JA, Fotino M, Stubenbord WT, Rubel AL: Renal transplantation between HLA identical siblings: comparison with transplants from HLA semi-identical donors. N Engl J Med 296:1030, 1977.

Dausset J: The major histocompatibility complex in man. Science 213: 1469, 1981.

Ferrone S, Curtoni ES, Gorini S: HLA Antigens in Clinical Medicine and Biology. New York, Garland/STM Press, 1983.

Gray I, Russell PS: Donor selection in human organ transplantation. Lancet 2:863, 1963.

Morris PJ: Histocompatibility in organ transplantation in man. *In* Joachim HL (ed): Pathobiology Annual 1973. New York, Appleton–Century–Crofts, 1973.

Myburgh JA, Shapiro M, Maier G, Myers AM: HL-A and cadaver kidney transplantation. 7 years experience of Johannesburg General Hospital. S Afr Med J 50:1279, 1976.

Rappaport FT, Converse JM, Billingham RE: Recent advances in clinical and experimental transplantation. JAMA 27:2835, 1977.

Russell PS, Monaco AP: The biology of tissue transplantation. N Engl J Med 271:502, 553, 610, 664, 718, 776, 1964.

Salvatierra O, Feduska NS, Cochrum KC, Najarian JS, Kountz SL, Belzer FO: The impact of 1,000 renal transplants of one center. Ann Surg 186:424, 1977.

Simmons RL, Van Hook EJ, Yunis EJ, Noreen H, Kjellstrano CM, Condie RM, Mauer SM, Buselmeier TJ, Najarian JS: 100 sibling kidney transplants followed 2 to 7½ years: a multifactorial analysis. Ann Surg 185:196, 1977.

Teraski PI, Mickey MR, Singal DP, Mitalli KK, Patel R: Serotyping for transplantation. XX. Selection of recipients for cadaver donor transplants. N Engl J Med 279:1101, 1968.

Thorsby E: The human major histocompatibility system. Transplant Rev 18:51, 1974.

Thorsby E: Histocompatibility antigens: immunogenetics and role of matching in clinical renal transplantation. Ann Clin Res 13:190, 1981.

Wilson RE, Henry L, Merrill JP: A model system for determining histocompatibility in man. J Clin Invest 52:1497, 1963.

Van Rood JJ, Eernisse JG: The detection of transplantation antigens in leukocytes. Prog Surg 7:217, 1967.

HLA and Disease Susceptibility

Arnett FC: HLA and genetic predisposition to lupus erythematosus and other dermatologic disorders. J Am Acad Dermatol 13:472, 1985.

Braun WE: HLA and Disease: A Comprehensive Review. Boca Raton, Fla., CRC Press, 1979.

Brewerton DA: HLA-B27 and the inheritance of susceptibility to rheumatic disease. Arthritis Hematol 19:656, 1976.

Brewerton DA, Caffrey M, Hart FD, James DCO, Nichols A, Sturrock RD: Ankylosing spondylitis and HL-A27. Lancet 1:904, 1973.

Brewerton DA, Caffrey M, Nichols A, Walters D, James DCO: Acute anterior uveitis and HL-A27. Lancet 2:994, 1973.

Brewerton DA, Caffrey M, Nichols A, Walters D, Oates JK, James DCO: Reiter's disease and HL-A27. Lancet 2:996, 1963.

Calin A: HLA-B27: To type or not to type. Ann Intern Med 92:208, 1980.

Calin A, Fries JF: An "experimental" epidemic of Reiter's syndrome revisited. Ann Intern Med 84:564, 1976.

Fitzmann SE: HLA patterns and disease association. JAMA 236:2305, 1976.

McDevitt HO: The HLA system and its relation to disease. Hosp Pract 20:57, 1985.

McMichael A, McDevitt HO: The association between the HLA system and disease. Prog Med Genet 2:39, 1977.

Morris PJ: Histocompatibility systems, immune response and disease in man. *In* Cooper MD, Warner NL (eds): Contemporary Topics in Immunobiology, Vol 3. New York, Plenum, 1974, p141.

Noer RN: An "experimental" epidemic of Reiter's syndrome. J Am Med Assoc 197(7):117, 1966.

Rachelefsky GS, Terasaki PI, Katz R, Steim ER: Increased prevalence of W27 in juvenile rheumatoid arthritis. N Engl J Med 290:892, 1974.

Sasazuki T, McDevitt HO: The association between genes in the major histocompatibility complex and disease susceptibility. Annu Rev Med 28:425, 1977.

Schaller JG, Hansen JA: HLA relationship to disease. Hosp Pract 16:41, 1981.

Tiilikainen A: On the way to understanding the pathogenesis of HLA associated diseases. Med Biol 58:53, 1980.

Zinkernagel RM: Association between major histocompatibility antigens and susceptibility to disease. Annu Rev Microbiol 33:201, 1979.

10 | The Immune Response

During an immune response to an immunogen, a series of cellular changes occurs in the responding animal that results in the production of serum antibody or specifically sensitized T cells. In addition to the "positive" effects of immunity, that is, the production of protective antibody or sensitized cells, immune responses are also controlled or limited so that overproduction of a particular antibody or population of sensitized cells does not occur. In this chapter, an overview of the cell interactions during induction of immunity and control of the response is presented.

Cellular Interactions in the Induction of Antibody Formation

T Cell–B Cell Collaboration

At least three distinct cell types are required for maximal antibody production to most antigens: T cells, B cells, and macrophages (Fig. 10-1). Macrophages in most instances (or other antigen-presenting cells) are required for stimulation of T helper cells; T helper cells produce growth and differentiation factors for B cells; and B cells are precursors that differentiate into antibody-producing and -secreting plasma cells. The necessity for T cells and B cells to cooperate during antibody formation was first demonstrated by passive transfer of thymus, bone marrow, and spleen cells to irradiated mice, followed by antigen challenge (Fig. 10-2). Mixtures of thymus and bone marrow cells were effective, whereas thymus or bone marrow cells alone were not. Cell suspensions from the spleen include both T and B cells, so that transfer of spleen cells alone was effective. In vitro studies using mixtures of purified cell populations also demonstrated that mixtures of T cells and B cells are required for induction of antibody formation.

Accessory Functions of Macrophages during Induction of Immune Responses

In addition to T and B cell collaboration during induction of antibody formation, there is a requirement for antigen processing by macrophages or other cell types (Fig. 10-3). Macrophages do not recognize antigens specifically but enhance T

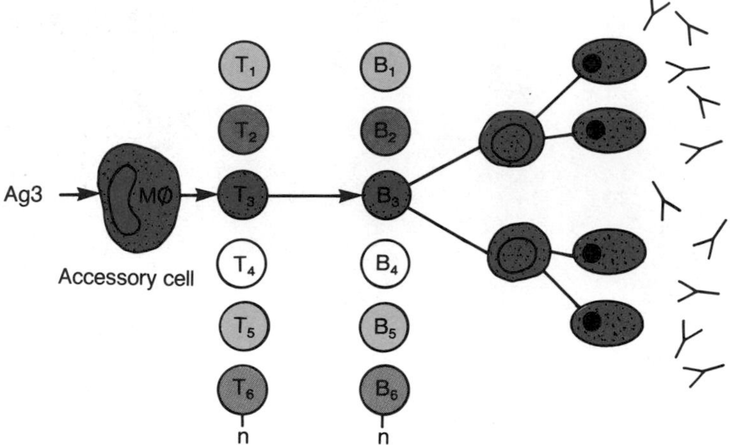

Figure 10-1. Simplified three-cell-population cooperation in induction of antibody formation: macrophages, T cells, and B cells. Macrophages do not recognize antigen specifically but process the antigen and present it to T and/or B cells. Specific antigen recognition (in this case, antigen 3) occurs at the level of T and B cells, by selection of cells with specific cell surface receptors for the antigen, T_3 and B_3. T cells help stimulate B cells to proliferate and differentiate into plasma cells that synthesize and secrete specific antibody.

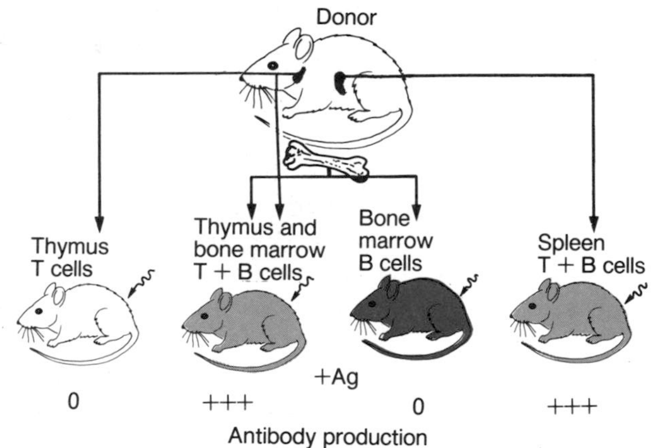

Figure 10-2. Thymus–bone marrow collaboration in induction of antibody formation. The demonstration of the requirement of two cell types (T and B cells) in induction of antibody was accomplished by Henry Claman. Cells from the spleen, thymus, and bone marrow were passively transferred separately or admixed before being transferred into irradiated recipients. The recipient was then challenged with antigen. The doses of radiation used were high enough to eliminate T and B cell functions in the recipient animal. Splenic cells alone produced high responses, whereas bone marrow or thymus cells alone produced no response. On the other hand, mixtures of thymus and bone marrow cells were capable of producing a strong response. The role of the macrophage was not identified in these experiments, because macrophages are relatively radioresistant and are functionally active in the irradiated recipients. Some antigens are "T independent" and can stimulate B cells without T cell help (see below).

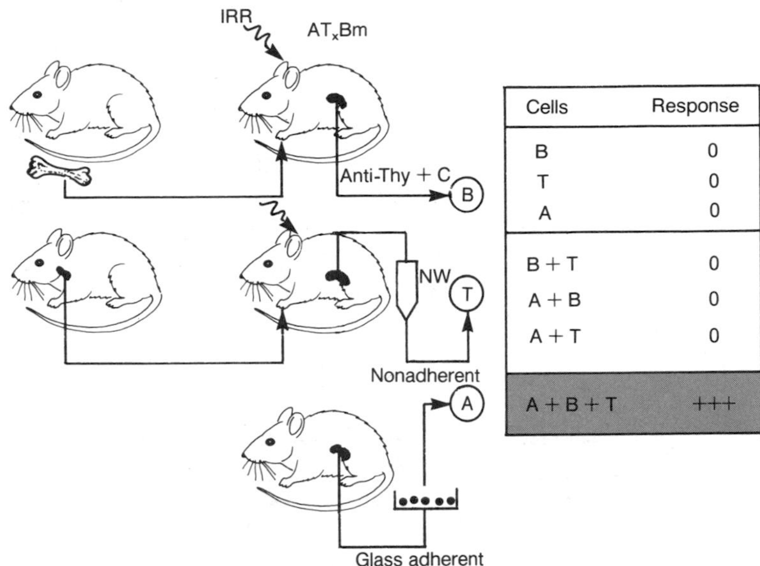

Cells	Response
B	0
T	0
A	0
B + T	0
A + B	0
A + T	0
A + B + T	+++

Figure 10-3. Demonstration of the requirement of "accessory" macrophages for induction of antibody formation in vitro. In this experimental model, B cells are obtained from the spleens of adult mice that have been injected with bone marrow cells from a normal adult donor following thymectomy and radiation treatment (ATxBm). T cells are obtained from the spleens of mice previously injected with thymus cells of a normal donor following radiation. Accessory cells (A) are obtained from the spleen cells of normal mice that are allowed to adhere to a glass surface. Nonadherent cells include T and B cells, whereas the adherent population is composed mainly of macrophages. Any one, or mixture of two, of these cell populations is not able to respond optimally to antigen stimulation in vitro. However, a mixture of the three cell populations does respond.

cell–B cell collaboration via antigen presentation. Such cellular cooperation experiments require the proper proportions of T cells, B cells, and accessory macrophages. For instance, too few or too many accessory cells may result in suboptimal conditions for antibody production.

Macrophage–T Cell–B Cell Cooperation

A model of the cellular interactions in induction of antibody formation is illustrated in Figure 10-4. An immunogen is first processed by a macrophage. The macrophage does not have a specific receptor for the antigen, although some macrophages may carry specific receptors transferred from T or B cells (cytophilic antibody). The macrophages concentrate or process the immunogen and facilitate T and B cell interactions. Analysis of peptide molecules that react with and activate T helper cells to proliferate has suggested that stimulating antigenic peptides contain two domains: an *epitope* that reacts with the paratope of the T cell receptor and an *aggretope* that reacts with an antigen-presenting class II MHC molecule. The epitope is

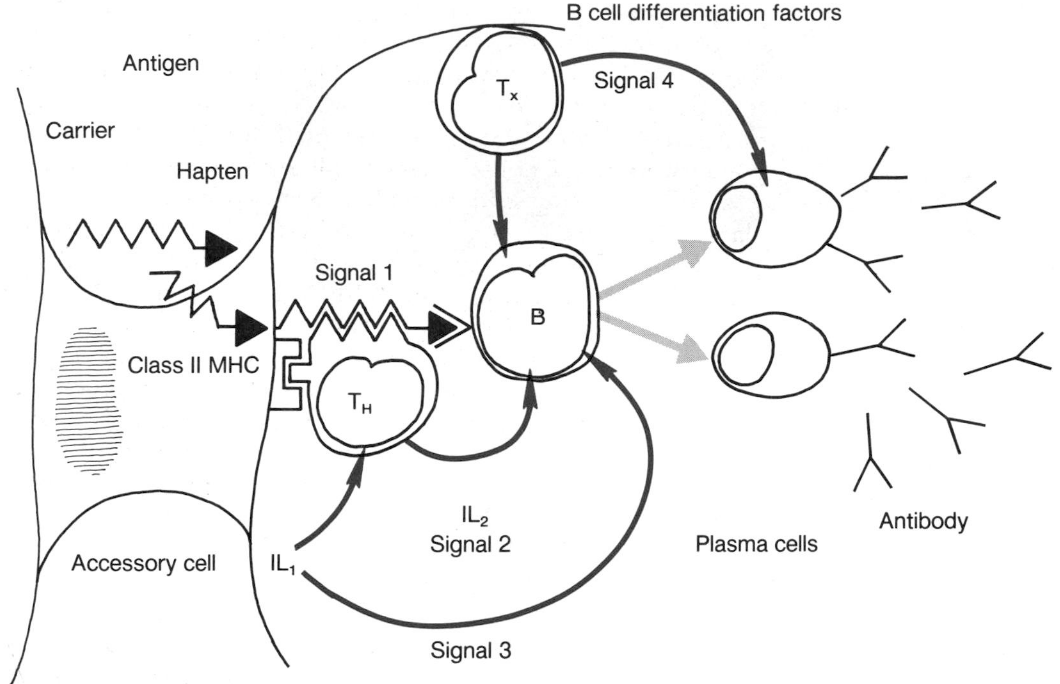

Figure 10-4. Macrophage–T cell–B cell cooperation in induction of antibody formation to haptens. Macrophages process the antigen nonspecifically and provide activation signals to T and B cells. T cells recognize the immunogenic carrier molecule in association with class II MHC markers (see Chapter 9), whereas B cells recognize the hapten. The reaction of the B cell with the hapten in the presence of the reaction of the T cell with the carrier along with the macrophage provides the required set of signals for B cell stimulation. It is postulated that at least three signals are required to stimulate B cells: one signal supplied by the antigen (hapten), one by the macrophage, and one by the T cell. Further signals are required to induce differentiation of B cells (see Fig. 10-5). During induction of these responses, antibodies to the carrier antigen are also produced (i.e., B cells to the carrier as well as to the hapten are stimulated), as are memory B cells.

the classic hydrophilic antigenic determinant; the aggretope is a hydrophobic domain that has affinity for the lipid bilayer of the antigen-presenting cell. Macrophages *process* the antigen, presumably by inserting the hydrophobic aggretope domains of the antigen into membrane structures containing the class II (I-A) molecules. This processed antigen then reacts with T cell receptors that recognize both the epitope and the class II marker of the processed antigen (see Fig. 10-12). The subject of activation of T cell subsets is presented in more detail below. T helper cells are activated by reaction with antigen and interleukin 1 (IL1), a factor produced by activated macrophages, and, in turn, produce interleukin 2 (IL2).

B cells are activated by a combination of signals, one specific (reaction of B cells with antigen) and others antigenically nonspecific (macrophage or T cell mediation). Activated lymphoid cells produce and secrete factors that are critical for the activation of proliferation and differentiation of cells in the immune response. These factors are termed *interleukins*. The properties of interleukins are presented in more detail below. For activation of B cells, T helper cells are activated by reaction with antigen processed by macrophages in association with class II MHC restriction elements. IL2 produced by activated T cells acts as a "second" signal for B cell activation and further T cell activation. Once the B cell is "turned on," it passes through a series of maturation divisions, resulting in the appearance of antibody-producing plasma cells. Continued presence of antigen in some form may be required to complete the proliferation–maturation phase. In addition, a number of B cell proliferation and differentiation factors are required to achieve full B cell expansion and differentiation into antibody-secreting cells (see below).

B cells may be stimulated in the absence of macrophages or T cells by "thymus-independent" antigens or B cell mitogens. Thymus-independent antigens stimulate B cells directly, are usually polymeric, and are believed to activate B cells by extensive cross-linking of surface receptors for antigen. T-independent antigens bypass the two or three signal mechanisms required for thymus-dependent antigens. Such antigens may be able to stimulate the specific antigen receptor of the B cells as well as stimulate proliferation, that is, be immunogens as well as mitogens.

Proliferation and Differentiation of Activated B Cells

Factors secreted by lymphoid cells during induction of an immune response appear to play a major role in proliferation and differentiation of activated B cells. A current model is presented in Figure 10-5. This model is based largely on in vitro studies. The model incorporates a combination of specific and nonspecific signals involving T cells, accessory cells, and B cells. Different T cell populations in the T helper series may be active at different stages of B cell activation and differentiation, or one T cell population may mature and acquire another function as the immune response proceeds. Both activation and differentiation of B cells require specific recognition of antigen provided through macrophage–T helper cell–B cell interaction and the effect of up to 10 or more B cell growth and differentiation factors released by lymphoid cells (interleukins).

B Cell Growth and Differentiation Factors

A partial listing of soluble factors secreted by activated T helper cells that act on B cells to support proliferation and/or differentiation is given in Table 10-1. These factors are studied by adding supernates of T cell cultures activated by antigen or

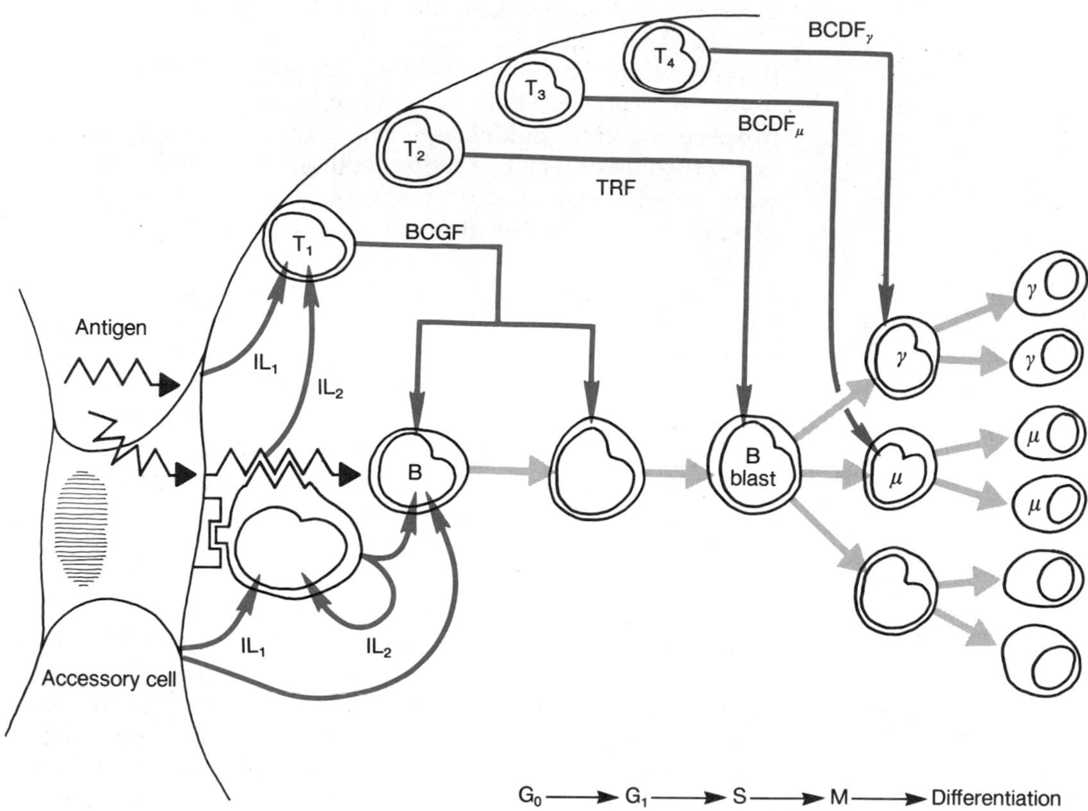

Figure 10-5. Scheme for activation and differentiation of B cells during induction of antibody formation. In this scheme T_H cells recognize antigen and class II self recognition markers on accessory cells that have processed the antigen. The macrophage accessory cell is stimulated to release interleukin 1 (IL1). IL1 acts on other T helper cells (T_1, T_2, T_3, and T_4), which have also reacted with antigen. IL1-activated helper T cells produce a second interleukin (IL2). IL1 acts on other T helper cells (T_1-T_4) that have been activated by antigen so that there are more receptors on these cells for IL2. IL2 also acts on the cells that produce it to stimulate the further activation of the cell (autocrine effect). T helper cells activated by IL2 stimulate proliferation of B cells that have been activated by specific cell surface reaction with antigen presented by the accessory cell and the action of IL1 and IL2. The activated B cells are then further stimulated to proliferate, through the action of B cell growth factors (BCGF), or to differentiate into antibody secreting plasma cells, by B cell differentiation factors (BCDF). These factors are also produced by T helper cells that have in turn been activated by reaction with antigen, IL1, and IL2.

mitogens, or supernates of T cell lines, to B cells in vitro. Because the in vitro culture conditions are selected to emphasize the effects of different culture supernates, it is not clear whether or not the effects noted in vitro have a physiological significance in vivo. In general these factors increase the proliferation or immunoglobulin (antibody) synthesis of B cell cultures activated by mitogens or by antigens and T helper cells.

Table 10-1. B Cell Growth and Differentiation Factors

Name	Function
BCGF I	Stimulates activated B cells to proliferate
BCGF II (T cell replacing factor)	Stimulates activated B cells to proliferate
BCDF	Differentiation of B cells
BCDF μ	Differentiation of μ-producing B cells
Isotype (Ig class) specific BCDF ϵ, δ, α	Induce isotype specific B cell line ϵ, δ, or α
LBCDF	Induces terminal differentiation of B cells
Interferon	Synergizes with interleukin 1 and 2
Interleukin 2	Synergizes with interleukin 1
Interleukin 4 (BSF1)	Stimulates activated cells

BCGF, B cell growth factor; BCDF, B cell differentiation factor.

Cellular Interactions in the Induction of Immune T Cells

As discussed in Chapter 8, in addition to providing help for T-dependent antibody production, T cells have many other major functions. These include suppressor cells (T_S), which serve to limit or control immune responses, T cytotoxic cells (CTL or T_K), which are capable in vitro of lysing target cells to which they are sensitized, and T_D cells, which mediate delayed hypersensitivity (DTH) in vivo through reaction with specific antigen and release of lymphokines. These functional subpopulations of T cells bear different cell surface markers (see Chapter 4).

T Cell–T Cell Cooperation

Functional T cell subpopulations are activated by a complicated set of interactions. Our present understanding of these cellular interactions depends upon separating lymphocyte subpopulations on the basis of surface markers and reconstituting function by mixing back together different cells. The functional subpopulations include helper/inducer cells capable of helping the expansion of B cells and their differentiation into antibody-secreting plasma cells, as well as other T inducer cells capable of expanding T cell precursors and stimulating them to differentiate into functionally mature T cells. These mature effector cells include CTL and DTH T cells as well as T_S cells. The T_S cells can function as a negative feedback arm to turn off inducer function or precursor responses. Experimentally, it takes an inducer cell plus a precursor cell in culture to generate an effector CTL, just as it requires a helper cell plus a B cell to generate antibody-producing plasma cells from B cells. Some of these inducer or suppressor interactions require direct cell-to-cell contact, whereas others are regulated via soluble factors released into the culture medium. Some of these factors (such as IL2) have been purified to homogeneity, cloned by recombinant methods, and found to bind to specific receptors on the surface of precursor cells. A diagram of the interactions is provided in Figure 10-6. It must be stressed that this scheme is based on in vitro systems that are subject to different interpretations.

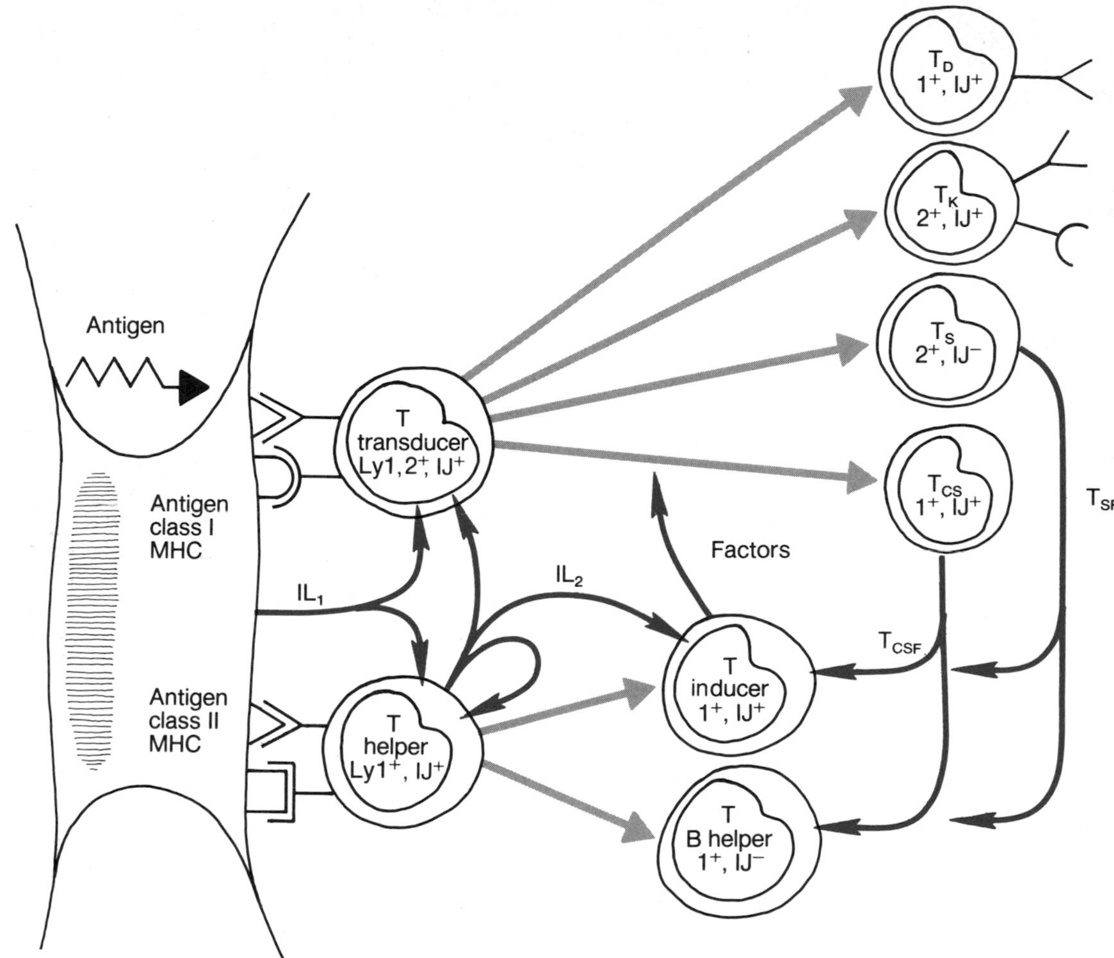

Figure 10-6. Hypothetical scheme of T cell interactions during an immune response in mice. This scheme is based on a composite of data from different systems. T cells are stimulated by antigen plus class II MHC markers on accessory cells to differentiate into the *inducer* series, or are stimulated by antigen plus class I MHC markers to differentiate into the *transducer* series. The inducer cells are capable of helping in the expansion of transducer precursor cells and the subsequent maturation into effector cells, such as CTL, DTH cells, or suppressor T cells. These inducer T cells may work through a soluble factor (IL2) or through direct cell-to-cell contact, which shows MHC restriction. The inducer cells may differentiate into functional T helper cells, aiding in the expansion of specific B cells in response to antigen. As with B cell specificities, the precursor T cells are already committed to a single specificity by rearrangement of V region genes of the T cell receptor for antigen. It is the critical role of the inducer T cells to stimulate clonal expansion of specific clones after selection by antigen.

Table 10-2. Interleukins Involved in T Cell Interactions of Mice

Name	Molecular Weight	Source	Target Cell	MHC Restriction	Function
Interleukin 1 (lymphocyte-activating factor)	15,000	Activated accessory macrophage	T cells, many other cells	None	Enhances T cell proliferation, IL2 production, B cell activation
Interleukin 2 (T cell growth factor)	30,000–35,000	Activated T cells	Activated T cells	None	Stimulates T cell proliferation and differentiation of activated T cells, binds to a specific receptor that is expressed after activation
Interleukin 3	40,000	Activated T cells	Activated T cells	None	Induces 20α-hydroxysteroid dehydrogenase in spleen cells, stimulates differentiation of activated T cells
Interleukin 4 (BSF1)	20,000	Cultured thymocytes	T and activated B cells	None	Stimulates resting T cells, anti-Ig activated B cells
Interferon α	25,000	T cells	NK cells	None	Stimulates IL1 production and NK activity, suppresses growth of certain viruses
Interferon γ (immune interferon)	20,000–25,000	T cells	T cells, NK cells	None	Stimulates NK and TK activity, enhances B cell differentiation (see Table 10-4)
T suppressor factor	70,000, single chain	T cells	T_S cells	Class I, V_H, antigen	Inhibits T helper cells

Data from Smith KA: Annu Rev Immunol 2:319, 1984; Howard M, Paul W: Annu Rev Immunol 1:307, 1983; Green DR, et al.: Annu Rev Immunol 1:439, 1983; Robb RJ: Immunol Today 5:203, 1984; Ihle JN, et al, *in* Lymphokines and Thymic Hormones, New York, Raven Press, 1981; Kishimoto T: Annu Rev Immunol 3:133, 1985.

Interleukins

Interleukins are produced by cells that are activated during immune responses, and are critical for induction, maintenance and control of an immune response. The major factors are interleukin 1 (IL1) and interleukin 2 (IL2). Interleukin 1 was first called *lymphocyte-activating factor* because of its ability to induce resting T cells to proliferate. IL1 is produced by macrophages activated either by nonspecific activators, such as latex beads and phorbol esters, or by reaction with products of mitogen-stimulated T cells or T cells that have reacted with antigen and class II MHC associated antigen on macrophages (macrophage activating factors). IL1 in turn acts on T helper/inducer cells that have reacted with antigen to stimulate the production of IL2. IL2 stimulates the proliferation of T cells that have been "activated" by reaction with IL1 and antigen. Such "activated" cells have increased IL2 receptors that can be demonstrated by the monoclonal antibody anti-TAC. The IL2 receptor is a cell surface glycoprotein of molecular weight 55,000 with a high affinity for IL2 binding. T cell subpopulations activated by antigen, IL1, and IL2 may produce a number of B cell growth and differentiation factors (see below). IL1 may also activate B cells that have reacted with antigen and T helper cells, but the evidence for this is not conclusive. Other interleukins and their putative actions are listed in Table 10-2.

Interferons

The term *interferon* is used for a family of proteins produced by virus-infected cells that interfere with virus replication. *Viral interference* refers to the phenomenon in which infection of cells with one virus inhibits multiplication in the cells of a second virus. Interferon production may also be stimulated by treating cells with synthetic polyribonucleotides or by activating lymphocytes (primarily T cells) with antigens or mitogens. The three major interferons are listed in Table 10-3. Interferons

Table 10-3. Interferon Nomenclature

New	Old
IFN - α	Type I, leukocyte, pH 2 stable
IFN - β	Type I, fibroblast, pH 2 stable
IFN - γ	Type II, immune, pH 2 labile

produced by cultured cell lines or by recombinant DNA in bacteria are now available in industrial quantities.

Interferons act at the cell surface via receptors and inhibit translation of viral mRNA by stimulation of protein kinase (which phosphorylates initiation factor) and of a ribonuclease that destroys viral mRNA. As noted above, immune interferon (IFN - γ) or type II interferon is produced by activated T cells and may have a more important immunoregulatory role than IFN-α or IFN-β. IFN-γ may be produced by either helper or suppressor T cells, after stimulation by antigens or mitogens, and is also produced by activated NK cells. IFN-γ is a single polypeptide chain of MW 20,000–25,000 depending on the degree of glycosylation, and has a number of activities in immune responses (Table 10-4). At present there is interest in the application of interferons for treatment of cancer and/or virus infections, but the results of extensive clinical trials have been disappointing.

Table 10-4. Some Activities of IFN-γ

Inhibits growth of normal and neoplastic cells
Synergizes with lymphotoxins
Induces proliferation and differentiation of NK/K and T_K (CTL)
Increases Class I and Class II MHC antigen expression in different cell types including macrophages, endothelial cells, and tumor cells
Increases expression of Fc receptor of myelomonocytic cells
Induces differentiation of myeloid cells and activates macrophages
Synergizes with BCDF to stimulate B cell differentiation and increase Ig production by B cells

Data from Trinchieri and Perussia: Immunol Today 6:131, 1985.

MHC Restriction of T_K Cytotoxicity

As presented in Chapter 8, CTL (T_K) can recognize and kill foreign cells, such as those provided by xeno- or allografts, and cells bearing "foreign antigens," such as tumor antigens or viral antigens. However, the recognition and killing of autologous cells that bear foreign antigens, such as virus-infected cells, also require self recognition. The CTL receptor for foreign antigen also carries specificity for self class I MHC markers. If an individual becomes infected with a virus that produces a cell surface antigen or develops a tumor that expresses a tumor antigen, the altered cells may be rejected by CTL that recognize both the new cell surface antigens and the self markers of the infected cells (see Figure 10-6).

MHC Antigens and T Cell Killing

The relationship of mouse MHC antigens to the specificity of virus cytotoxicity may be demonstrated using in vitro systems for killing of virus-infected target cells. Cytotoxic T cells from mice immunized to virus are cytotoxic for target cells containing the viral antigen only if the cells also have the same MHC type as the killer cells. Thus, cytotoxic spleen lymphocytes obtained from a virus immune donor of strain A will kill other virus-infected target cells of strain A origin, but not of strain B origin, and vice versa. CTL from $(A \times B)F_1$ donors will kill both A and B infected targets, but not those of another strain (Fig. 10-7). Cloned CTL from $(A \times B)F_1$ immune donors will kill either the A or the B infected cells, but not both, because each clone has a single receptor specificity for class I MHC markers. Interestingly some CTL clones are specific for hybrid MHC markers formed in the F_1 and not in either A or B parental

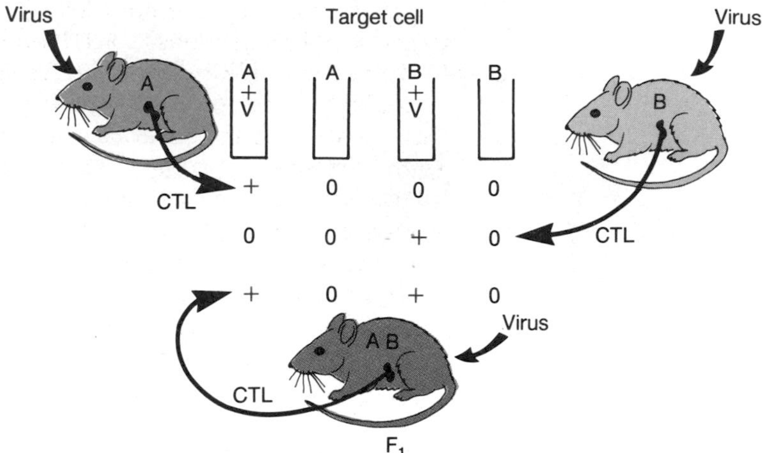

Figure 10-7. Histocompatibility restriction of cell-mediated cytotoxicity. Sensitized T cytotoxic cells of mice of a given MHC (histocompatibility) type are capable of lysing only virus-infected target cells that also have the same MHC type. +, Lysis of target cells; O, no lysis.

strains, such as $A_\alpha{}^A A_\beta{}^B$ or $A_\alpha{}^B A_\beta{}^A$. Antisera to MHC class I mouse H-2D or H-2K regions will inhibit killing of target cells by CTL by blocking the H-2K or H-2D determinants on the target cell. Presumably these antisera block the self recognition required for lysis of tumor target cells by immune specific T cytotoxic cells.

Mechanism of MHC Restriction of Cytotoxicity

The mechanisms of MHC-restricted antigen recognition by CTL are not clearly understood. Three concepts have been offered: dual recognition; composite single receptor; and single receptor, altered self (Fig. 10-8). According to the dual recognition

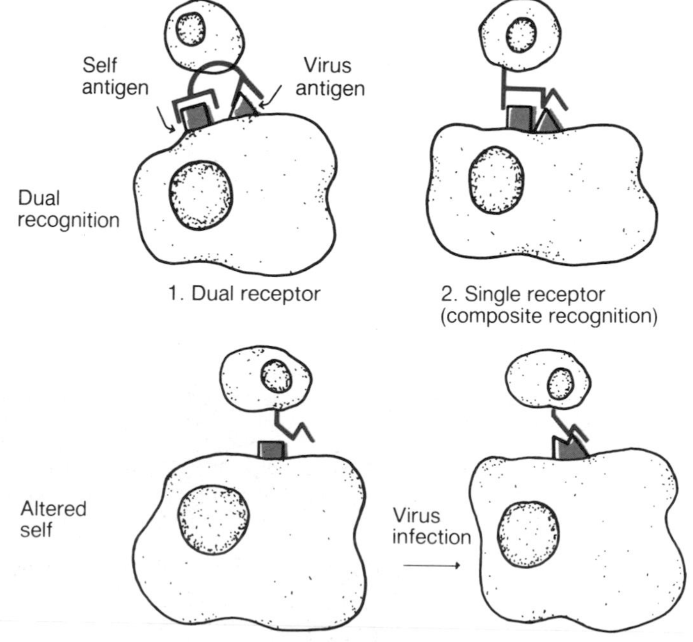

Figure 10-8. Self recognition in target cell killing. T cytotoxic cells must be able to recognize self markers as well as foreign antigens in order to kill the target cell. Several possible models of this recognition have been proposed: (1) Dual receptor: The killer cell possesses two separate receptors, one for self, another for the foreign antigen. (2) Composite single receptor: There is a single T cell receptor that can recognize both self and foreign antigen. (3) Altered self: There is a single receptor that can recognize an altered self cell surface marker. Model 2 appears most likely on the basis of DNA transfection (see text), but model 3 is also possible.

hypothesis, two receptors are required for cell killing, one reacting with self class I MHC and the other with the foreign (virus) antigen. Reaction of both receptors with the target cell is required for cell killing. The composite single receptor hypothesis postulates a single receptor that recognizes both viral antigen (epitope) and class I MHC aggretope. The altered self hypothesis defines a single receptor that recognizes the viral antigen (epitope) as part of an MHC cell surface complex; the viral antigen is incorporated into the cell surface as part of or associated with the class I MHC cell surface molecules (aggretope). The virus–self interaction results in a structure recognized by the reacting cell that is not provided by either virus or self alone. Evidence supporting each model is available.

Recently, a single receptor with dual specificity has been confirmed, at least for some T cells. Transfer by DNA transfection of the T cell receptor alpha and beta donor genes for a known antigen and MHC specificity into a new cell gives the new cell the same antigen and MHC specificity as the donor cell. Thus, the two chains of a single T cell receptor carry the specificity for both antigen and MHC recognition (model 2 or 3, Fig. 10-8). Whether the antigen and MHC also combine to form an "altered self" complex prior to binding the T cell receptor remains controversial (model 3).

Adaptive Differentiation of Self Recognition

The ability of T cells to recognize the self class I MHC markers on target cells depends on the environment in which the CTL precursors develop (i.e., the MHC type of the thymus) and not on the genotype of the precursor cells (Fig. 10-9). Thus, if F_1

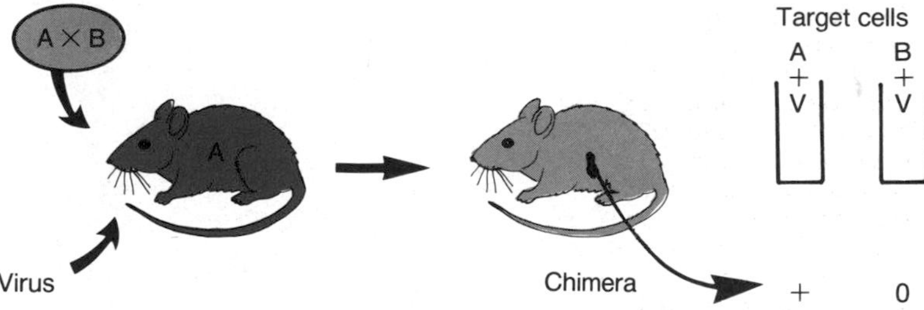

Figure 10-9. Adaptive differentiation of self recognition. The ability to recognize self on target cells is an inherited genetic property of the effector cells, but phenotypic expression is controlled by the environment in which recognition of the foreign antigens takes place. Thus, AB-type T cells transferred to A recipients will not recognize B as self on virus-infected target cells. In the example illustrated, (A × B) F_1 T cells exposed to virus in a parental A-type recipient are able to recognize virus on A target cells, but not on B target cells. However, thymus education of T cell self recognition is not absolute; some recognition of B class I MHC by A × B cells that have differentiated in A thymus is also seen.

(AB) stem cells are injected into a parental irradiated recipient (A), the T cytotoxic cells that develop in the A-type thymus are capable of killing A, but not B, virus-infected cells. If the (A × B)F_1 stem cells had matured in their own F_1 thymus, they would have acquired the ability to kill either A or B infected cells. It is postulated that the CTL develop receptors for self in the environment of the thymus. Since the A and B CTL develop in an A thymus environment, only A target cells are recognized (self A receptors but not self B receptors are produced). The epithelial cells of the thymus express class I MHC markers and may be capable of "educating" the precursors of CTL during thymic maturation to recognize self class I MHC.

MHC Restrictions in Induction of Cytotoxic T Cells

Whereas the thymus limits the range of what the T cells will see as self, the expansion of the T cell clones of a given specificity depends on the MHC type of the antigen-presenting cell. Interaction of T inducer cells with precursors of CTL is activated by infected immunogenic cells bearing class I and II MHC markers. This is the critical step in ensuring that antigen-specific CTL will be available to combat specific virus infections. Infected host cells specifically are killed; other host cells are not killed, and limitation of virus infection is achieved with minimal damage to noninfected cells.

A schematic presentation of the cellular interactions involved in generation of human CTL is given in Figure 10-10. The activation of T helper/inducer cells for CTL is restricted by antigen on the presenting cell and class II MHC products. The activation of CTL is restricted by antigen and either class I or class II MHC products.

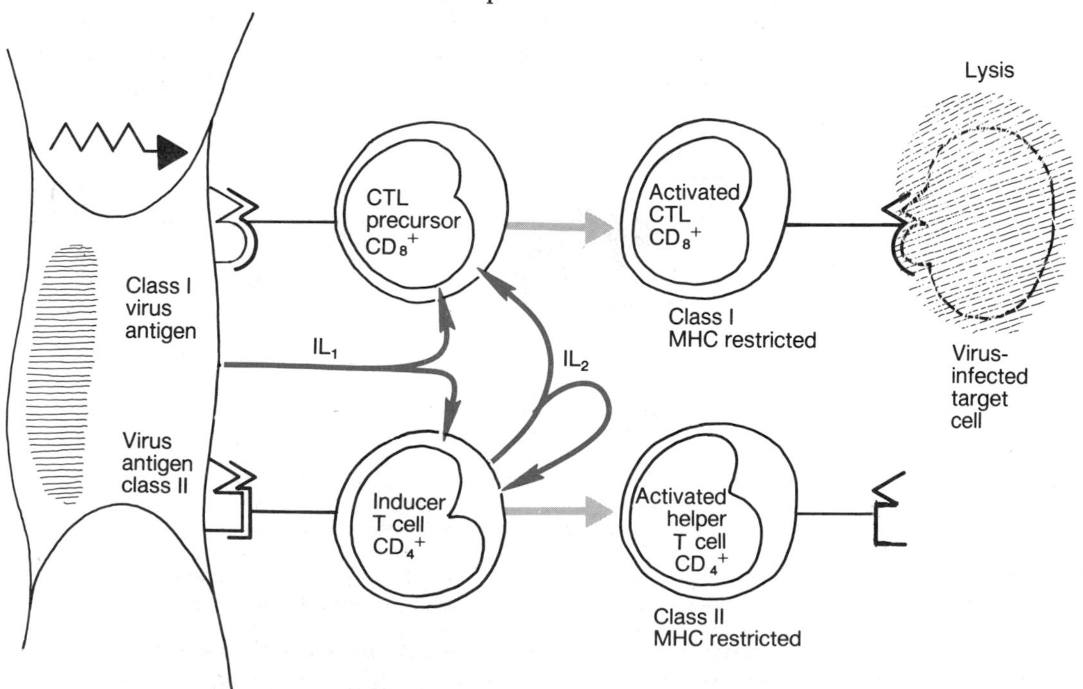

Antigen and MHC Recognition Structure of T Cells (T Cell Receptor)

The T cell surface receptor complex involved in antigen and MHC recognition is characterized in Table 10-5. The variable regions of the α- and β-chains form the antigen-binding site and

Table 10-5. Surface Structures Involved in Antigen Recognition by Human T Lymphocytes

Chains	Molecular Weight Nonreduced	Molecular Weight Reduced	Function
A. T cell receptor complex α and β	90,000	41,000–43,000 (two chains)	Dual recognition of antigen and MHC
"T_3 complex"—δ	23,000	23,000	Phosphorylated during cell activation
γ	20,000–23,000	20,000–23,000	Unknown
ϵ	20,000	20,000	Phosphorylated during cell activation
ζ	32,000	16 (two chains)	Unknown
B. T_4 (CD4)	62,000	62,000	MHC class II recognition
C. T_8 (CD8)	76,000	31,000 + 33,000	MHC class I recognition

also determine the MHC specificity. In the presence of antigen and MHC, the T cell is activated. This results in phosphorylation of at least two subunits of the receptor complex, the δ- and ϵ-chains. By analogy with other receptors, one of these subunits may act as a regulatory protein for another enzyme system, which generates an internal "second signal" for T cell activation. Current work focuses on the possibility that phosphodiesterase is activated, resulting in the release of diacylglycerol, which in turn activates protein kinase C. In addition, the other product of phosphodiesterase action, inositol trisphosphate, may serve to mobilize calcium stores, resulting in further activation of protein kinase C. The observed phosphorylation of some of the subunits of the T cell receptor complex may reflect the function of protein kinase C during T cell activation.

Antigen binding can be mimicked by monoclonal antibodies to the T cell receptor α- and β-chains or to the δ-chains. By immobilizing the antibodies on beads, cross-linking of receptors by the antibody is enhanced, and T cell activation by either type of antibody bound to beads is facilitated. Similarly, when

◀ **Figure 10-10.** Generation of class I MHC restricted CTL (T_K cells). A T_8^+ human precursor cell is activated by reaction with antigen, MHC class I products, and IL1. Differentiation into an activated killer occurs under the influence of IL2 from T_4^+ helper cells. The cytotoxic T cells produced require reaction with both antigen and class I markers on target cells in order to effect lysis of the target cell. It should be emphasized that functions of T_4 (CD4) cells are MHC class II restricted and that functions of T_8 (CD8) cells are MHC class I restricted.

OKT_3 monoclonal antibody is used to modulate off the δ-chain, the other chains of the receptor complex are found to modulate as well; and when antibody to the α- and β-chains is used, the δ-chain also modulates.

Two other chains on the T cell surface, T_4 (CD4) and T_8 (CD8), are associated with the recognition of class I or class II only, without interacting with antigen at all. They are thought to work by binding nonpolymorphic (constant) determinants on class I or class II antigens of the antigen presenting cell. Whether these molecules are associated with the T cell receptor complex is not certain at this time. Ti, the T cell receptor responsible for antigen recognition, is associated strongly with T_3, the common T cell marker. A theoretical scheme for T cell recognition is given in Figure 10-11.

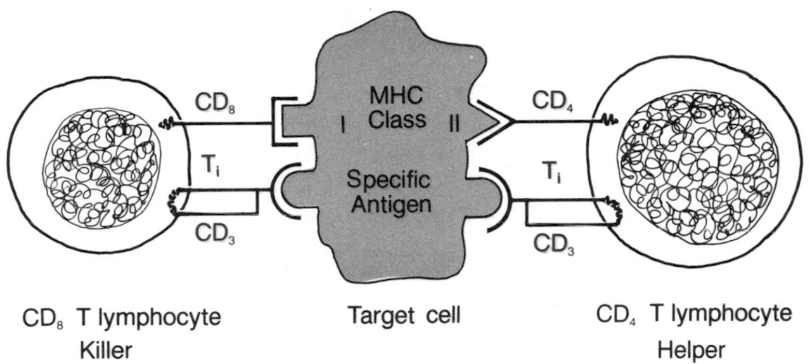

Figure 10-11. Model of antigen recognition by human T lymphocytes. Each T lymphocyte possesses two types of recognition structures. The T_8 and T_4 glycoproteins bind to nonpolymorphic regions of class I and class II MHC gene products, respectively. In contrast, T_3–Ti recognizes specific antigen in the context of a polymorphic MHC gene product.

Significance of MHC Restriction of Killing

The significance of MHC restriction of killing in human immune responses remains uncertain. It seems unlikely in humans that immune lymphocytes will be faced with viral antigens presented on histoincompatible cells. However, in vitro studies have demonstrated how recognition occurs and which surface molecules are important. Also, rejection of MHC-different grafts may occur without self recognition as part of the graft rejection mechanism. Organ grafts between an MHC-incompatible donor and recipient are rapidly rejected. It is possible that foreign MHC markers are recognized as "altered self."

Major histocompatibility complex markers may act to focus the effect of T cytotoxic cells on virus-infected cells. The function of T killer cells is to kill other cells. It is well known that cellular immune mechanisms play a major role in defense against virus infections. Since T killer cells do not bind free virus but can act only on viral antigens associated with MHC on a cell surface, MHC restriction prevents diversion of T_K cells and focuses their effects on cells. Thus MHC restriction may provide an effective means of concentrating the effects of T killer cells on virus-infected cells.

It is also possible that self recognition MHC restriction of killing may play a role in recognition of neoantigens that may appear in developing or incipient tumors. Thus, altered self may be recognized and the altered tumor cells eliminated before frank cancer develops. This concept, termed *immune surveillance,* has been considered by some to play an important role in preventing tumor development.

Summary of MHC Restrictions during Activation of T Cells

A summary of MHC and antigenic restrictions in generation of immune reactive T cells is given in Table 10-6. T helper cell activation and delayed hypersensitivity effector cells are antigen and class II MHC restricted; CTL activities are antigen and class I or class II MHC restricted. Suppression can be class I restricted or unrestricted. Surface phenotype (CD4 or CD8) correlates mainly with MHC recognition of class II ($CD4^+$) or class I ($CD8^+$).

Table 10-6. Restrictions on Lymphoid Cell Activation

Function	Surface Phenotype	Restriction
T helper	$CD4^+CD8^-$	Class II MHC + antigen
DTH	$CD4^+CD8^-$	Class II MHC + antigen
CTL	$CD4^-CD8^+$ or $CD4^+CD8^-$	Class I or II MHC + antigen
Suppressor	$CD4^-CD8^+$	Class I MHC

Considering the important regulatory role of class II restricted inducer cells (all of which are $CD4^+$), it is not surprising that a virus such as the AIDS-related virus, which infects T cells through the CD4 marker and thus selectively depletes the CD4 population, can cause the severe immune suppression and other abnormalities of lymphocyte growth seen in AIDS patients.

Lymphoid Cell Interactions in Vivo

The anatomic location of macrophage – T cell – B cell interactions in vivo is the cortex of the lymph node and the white pulp of the spleen (see Chapter 3). T and B cells may start out anatomically separated but come together during the induction of a primary antibody response. A special mechanism may exist to permit circulating T lymphocytes to lodge not only in thymus-dependent areas but also in B cell areas such as lymph node follicles or within splenic follicles, thus providing an anatomic focus for the direct cellular interaction of T and B cells (see Fig. 10-5). Lymphoid cell interactions may occur dynamically during induction of a primary immune response, as illustrated by the morphologic events that occur in the spleen leading to the production of germinal centers in the white pulp (Fig. 10-12). Labeled antigen localizes in dendritic macrophages that lie along the penicilli arterioles. These macrophages migrate to

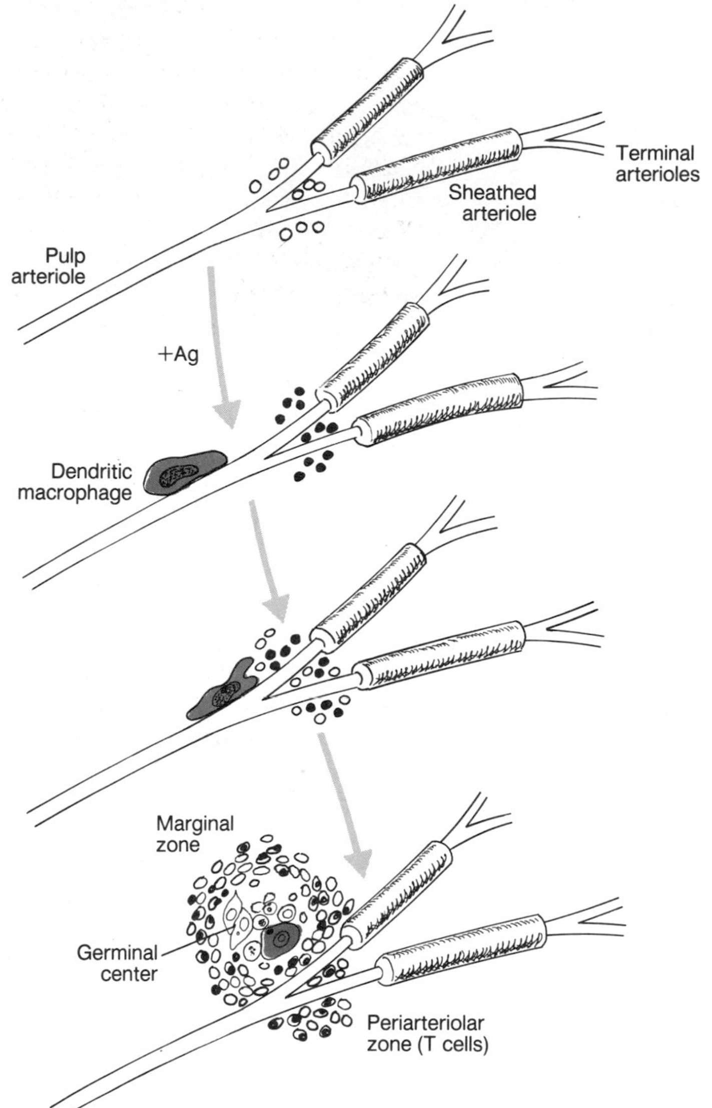

Figure 10-12. Formation of germinal centers in the splenic white pulp following immunization. Penicilli arterioles of the spleen may be divided into three segments: the pulp arteriole, the sheathed arteriole, and the terminal arteriole. Injected antigen is taken up by dendritic macrophages located adjacent to penicilli arterioles and germinal centers formed at the bifurcation of the arteriole after migration of the periarteriolar macrophage. The antigen-localizing macrophage may serve as a nucleus around which T and B cells interact, resulting in formation of a mature germinal center. Antibody-secreting plasma cells are produced by proliferation and differentiation of B cells and migrate into the cords of the splenic red pulp.

the point of bifurcation of the arteriole, where other lymphoid cells accumulate, leading to the production of a "germinal center." By 4 days after injection, antigen-containing macrophages may be observed in the periarteriolar sheath, and by 6 days, in the germinal center. It is not clear just how macrophages, T cells, and B cells migrate together during the primary antibody response in vivo, but structures such as the white pulp of the spleen may facilitate housing of different cell types, permitting cellular interactions to take place. The dendritic macrophages of lymphoid organs may act to bring together T cells and B cells, with proliferation of the B cells resulting in the formation of germinal centers.

Immune Memory

Following stimulation by antigen, the responding B and T lymphocytes undergo proliferation and differentiation, respectively, into plasma cells that synthesize and secrete antibody (humoral immunity) or into T lymphocytes (specifically sensitized cells) that have the ability to react directly and specifically with antigen (cellular immunity). In addition, long-lived cell lines with the ability to react upon second contact with the original antigen by a more rapid and increased proliferation and differentiation are also produced for both T cell and B cell function (memory cells or antigen-primed cells). A second contact with the same or a closely related antigen stimulates a more rapid reaction, with the production of a greater specific immune response. This anamnestic, or secondary, response is believed to be the result of the memory cells elicited by the preceding antigenic stimulation. Memory is expressed by both T and B cells. In certain situations where two different but related antigens share some antigenic determinants in common but also have determinants that are unique for each antigen, exposure to the second related antigen (after previous exposure to the other antigen) results in an anamnestic response both to the shared determinants and to the unique determinants of the first antigen even though the second antigen does not contain such determinants ("original antigenic sin").

The antibody formed as a result of the secondary response differs not only in quantity but also in quality from that formed as a result of the primary response. There are two main differences: the immunoglobulin class of antibody produced and the strength of binding to the antigen (avidity). The initial antibody is of the IgM class; that of the secondary response is usually IgG.

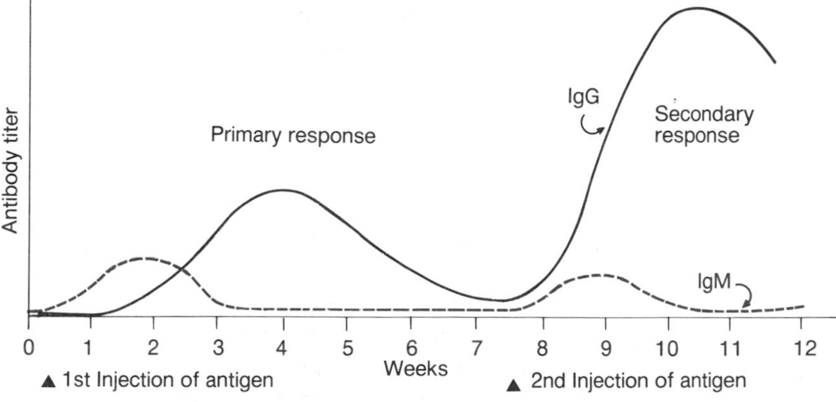

Figure 10-13. Primary and secondary antibody responses. Serum levels of IgM and IgG after primary (Day 0) and secondary (Week 8) immunization with the same antigen. In a primary response, IgM antibody precedes IgG antibody. In a secondary response, IgM and IgG both appear early and the IgG response is much greater. Not only is the titer of the IgG antibody elevated to a much higher titer more rapidly during a secondary response as compared with the primary response, but the avidity of the secondary response antibody is also much higher.

A secondary response usually results in more antibody with stronger binding affinity for the immunizing antigen than the primary response. However, a number of variables, such as antigen dose, route of exposure, and length of time between the primary and secondary immunizations, determine the nature of a secondary response.

Control of Antibody Production

Regulatory mechanisms are important in controlling the size, nature, and duration of an immune response. If the response were not controlled, antigen stimulation of proliferation would lead to an overgrowth of body tissues similar to that seen with lymphoid tumors, such as multiple myeloma (plasma cells), lymphoma, or leukemia. Following primary or secondary immunization, there is a burst of antibody production that peaks in a few days. Serum antibody titers then fall off gradually owing to a decreasing number of antibody producing cells and catabolism of the antibody formed. Further antibody formation occurs at a very low rate and may eventually be undetectable if no reexposure to the antigen occurs. After a primary immunization, there is a refractory period during which reinjection of antigen will not produce a further increase in the immune response. The number of antibody-forming cells produced and the serum titer of antibody formed upon secondary immunization is directly related to the time between the first and second immunizations with the same antigen (Fig. 10-14). The extent of

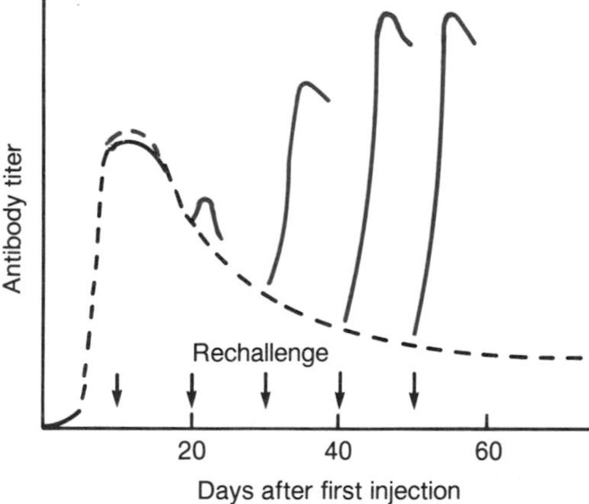

Figure 10-14. Relationship between the magnitude of a secondary antibody response and the interval between first and second exposure to an antigen. The magnitude of an antibody response to a second exposure to the same antigen depends upon the time between the first and second exposures. Although a secondary response is usually greater than the primary, there is a refractory period during the primary response when exposure to a second antigen has little effect. ---, primary response; —, secondary response. The arrows indicate the time of the second injection of antigen.

antibody production by B cells is regulated by at least three possible mechanisms: a humoral antibody feedback mechanism, T suppressor action, and idiotype control networks (Fig. 10-15).

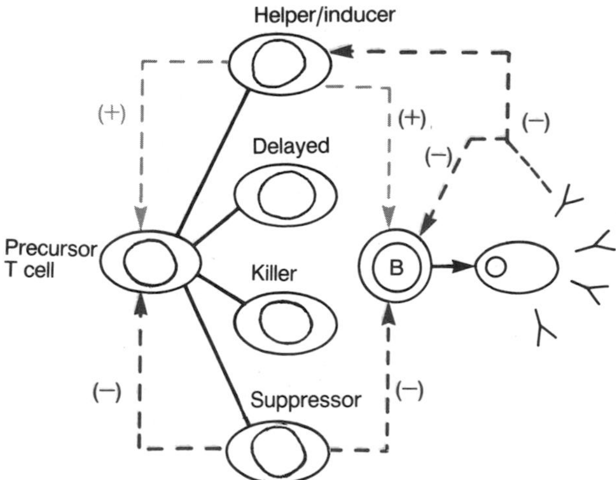

Figure 10-15. Immune response control mechanisms. T helper and T suppressor cells act on both T and B cell generating systems to control the extent of an immune response. T helper cells collaborate with B cells during the induction of T cell–dependent antibody responses, and with T inducer cells for the development of effector T cell populations, such as T_D, T_K, and T_S cells. T suppressor cells act on both B cells and T cells to limit the development of antibody-producing cells or T effector cells. In addition, immunoglobulin antibody inhibits antibody production by action on T and/or B cells, possibly through an idiotype network.

Feedback Inhibition by Passive Antibody

Passive administered specific antibody can suppress the induction of an immune response to the specific antigen without affecting responses to other antigens. The mechanism of action of the specific antibody in this situation is unknown, but the observation supports the concept that specific antibody inhibits further production of antibody of the same specificity by a feedback control system. Continued antibody production most likely requires the steady recruitment of antigen-reactive B cells to differentiate into antibody-secreting plasma cells. The presence of specific antibody may block antigenic stimulation of most of the reactive B cells.

T Suppressor Cells

During induction of an immune response, T_S cell activity is also stimulated, and it is likely these cells play a critical role in limiting the extent of antibody production. T_S cells are believed to act by mediation of a suppressor factor (T_sF) on T helper cells or on B cell differentiation (see above). During a primary or secondary immune response, T_H cells dominate during the inductive and productive phases, but T_S cells dominate during a refractory period following a primary immune response. This dominance is short-lived. Thus, a secondary injection of antigen shortly after a primary response may produce little or no additional reaction, whereas a secondary injection given weeks later will produce a rapid and extensive secondary response (see Fig. 10-14). The loss of suppression may be due to a decline in T_S cells or to the development of contrasuppressor cells, which counteract the effect of suppressor cells. However, the role and existence of contrasuppressor cells are controversial.

Idiotype Networks

The essence of the idiotype network as hypothesized by Niels Jerne is shown in Figure 10-16. Jerne postulated that each anti-

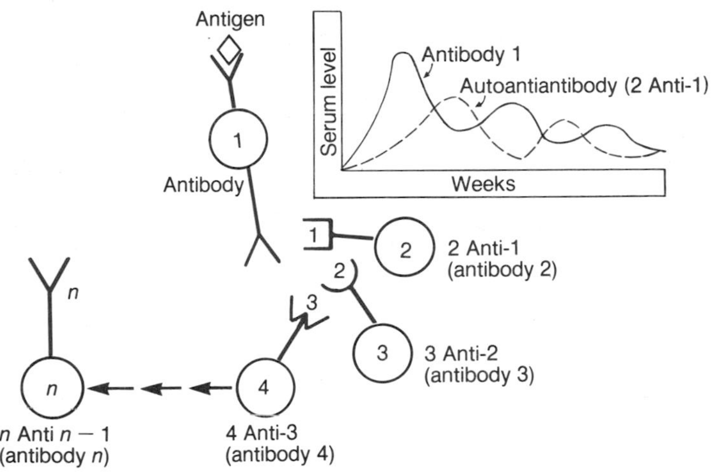

Figure 10-16. The network theory. The network theory postulates a circular set of antibodies to idiotypes (receptors) that interact to limit immune responses. It is further postulated that for each antibody produced, an anti-idiotype response is also produced. Thus if an antigen stimulates a B cell receptor (idiotype), the antibody produced will stimulate an anti-idiotype. This anti-idiotype, in turn, will stimulate a second anti-idiotype. Such a system provides a step-down mechanism to turn off the ongoing response. Thus the 2 anti-1 idiotype turns off the 1 anti-antigen; the 3 anti-2 turns off the 2 anti-1; etc. It is postulated that each step requires less anti-idiotype, so that eventually the system absorbs the stimulus and restores the series of anti-idiotype responses to "normal levels." In this manner a "dynamic equilibrium" is maintained. The inset depicts the cyclic appearance of primary antibody (solid line) and auto-anti-idiotype (2 anti-1) to this antibody following immunization.

body is itself looked upon by the immune system as an antigen with unique determinants (idiotype). Antibody produced in response to a foreign antigen elicits an anti-idiotypic antibody, which serves to control the further production of more idiotype-containing antibody. Anti-idiotypic antibodies have been demonstrated to appear in a cyclic manner following an antibody response, and the levels fluctuate immensely with the levels of the original antibody (idiotype). However, the exact mechanism whereby anti-idiotype controls the production of idiotype is not known.

The Immune System–Nervous System Relation

Several circumstantial observations have linked the extent of an immune response to control by the nervous system. These observations are:

1. There are sympathetic nerve fibers in lymphoid organs.
2. Lymphocytes have receptors for sympathetic mediators (norepinephrine, epinephrine).
3. Sympathectomy increases the density of β-adrenergic receptors on T and B lymphocytes and increases antibody responses by spleen cells.
4. Diminished norepinephrine levels are found in rat spleen during the primary immune response.
5. Stress, which increases sympathetic mediators (norepinephrine), decreases immune response.
6. Experimental animals may be "conditioned" to exhibit lower-than-normal immune responses by taste aversion learning.

These findings suggest that sympathetic–parasympathetic balance can affect the immune response and perhaps the immune response can be influenced by the central nervous system. Sympathetic dominance decreases immune responsiveness. Further understanding of the potential of this controlling mechanism is anticipated with intense interest.

Theories of Antigen Recognition

Historically, two mechanisms of specific induction of an immune response have been proposed: instructive and selective (Fig. 10-17).

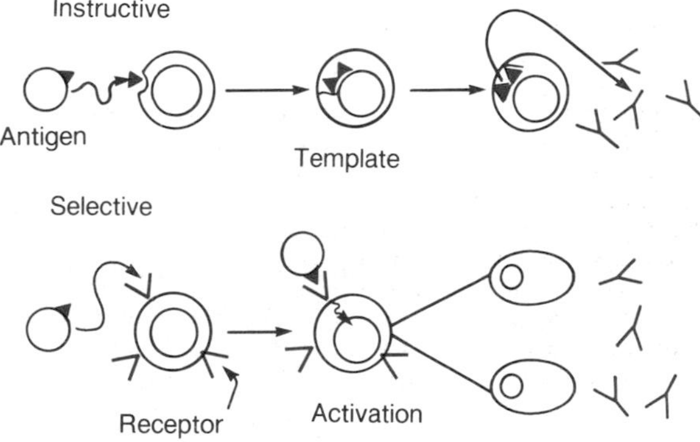

Figure 10-17. Theories of antigen recognition. Two major theories of antigen recognition have been proposed: instructive and selective. The instructive theory implies that the antigen in some way supplies specific structural information to the responding cell. Selective theories hold that the responding cells already contain in their genome the information required to produce specific antibody. The antigen reacts with specific receptors on the cell surface (preformed antibody) and thus selects a population of cells with the specific receptor to proliferate and differentiate into antibody-secreting cells.

Instructive

Instructive theories of antibody formation are included for historical interest only, as they are no longer considered plausible. Instructive theories state that antigen serves as a template upon which antibody molecules are folded to impose an antigen combining site. This theory was in vogue in the early part of the twentieth century and was supported by the findings of Linus Pauling, who denatured antibody and then tried to recover activity by renaturation of the antibody. He was unable to do so in the absence of antigen. It is now known that the tertiary structure of antibody can be destroyed by breaking the disulfide bonds of the molecule, but when these bonds are rejoined correctly, the antigen-binding activity of the antibody is restored even in the absence of antigen. The primary structure of a protein determines the folding of the molecules (tertiary structure), and therefore the antigen-binding specificity of an antibody must be dictated by the amino acid sequence of the antibody molecule. Most immunologists now agree that instructive theories are no longer tenable in the light of our present knowledge of molecular biology. Instead of "instructing" the cell regarding the structure of the antibody to be produced, the role of antigen is now known to be selecting cells already expressing a receptor for the antigen.

Selective

Selective theories state that the coding for antibody specificity is genetically determined and already present in the responding cell; contact of the cell with antigen serves to stimulate the expression of the preexisting potential. There are two variations of selective theories: germ line and somatic mutation. The germ line selective theory postulates that vertebrates have a separate gene for each polypeptide chain that has developed with evolution of the species. The somatic mutation theory postulates that the evolution of immune cells occurs within the lifetime of the individual by mutation or modulation of a much smaller number of inherited cistrons.

Germ Line

In 1900, Paul Ehrlich presented his side-chain theory, in which he stated that all cells, not just lymphoid cells, had a variety of side chains (termed *haptophores*) that had evolved in the germ line. These side chains normally functioned as receptors for metabolites, but could also react with antigens. As a result of reaction with antigen, there was a compensatory synthesis of new side chains. This synthesis resulted in an excess of side chains, so that many were released into the circulation and became detectable as antibodies.

In 1955, Jerne postulated the natural selection theory, which took into account some of the information that had accumulated during the preceding 50 years. Jerne postulated that the production of specific antigen receptor molecules by lymphoid cells was random. The number of antigenic specificities that each of these receptor molecules would recognize was finite and dictated by the genome of the individual. Receptor molecules were released from the cells (natural antibody), and antigen served to select the specific circulating receptors with which it reacted (natural selection). The receptor that had reacted with antigen was then carried back to the cell with the potential to produce antibody, and the antigen–receptor molecule complex in some way stimulated the cell to proliferate, differentiate, and produce more receptor molecules (antibody). Szilard, in 1960, postulated that there was a separate gene that coded for each antibody and that the complete array of genes required for all antibodies was present in each potentially reacting cell. Antigen served to induce cell differentiation, fix the specificity of the reacting cell, and stimulate production of antibody. Both Jerne and Szilard said that the precursor of the antibody-producing cell was omnipotent and could generate separate cells that collectively recognize all immunogens.

Somatic

Burnet was the first to postulate that the immune potential was the result of somatic mutation. He reasoned that the immune response to a specific antigen originated in a few omnipotent stem cells that were highly mutable. During somatic development, individual precursor cells that had the capacity to respond to one or a very limited number of antigens were differentiated. Upon contact with the specific antigen, these precursors were stimulated to proliferate, and the progeny constituted a clone of cells producing the specific antibody (clonal selection). Burnet's clonal selection theory stimulated a vast amount of important research. A number of workers have extended Burnet's theory and have implicated various genetic mechanisms as occurring during somatic development to explain the amino acid structure of immunoglobulins. However, somatic mutation on a random basis as a means of creating the diversity needed for recognition of many different antigens implies uncontrolled production of information with a high rate of nonsense mutations (wastage). Recent observations suggest that somatic mutation occurs mainly during the maturation of an ongoing antibody response and may result in antibodies of high affinity during the secondary response.

* * *

The most pressing questions to be examined by any theory are: (1) How does an immunologically reactive cell recognize antigen? (2) How does this recognition stimulate antibody production? (3) How does an individual develop the capacity to recognize so many different antigenic specificities (generation of diversity)?

Immunologically reactive cells recognize antigens by means of specific receptor molecules present on their surface. The process whereby this reaction of antigen with a reactive or precursor cell stimulates the cell to proliferate is related to the ability of the antigen to activate the cell through reaction with cell surface receptors, and is incompletely understood. Generation of diversity may occur by germ line evolution or by somatic mutation. Each reactive cell has the capacity to recognize one or very few antigens (i.e., is restricted). There must be a very active selective mechanism capable of finding the rare T or B cell specific for each antigen. It is known that each differentiated antibody-producing plasma cell is restricted to producing antibody of one specificity and immunoglobulin of one type, but the potential of the recognition cell or precursor cell is not clearly defined. It is possible that restriction may occur during differentiation of a given cell line by rearrangement of receptor genes. There is evidence the unrearranged Ig genes may be expressed in very early B cell differentiation. V_H-to-VDJ rearrangement in a heavy chain gene enhances Ig secretion in mature cells.

Summary

Antigen recognition leading to an immune response involves different functional cell populations (Fig. 10-18). Immunogens

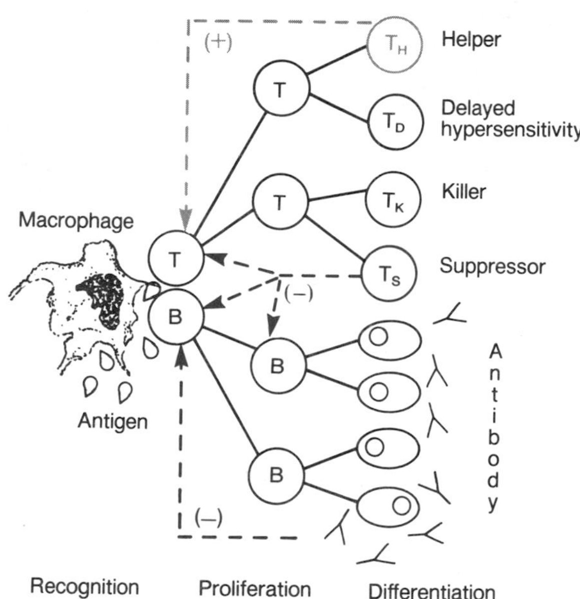

Figure 10-18. Cellular interactions in the immune response. The immune response involves the interaction and differentiation of a number of different cell populations from immature precursor cells to mature effector cells. During the early steps of development, precursor cells acquire specificity through gene rearrangement and production of specific receptors. Antigen specifically selects receptor cells at a later step and selectively stimulates the appropriate cells to proliferate and differentiate into functional effector cells. Controlling mechanisms are also activated that turn off the proliferation of reactive cells and limit the extent of the response. (For details see Summary.)

are processed by macrophages that present the antigen to specifically reactive T and B cells. Antigen processing by macrophages results in association of the antigen with class II MHC gene products (I-A). T cells recognize antigen and I-A simultaneously, so that most immune responses are class II MHC restricted. Activated macrophages produce interleukin 1, which activates T cells in the presence of antigen. In turn, activated T helper/inducer cells secrete interleukin 2, which supports proliferation of activated T and B cells. B cells are stimulated by antigen and other T cell factors (interleukins) to proliferate and differentiate into plasma cells, which secrete specific immunoglobulin antibodies. T cells proliferate and differentiate into at least four functional populations: helper/inducer cells (T_H), cells that effect delayed hypersensitivity reactions (T_D), cytotoxic killer cells (T_K), and suppressor cells (T_S). T_H cells cooperate with B cells during induction of antibody formation, and T_S cells provide a mechanism for limiting the extent of an immune response. Another T cell population, T contrasuppressor cells, may modulate the effect of T suppressor cells in mice, but such an activity in humans is controversial. In addition, T and B memory cell populations are produced that permit the primed individual to respond more rapidly to a second exposure of the same antigen. Thus, immunization results in the establishment of a new state of awareness in the responding individual via the generation of a complex of new cell populations. The immune response provides not only specifically sensitized cells and immunoglobulin antibody but also an inherent control system that limits the extent of the response. It is now generally accepted that the germ line receptor genes provide the basic structures needed to encode for antigen receptors and that further diversity may be added by somatic mutation.

References

Cell Interactions in the Induction of Antibody Formation

Altman A, Katz DH: The biology of monoclonal lymphokines secreted by T cell lines and hybridomas. Adv Immunol 33:73, 1982.

Dinarello CA: An update on human interleukin-1: from molecular biology to clinical relevance. J Clin Immunol 5:287, 1985.

Durum SK, Schmidt JA, Oppenheim JJ: Interleukin 1: an immunological perspective. Annu Rev Immunol 3:263, 1985.

Henry C, Trefts PE: Helper activity in vitro to a defined determinant. Eur J Immunol 4:824, 1974.

Katz DH: Lymphocyte Differentiation, Recognition, and Regulation. New York, Academic Press, 1977.

Makela O, Cross A, Kosunen TV (eds): Cell Interactions and Receptor Antibodies in Immune Responses. New York, Academic Press, 1971.

Miller JFAP, Basten A, Sprent J, Cheers C: Interaction between lymphocytes in immune response. Cell Immunol 2:469, 1971.

Miller JFAP, Mitchell FG: Cell to cell interaction in the immune response. I. Hemolysin forming cells in neonatally thymectomized mice reconstituted with thymus or thoracic duct lymphocytes. J Exp Med 128:801, 1968.

Mitchison NA: The carrier effect in the secondary response to hapten–protein conjugates. II. Cellular cooperation. Eur J Immunol 1:18, 1971.

Moller G (ed): Role of macrophages in the immune response. Transplant Rev 40, 1978.

Moller G (ed): Interleukins and lymphocyte activation. Immunol Rev 63, 1982.

Moiser DE, Coppleson LW: A three-cell interaction required for the induction of the primary response in vitro. Proc Nat Acad Sci USA 61:542, 1968.

Mosier DE, Johnson BM, Paul WE, McMaster PRB: Cellular requirements for the primary in vitro antibody response to DNP-Ficoll. J Exp Med 139:1354, 1974.

Nelson DS (ed): Immunobiology of the Macrophage. New York, Academic Press, 1976.

Rosenthal AS: Regulation of the immune response: role of the macrophage. N Engl J Med 303:1153, 1980.

Schwartz RS, Ryder RJW, Gottlieb BAA: Macrophages and antibody synthesis. Prog Allergy 14:81, 1970.

Sercarz EE, Metzger DW: Epitope specific and idiotype specific cellular interactions in a model protein antigen system. Springer Semin Immunopathol 3:145, 1980.

Shevach EM, Rosenthal AS: Function of macrophages in antigen recognition by guinea pig T lymphocytes. II. Role of the macrophage in the regulation of genetic control of the immune response. J Exp Med 138:1213, 1974.

Singer A, Hodes RJ: Mechanisms of T-cell B-cell interaction. Annu Rev Immunol 1:211, 1983.

Taylor RB, Iverson GM: Hapten competition and the nature of cell cooperation in the antibody response. Proc R Soc Lond [Biol] 176:393–418, 1971.

Unanue ER: Cooperation between mononuclear phagocytes and lymphocytes in immunity. N Engl J Med 303:977, 1980.

Weinbaum FI, Butchko GM, Lerman S, Thorbecke GJ, Nisonoff A: Comparison of cross-reactivities between albumins of various species at the level of antibody and helper T cells—studies in mice. J Immunol 113:257, 1974.

B Cell Differentiation

Aarden LA, et al: Revised nomenclature for antigen non-specific T cell proliferation and helper factors. Mol Immunol 17:641, 1980.

Abney E, et al: Sequential expression of immunoglobulin on developing B lymphocytes: a systematic survey that suggests a model for the generation of immunoglobulin isotype diversity. J Immunol 120:2041, 1978.

Byers VS, Sercarz EE: The X–Y–Z scheme of immunocyte maturation. IV. The exhaustion of memory cells. J Exp Med 127:307, 1968.

Cantor H, Boyse EA: Lymphocytes as models for the study of mammalian cellular differentiation. Immunol Rev 33:105, 1976.

Cebra JJ, Komisar JL, Schweitzer PA: C_H isotype "switching" during normal B-cell development. Annu Rev Immunol 2:493, 1984.

Dutton RW: Separate signals for the initiation of proliferation and differentiation in the B cell response to antigen. Transplant Rev 23:66, 1975.

Gearing AJH, Johnstone AP, Thorpe R: Production and assay of the interleukins. J Immunol Methods 83:1, 1985.

Hamaoka T, Ohno S: Regulation of B cell differentiation: interactions factors and corresponding receptors. Annu Rev Immunol 4:167, 1986.

Hanleyhyde JM, Lynch RG: The physiology of B cells as studied with tumor models. Annu Rev Immunol 4:621, 1986.

Howard M, Paul WE: Regulation of B-cell growth and differentiation by soluble factors. Annu Rev Immunol 1:307, 1983.

Kishimoto T: Factors affecting B-cell growth and differentiation. Annu Rev Immunol 3:133, 1985.

Makinodan T, Albright JF: Proliferative and differentiative manifestations of cellular immune potential. Prog Allergy 10:1, 1967.

Mather EL, et al: Mode of regulation of immunoglobulin μ- and γ-chain expression varies during B-lymphocyte maturation. Cell 36:329, 1984.

Melchers F, Anderson J: Factors controlling the B cell cycle. Annu Rev Immunol 4:13, 1986.

Moller G (ed): Effects of Anti-Immunoglobulin Sera on B Lymphocyte Function. Immunol Rev 52, 1980.

Moller G (ed): B Cell Differentiation Antigens. Immunol Rev 69, 1983.

Moller G (ed): B Cell Growth and Differentiation Factors. Immunol Rev 78, 1984.

Rajewsky K, Takemori T: Genetics, expression and function of idiotypes. Annu Rev Immunol 1:569, 1983.

Robertson SM, et al: Antiarsenate antibody response: A model for studying antibody diversity. Fed Proc 41:2502, 1982.

Sell S: Development of restriction in the expression of immunoglobulin specificities by lymphoid cells. Transplant Rev 5:19, 1970.

Vitetta ES, Uhr JW: Immunoglobulin-receptors revisited: a model for the differentiation of bone marrow lymphocytes is discussed. Science 189:964, 1975.

Waldemann TA, Broder S: Polyclonal B-cell activators in the study of the regulation of immunoglobulin synthesis in humans. Adv Immunol 32:1, 1982.

Wall R, Kuehl M: Biosynthesis and regulation of immunoglobulins. Annu Rev Immunol 1:499, 1983.

Whitlock C, et al: In vitro analysis of murine B cell development. Annu Rev Immunol 3:213, 1985.

Yancopoulos CP, Alt FW: Regulation of the assembly and expression of variable region genes. Annu Rev Immunol 4:339, 1986.

T Cell Activation and Differentiation

Ashwell JD, et al: Can resting B cells present antigen to T cells? Fed Proc 44:2475, 1985.

Atassi MZ, et al: Immune recognition of serum albumin. XIV. Cross reactivity of T lymphocyte proliferation of subdomains 3, 6 and 9 of bovine serum albumin. Mol Immunol 19:313, 1982.

Barth RK, et al: The murine T cell receptor uses a limited repertoire of expressed V_β gene segments. Nature 316:517, 1985.

Binz H, Wigzell H: Antigen binding idiotypic T-lymphocyte receptors. Contemp Top Immunobiol 7:113, 1977.

Cantor H, Asofsky R: Synergy among lymphoid cells mediating the graft-versus-host syndrome. II. Synergy in G. v H. reactions produced by Balb/c lymphoid cells of differing anatomic origin. J Exp Med 131:235, 1970.

Cantrell PA, Smith KA: The interleukin-2 T-cell system: a new cell growth model. Science 224:1312, 1984.

Fitch FT: Cell clones and T cell receptors. Microbiol Rev 50:50, 1986.

Goodman JW, et al: The complexity of structures involved in T-cell activation. Annu Rev Immunol 1:465, 1983.

Grey HM, Chesnut R: Antigen processing and presentation to T cells. Immunol Today 6:101, 1985.

Kreiger JI, et al: Antigen presentation by spleen B cells: Resting B cells are ineffective, whereas activated B cells are effective accessory cells for T cell responses. J Immunol 135:2937, 1985.

Leskowitz S, Jones VE, Zak SJ: Immunochemical study of antigenic specificity in delayed hypersensitivity. V. Immunization with monovalent low molecular weight conjugates. J Exp Med 123:229, 1966.

Marchalonis JJ: Lymphocyte surface immunoglobulins: molecular properties and functions as receptors for antigens are discussed. Science 190:20, 1975.

McNamara M, Gleason K, Kohler H: T cell helper circuits. Immunol Rev 79:87, 1984.

Moller G (ed): Lymphocyte activation by mitogens. Transplant Rev 11, 1972.

Moller G (ed): Interleukins and lymphocyte activation. Immunol Rev 63, 1982.

Paul WE: Functional specificity of antigen-binding receptors of lymphocytes. Transplant Rev 5:130–166, 1970.

Paul WE, Benacerraf B: Functional specificity of thymus-dependent lymphocytes: a relationship between the specificity of T lymphocytes and their function is proposed. Science 195:1293, 1977.

Robb RJ: Interleukin 2: the molecule and its function. Immunol Today 5:203, 1984.

Tigelaar RE, Asofsky R: Synergy among lymphoid cells mediating the graft-versus-host response. V. Derivation by migration in lethally irradiated recipients of two interacting subpopulations of thymus derived cells from normal spleen. J Exp Med 137:239, 1973.

Weiss A, et al: The role of the T3/antigen receptor complex in T cell activation. Annu Rev Immunol 4:593, 1986.

Cellular Reactions in Vivo

Gutman GA, Weissman IL: Lymphoid tissue architecture: experimental analysis of the origin and distribution of T-cells and B-cells. Immunology 23:465, 1972.

Humphrey JG, Frank MM: The localization of non-microbial antigens in the draining lymph nodes of tolerant, normal and primed rabbits. Immunology 13:87, 1967.

Mitchell J: Lymphocyte circulation in the spleen. Marginal zone bridging channels and their possible role in cell traffic. Immunology 24:93, 1973.

Moller G (ed): Accessory cells in the immune response. Immunol Rev 53, 1980.

Nossal GJV, Ada GL: Antigens, Lymphoid Cells and the Immune Response. New York, Academic Press, 1971.

Nossal GJV, Ada GL, Austin CM: Antigens in immunity. IV. Cellular localization of ^{125}I-labeled flagella in lymph nodes. Aust J Exp Biol Med Sci 42:311, 1964.

Parrott DM, DeSousa MA: Thymus dependent and thymus independent populations, origin, migratory patterns and lifespan. Clin Exp Immunol 8:663, 1971.

Sertl K: Dendritic cells with antigen-presenting capacity reside in airway epithelium, lung parenchyma and visceral pleura. J Exp Med 163:436, 1986.

Silveira NPA, Mendes NF, Tolnai MEA: Tissue localization of two populations of human lymphocytes distinguished by membrane receptors. J Immunol 108:1456, 1972.

Stingl G, et al: Analogous functions of macrophages and Langerhans cells in the initiation of the immune response. J Invest Dermatol 71:59, 1978.

Tew JG, Mandel TE, Burgess AW: Retention of intact HSA for prolonged periods in the popliteal nodes of specifically immunized mice. Cell Immunol 45:207, 1979.

White RG: Functional recognition of immunologically competent cells by means of fluorescent antibody technique. *In* Wolstenholme GEW, Knight J (eds): The Immunologically Competent Cell. London, Churchill, 1963.

White RG, French VI, Stark JM: Germinal center formation and antigen localization in Malpighian bodies of the chicken spleen. *In* Cottier H (ed): Germinal Centers in Immune Responses. Berlin, Springer, 1966, pp131–142.

MHC Restriction of Cell Interactions

Cone RE: Molecular basis for T cell recognition of antigen. Prog Allergy 29:182, 1981.

Feeney AJ, et al: T helper cells required for the in vitro primary antibodies response to SRBC are neither SRBC-specific nor MHC restricted. J Mol Cell Immunol 1:211, 1984.

Haskins K, Kappler J, Marrack P: The major histocompatibility complex–restricted antigen receptor on T cells. Annu Rev Immunol 2:51, 1984.

Katz DH, Hamaoka T, Dorf ME, Benacerraf B: Cell interactions between histoincompatible T and B lymphocytes. The H-2 gene complex determines successful physiologic lymphocyte interactions. Proc Nat Acad Sci USA 70:2624–2628, 1973.

Malissen B, et al: Gene transfer of H_2 class II genes: antigen presentation by mouse fibroblast and hamster B cell lines. Cell 36:319, 1984.

Moller G (ed): Acquisition of the T cell repertoire. Immunol Rev 42, 1978.

Moller G (ed): Structure and function of HLA-DR. Immunol Rev 66, 1982.

Nagy Z, et al: Ia antigens as restriction molecules in Ir gene controlled T-cell proliferation. Immunol Rev 60:59, 1981.

Rosenthal AS, Shevach EM: Function of macrophages in antigen recognition by guinea pig T lymphocytes. I. Requirement for histocompatible macrophages and lymphocytes. J Exp Med 138:1194, 1974.

Santos GW: Adoptive transfer of immunologically competent cells. III. Comparative ability of allogenic and syngeneic spleen cells to produce a primary antibody response in the cyclophosphamide treated mouse. J Immunol 97:587, 1966.

Schrader SW: Mechanism of activation of the bone marrow–derived lymphocyte. III. A distinction between a macrophage-produced triggering signal and the amplifying affect on triggered B lymphocytes of allogeneic interaction. J Exp Med 138:1466, 1973.

Schwartz RH: T lymphocyte recognition of antigen in association with gene products of the major histocompatibility complex. Annu Rev Immunol 3:237, 1985.

Shih WH, et al: Analysis of histocompatibility requirements for proliferation and helper T cell activity. T cell population depleted of alloreactive cells by negative selection. J Exp Med 152:1311, 1980.

Singer A, Hathcock KS, Hodes RJ: Cellular and genetic control of antibody responses. V. Helper T cell recognition of H-2 determinants on accessory cells but not on B cells. J Exp Med 149:1208, 1979.

Zinkernagel RM, et al: On the thymus in the differentiation of "H-2 self-recognition" by T cells. Evidence for dual recognition. J Exp Med 147:882, 1978.

Control of Immune Response

See Chapter 11.

Asherson GL, Colizzi V, Zembala M: An overview of T-suppressor cell circuits. Annu Rev Immunol 4:37, 1986.

Dorf ME, Benacerraf B: Suppressor cells and immunoregulation. Annu Rev Immunol 2:127, 1984.

Gershon RK, et al: Suppressor T cells. J Immunol 108:586, 1972.

Gershon RK, et al: Contrasuppression: A normal immunoregulatory activity. J Exp Med 153:1533, 1981.

Green DR, Flood PM, Gershon R: Immunoregulatory T-cell pathways. Annu Rev Immunol 1:439,1983.

Greene MI, et al: Regulation of immunity to the azobenzenearsonate hapten. Adv Immunol 32:253, 1982.

Hamaoka T, Yoshizawa M, Yamamoto H, Kuroki M, Kitagawa M: Regulatory functions of hapten-reactive helper and suppressor T lymphocytes. II. Selective reactivation of hapten-reactive suppressor T cells by hapten-nonimmunogenic copolymers of C-amino acids, and its applications to the study of suppressor T-cell effect on helper T-cell development. J Exp Med 146:91, 1977.

Hausman PB, Sherr DH, Dorf ME: Anti-idiotypic B cells are required for induction of suppressor T cells. J Immunol 136:48, 1986.

Herzenberg LA, Tokuhisa T, Hayakawa K: Epitope specific regulation. Annu Rev Immunol 1:609, 1983.

Ishizaka K: Regulation of IgE synthesis. Annu Rev Immunol 2:159, 1984.

Jerne NK: The immune system: A network of V domains. Harvey Lect 70:93, 1975.

Katz DH: The allogeneic effect on immune responses: model for regulatory influences of T lymphocytes on the immune system. Transplant Rev 12:141, 1972.

Moller G (ed): Suppressor T lymphocytes. Transplant Rev 26, 1975.

Moller G (ed): Regulation of the immune response by antibodies against the immunogen. Immunol Rev 49, 1980.

Moller G (ed): Idiotype networks. Immunol Rev 79, 1984.

Rowley DA, Fitch FW, Stuart FP, Kohler H, Cosenza H: Specific suppression of immune responses. Science 181:1133, 1973.

Sterzl J: Factors and methods for the control of the immune response. *In* Rose N, et al (eds): International Convocation on Immunology. New York, Karger, 1969, p81.

Uhr JW, Moller G: Regulatory effect of antibody on the immune response. Adv Immunol 8:81, 1968.

Unanue EF: The regulatory role of macrophages in antigenic stimulation. Adv Immunol 15:95, 1972.

Unanue EF: The regulatory role of macrophages in antigenic stimulation. Part two: Symbiotic relationship between lymphocytes and macrophages. Adv Immunol 31:1, 1981.

Immune Memory

Bandilla KK, McDuffie FC, Gleich GJ: Immunoglobulin classes of antibodies produced in the primary and secondary responses in man. Clin Exp Immunol 5:627, 1969.

Celada F: Quantitative studies of the adaptive immunological memory in mice. II. Linear transmission of memory. J Exp Med 125:199, 1967.

Cerottini J-C, Trnka Z: The role of persisting antigen in the development of immunological memory. Int Arch Allergy 38:37, 1970.

Dutton DW, Eady JD: An in vitro system for the study of the mechanism of antigen stimulation in the secondary response. Immunology 7:40, 1964.

Fecsik AI, Butler WT, Coons AH: Studies on antibody production. XI. Variation in the secondary response as a function of the length of interval between the two antigenic stimuli. J Exp Med 12:1041, 1964.

Hege JS, Cole LJ: Antibody plaque-forming cells: kinetics of primary and secondary responses. J Immunol 96:559, 1966.

Jerne NK, et al: Plaque forming cells: methodology and theory. Transplant Rev 18:130, 1974.

Mason DW, Gowans J-L: Subpopulations of B lymphocytes and the carriage of immunological memory. Ann Inst Pasteur Ser C 127:657, 1976.

Nossal GJV, Austin CM, Ada GL: Antigens in immunity. VII. Analysis of immunological memory. Immunology 9:333, 1965.

Ovary Z, Benacerraf B: Immunological specificity of the secondary response with dinitrophenylated proteins. Proc Soc Exp Biol Med 114:72–76, 1963.

Paul WE, Siskind GW, Benacerraf B, Ovary Z: Secondary antibody responses in haptenic systems: cell population selection by antigen. J Immunol 99:760, 1967.

Sell S, Park AH, Nordin AA: Immunoglobulin classes of mouse antibody forming cells. I. Localized hemolysis-in-agar plaque forming cells belonging to five immunoglobulin classes. J Immunol 104:483, 1970.

Tada T, Takemori T, Okumura K, Nonaka M, Tokuhisa T: Two distinct types of helper T cells involved in the secondary response: independent and synergistic effects of Ia^- and Ia^+ helper T cells. J Exp Med 147:446, 1978.

Takaoki M: Transition in the character of immunological memory in mice after immunization. II. Memory in T and B cell populations. Jpn J Microbiol 20:475, 1976.

Tew JG, Mandel TE: The maintenance and regulation of serum antibody levels: evidence indicating a role for antigen in lymphoid follicles. J Immunol 120:1063, 1978.

Weigle WO: Cyclical production of antibody as a regulatory mechanism in the immune response. Adv Immunol 21:87, 1975.

The Immune System–Nervous System Relation

Adler R: Psychoneuroimmunology. Orlando, Fla., Academic Press, 1981.

Blalock JE, Bost KL, Smith EM: Neuroendocrine peptide hormones and their receptors in the immune system: production, processing and action. J Neuroimmunol 10:31, 1985.

Cohen N, Adler R: Antibodies and learning: a new dimension. *In* Sternberg CM, Lefkovits I (eds): The Immune System. Basel, Karger, 1981, p51.

Hall NR, et al: Immunoregulatory peptides and the central nervous system. Springer Semin Immunopathol 8:153, 1985.

Kerza-Kwiatecki AP: First international workshop on neuroimmunomodulation (NIM). J Neuroimmunol 10:9, 1985.

Livnat S, et al: Involvement of peripheral and central catecholamine systems in neuroimmune interactions. J Neuroimmunol 10:5, 1985.

Roszman TL, Brooks WH: Neural modulation of immune function. J Neuroimmunol 10:59, 1985.

Wybran J: Enkephalins and endorphins as modifiers of the immune system present and future. Fed Proc 44:92, 1985.

Theories of Antibody Formation

Burnet FM: Enzyme, Antigen, and Virus. London, Cambridge University Press, 1956.

Burnet FM: The Clonal Selection Theory of Acquired Immunity. London, Cambridge University Press, 1959.

Burnet FM: The Integrity of the Body: A Discussion of Modern Immunological Ideas. Cambridge, Harvard University Press, 1962.

Bretcher PA, Cohn M: A theory of self–non self discrimination. Science 189:1042, 1970.

Dreyer WJ, Bennett JC: The molecular basis of antibody formation: A paradox. Proc Nat Acad Sci USA 54:864, 1965.

Ehrlich P: An immunity with special reference to cell life. Proc Soc Lond [Biol] 66:424, 1900.

Finch LR: γ-Globulin operon: a hypothesis for the mechanism of the specific response in antibody synthesis. Nature 201:1288, 1964.

Habe E: Recovery of antigenic specificity of denaturation and complete reduction of disulphides in a papain fragment of antibody. Proc Nat Acad Sci USA 52:1099, 1964.

Haurowitz F: Antibody formation and the coding problem. Nature 205:847, 1965.

Hood L, Talmadge DW: Mechanisms of antibody diversity: germ line basis for variability. Science 168:325, 1970.

Jerne NK: The natural selection theory of antibody formation. Proc Nat Acad Sci USA 41:849, 1955.

Jerne NK: The somatic generation of immune recognition. Eur J Immunol 1:1, 1971.

Landsteiner K: The specificity of serological reactions, 2nd ed. Cambridge, Harvard University Press, 1945.

Lederberg IS: Genes and antibodies. Science 129:1649, 1959.

Pauling LA: A theory of the structure and process of formation of antibodies. J Am Chem Soc 62:2643, 1940.

Perlmann GE, Diringer R: The structure of proteins. Annu Rev Biochem 29:151, 1960.

Schweet R, Owen RD: Concepts of protein synthesis in relation to antibody formation. J Cell Physiol (Suppl) 50(1):199, 1957.

Smith T: Active immunity produced by so-called balanced or neutral mixtures of diphtheria toxin and anti-toxin. J Exp Med 11:241, 1909.

Smithies O, Poulik MD: Initiation of protein synthesis at an unusual position in an immunoglobulin gene. Science 175:187, 1972.

Szilard L: The molecular basis of antibody formation. Proc Nat Acad Sci USA 46:293, 1960.

Talmadge DW, Perlman DS: The antibody response: a model based on the antagonistic actions of antigen. J Theor Biol 5:321, 1963.

11 Immune Tolerance and Autoimmunity

The exposure of a responsive individual to a potential immunogen may result in an immune response or it may not. It is critical that an individual respond to foreign antigens for protection, but not to self antigens. Thus, exposure to foreign antigens should elicit immunity; exposure to self antigens should not. The lack of an immune response to a specific antigen when responses to other antigens are retained is termed *immune tolerance*. Tolerance is a specific example of the effect of control mechanisms on the immune response. Tolerance has been one of the most controversial areas in immunology and remains a phenomenon that must be explained by any theories of immunity. Sir MacFarlane Burnet first postulated immune tolerance to explain why an individual does not normally make an immune response to his own tissues, although his macromolecules may be immunogenic when they are given to a different individual. He further explained immune tolerance as a means of recognition of "self" and "nonself." He considered the mechanism of immune self recognition as not innate, but a process of maturation; that is, tolerance is acquired somatically. Loss of tolerance to self antigens would lead to the production of autoantibodies and autoimmune disease; thus the other side of the tolerance coin is autoimmunity (see below).

Natural Tolerance

Natural tolerance was postulated to develop during fetal life, when the individual does not yet have the capacity to produce an immune response. Contact with antigens at this time would affect the maturation of the immune system so that recognition of antigen and reaction of immune mechanisms to the antigen would not develop. Under usual conditions during intrauterine embryonic development the fetus contacts only its own antigens and therefore develops immune tolerance to them. However, Burnet predicted that if a foreign antigen were presented to the fetus before or during maturation of its immune system, specific immune tolerance could be produced to this antigen as well.

Burnet's theories were largely stimulated by Ray Owen's demonstration of tolerance to foreign antigens in dizygotic twins of cattle. Such twins are genetically different, but have a common circulation during fetal life so that there is a continuous exchange of proteins and blood cells. When mature, these twins tolerate and do not manifest an immune response to each other's antigens, although they display normal immunity to antigens that are foreign to both. Since Owen's observation, many other instances of immune tolerance to foreign antigens have been produced in experimental animals. Sir Peter Medawar demonstrated that if a potential foreign immunogen is introduced into an animal early in its life, instead of producing antibody or sensitized cells the animal develops specific immune tolerance to it. Upon second contact with the same antigen at an age when an immune response would be expected, the tolerant animal does not respond.

The successful induction of neonatal tolerance was demonstrated for foreign cells by Rupert Billingham. States of tolerance can be most easily induced in fetal and neonatal animals until a few days after birth. This is known as the "window" of tolerance induction. A few days after birth, exposure to an antigen no longer induces tolerance. At the same time it is known that in some circumstances the fetal animal can make an immune response to many antigens. As is discussed below, the induction of tolerance or immunity depends on a number of variables, but in general tolerance is much more readily induced in fetal than in adult animals. The induction of tolerance to self antigens is believed to take place during maturation of lymphoid cells, in both the fetus and the adult. In this chapter some of the characteristics of tolerance are described, and then the hypothetical mechanisms of tolerance and autoimmunity, as well as the breaking of tolerance, are presented. A single mechanism does not explain all the characteristics of the different states of tolerance. Different mechanisms may be responsible for different tolerance phenomena. Immune tolerance to nonself antigens is called *acquired* tolerance, in contrast to the developmental phenomenon of natural tolerance to self antigens.

Acquired Tolerance

A number of factors determine the type and extent of an immune response, because of activation of negative or positive arms of the immune response control system (see Chapter 10). Some of the factors include the age and immune status of the responding animal, the properties of the antigen (e.g., molecular weight, number of repeating units, solubility), the antigen dose and route of exposure, the genetic makeup of the responding animal, and the number of previous exposures to the same antigen or structurally related antigens. Because of these variables, a given individual may produce different amounts of different classes of antibody and different degrees of cellular reactivity or suppressor activity to the same antigen. Tolerance may be instituted in an adult animal by contact with antigen after exposure to systemic immunosuppressive events, such as the administration of irradiation or large doses of antimetabolic agents. An antigen that induces tolerance is called a tolerogen; the same antigen presented in different circumstances may stimulate an immune response (immunogen). A strong immunogen is by definition a poor tolerogen and vice versa. Some of the characteristics of the acquired tolerant state that have been discovered from experimental work are the following:

1. Tolerance is most easily induced by antigens that are closely related to those of the host; induction of the tolerant state becomes more difficult as the complexity and the number of antigenic determinants of the antigen increase. In other words, the ability to induce acquired tolerance to a given antigen is inversely related to the degree of immunogenicity of the antigen (Table 11-1).

Table 11-1. Relation of Degree of Immunogenicity to Source and Complexity of Antigen

Complexity of Antigen	Autogeneic (Same Individual)	Syngeneic (Genetically Identical Individual)	Allogeneic (Different Individual, Same Species)	Xenogeneic (Different Species)
Serum proteins	0	0	±[b]	++
Altered serum proteins[a]	+	+	+	++
Erythrocytes	0	0	++	++++
Tissue grafts	0	0	+++	+++++

0, no response; ±, inconsistent response, + weak response, ++ through +++++, rough indication of degree of immunogenicity.
[a] Denatured or conjugated with haptens.
[b] An immune response may occur to some serum proteins (see Allotypes, Chapter 6).

2. Tolerance is of finite duration, and the duration of the tolerant state depends upon the continued presence of antigen. Newborn rabbits made tolerant to an antigen so that no immune response can be elicited at 4 months of age may have an immune response to the same antigen at 12 months of age. If such animals are given repeated doses of the antigen, they remain tolerant at 12 months of age.
3. Either very high or very low doses of antigen may induce tolerance to an antigen that will elicit an antibody response when an intermediate dose is used (high- and low-dose tolerance).
4. The state of tolerance may be terminated by injection of

antigens that contain antigenic determinants (specificities) in common with the antigen to which the individual is tolerant but also contain antigenic determinants to which the same individual is not tolerant.

5. Both T cells and B cells may be made tolerant (Fig. 11-1). T

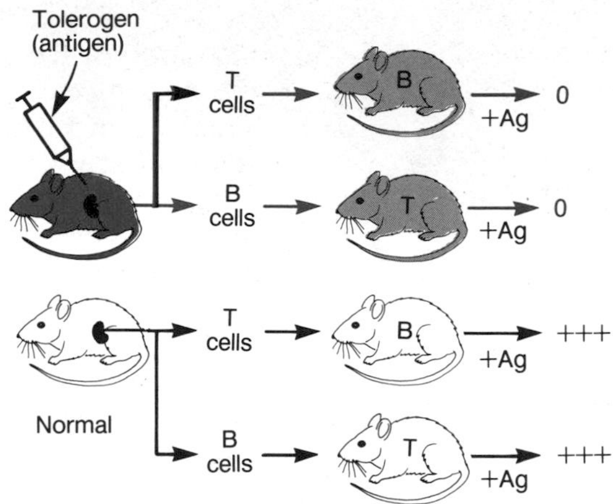

Figure 11-1. Demonstration of tolerance in T and B cells. Spleen cells from mice tolerant to a specific antigen are separated into T cells (nylon wool passage) and B cells (survive antithymocyte treatment). The T cells are injected into B cell mice (adult thymectomized, irradiated, and restored with normal bone marrow cells) and the B cells into T cell mice (irradiated and restored with normal thymus cells). Upon challenge with antigen (Ag), neither reconstituted mouse responds. However, injection of T or B cells from normal mice into B or T cell animals results in a responding animal. In addition, challenge with an antigen unrelated to the tolerogen results in an immune response to this second antigen. Similar results are obtained in vitro, when T or B cells from a tolerant animal are mixed with B or T cells from a normal animal.

cells are made tolerant for long periods of time by low doses of antigen, whereas B cells require higher doses of antigen. Tolerance of either T or B cells leads to tolerance in the animal. However, the B cells "recover" or are replaced by new B cells after a relatively short time, whereas T cells may remain tolerant for longer periods. B cells are more easily made tolerant early in development, at the stage when surface IgM first appears, than at later stages of maturation.

6. Transfer of cells from a tolerant donor to a normal syngeneic host may confer specific tolerance in the recipient. This effect is not produced if the T cells of the donor are killed prior to transfer. Cells transferred from a tolerant donor animal to an irradiated host (e.g., an animal whose own immune system has been destroyed) restore the general immune responsive state of the irradiated animal, except that tolerance to the specific antigen to which the original donor of the cells was tolerant is also transferred (adoptive tolerance).

The breaking of self tolerance by related antigens can be explained by a two-cell system (Fig. 11-2). Antigens that cross-

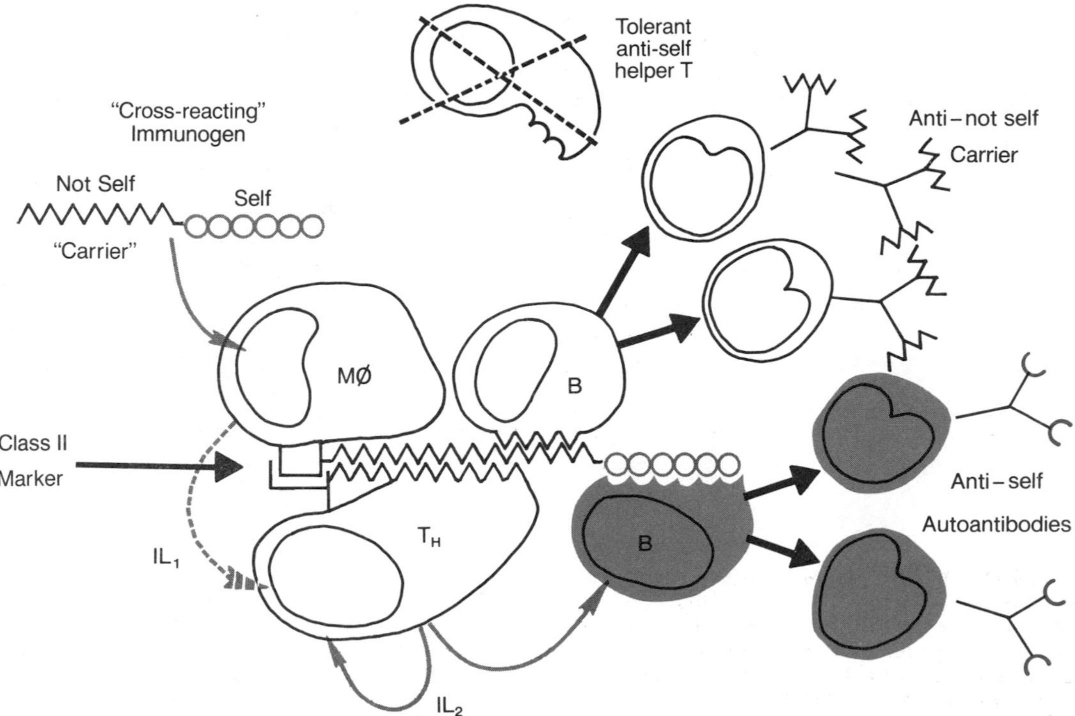

Figure 11-2. Interplay of T and B cells in "breaking" of B cell tolerance to self antigens. The immunogen contains two types of determinants: one set of foreign (nonself) determinants and one set of self determinants. T and B cells, each required for maximum primary antibody responses, contain individual cells or populations of cells that separately recognize these different determinants. Both T and B cells can become tolerant to these antigens, but experimental data show that T cells are made tolerant for much longer periods. Thus, recovery of responsiveness of B cells to self antigens may occur rapidly. However, T cells are needed to provide helper function to B cells for antibody production to occur. If an immunogen contains both self and foreign antigens, T cells specific for the foreign determinant can provide helper function for both self and foreign antigens to B cells. Thus, antibodies to both self and foreign antigens are produced.

react (i.e., contain some determinants in common) with the antigen used to induce tolerance are processed by the antigen-presenting macrophage and presented to cells that specifically recognize the foreign immunogenic epitopes of the antigen. These recognition cells are able to induce a response in self reacting responsive precursor lines that have recovered from the tolerant state. The recovery of cells from a tolerant state may result from the ongoing development from uncommitted stem cells of cells with the ability to react with the specific antigen, the resynthesis of receptor sites by cells whose sites have been blocked or destroyed, or the removal of some block to the development of a potentially reactive cell. T cells and B cells may become tolerant or lose tolerance as a result of different mechanisms.

Mechanisms of Tolerance

Tolerance may involve either positive or negative control systems entailing the interaction of cells during induction of an immune response. For many years the explanation of tolerance was based on the clonal selection of Burnet. Although this theory may still explain some types of tolerance, more recent studies have identified tolerant situations that require a different explanation. In general, tolerance may be explained by clonal deletion/anergy or by complex immunoregulatory systems involving suppressor T cells or antibody inhibition pathways. Six general mechanisms of immune tolerance are presented: clonal elimination/anergy, suppressor T cells, natural suppressor cells, blocking antibody, idiotype network, and antigen catabolism (processing).

Clonal Elimination/ Clonal Anergy

The clonal selection theory of Burnet postulates that the ability of an individual to recognize an immunogen lies in individual reactive cells or cell lines (clones) (Fig. 11-3). Upon contact with the antigen, the cells with the capacity to recognize the antigen are stimulated to multiply and differentiate. The property of antigen recognition is restricted in the sense that each reactive cell recognizes only one antigen. In fetal life or in special situations in adults, contact of the reacting cell with antigen causes the elimination of this cell and, therefore, loss of the ability of the individual to make an immune response to that antigen (tolerance). The death or loss of immunologically reactive precursor cells upon contact of these cells with the individual's own tissues in fetal life results in the establishment of natural tolerance. In adult animals, the establishment of acquired tolerance may be preceded by a brief period of antibody production. This is explained by antigen-driven differentiation leading to depletion of antigen recognition cells (exhaustive differentiation). The clonal selection theory of tolerance is unable to explain the observation that tolerance is often easily broken. Such experiments indicate that acquired tolerance depends not on the loss of immunologically reactive precursor cells but on an altered reactivity of cells that can be redirected to immune responsiveness by certain procedures. Thus, acquired tolerance is most likely due not to the elimination or failure of development of specifically reactive cells but to blocking of expression or temporary inactivation of cells required for a specific response, that is, *clonal anergy*.

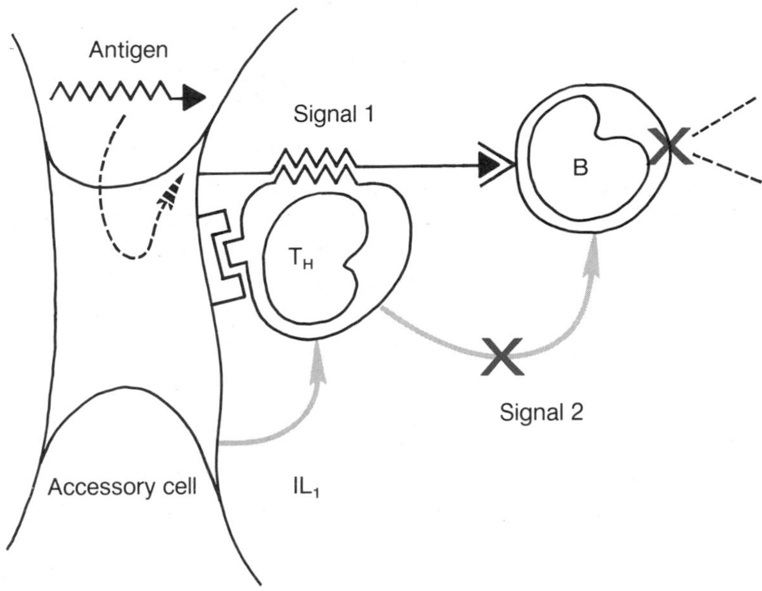

Figure 11-3. Clonal elimination or anergy. In this model of tolerance the responding immune cells are either eliminated or rendered inert. As depicted in this figure, B cells require at least two signals to be stimulated to proliferate. Signal 1 is provided by contact with antigen and signal 2 by factors (IL2, BCGF, etc.) produced by T helper cells. If the B cell receives the antigenic first signal in the absence of the second signal, it may be made tolerant. B cells are most easily made tolerant when they are in an immature (surface IgM only) IgD negative state. A similar mechanism may function if thymocytes or pre-T cells contact self antigens in the thymus while in an immature state. T cells require contact with antigen (signal 1), activation by IL1 (signal 2), and autostimulation by IL1 (signal 3). If T cells make contact with antigen without processing by macrophages or in the absence of IL1 or IL2 production, it is possible that elimination rather than stimulation may occur.

Suppressor Cells

The first clues to the presence of suppressor T cells came with the observations of Richard Gershon concerning the effects of transfer of normal or immune cells to tolerant hosts and of tolerant cells to normal hosts of the same MHC type. Gershon found that tolerance could be passively transferred using T cells from tolerant animals. This phenomenon was termed *infectious tolerance* and strongly implied a role for suppressor T cells in the induction and maintenance of tolerance (Fig. 11-4).

A number of additional findings support a role for suppressor T cells in controlling the response of B cells: (1) An increase in antibody production may be obtained after thymectomy. (2) Thymocytes from rats treated with antigen 48 hours previously, when transferred to syngeneic recipients, may specifically suppress the response of the recipients to the same antigen. (3) Anti-T cell treatment of young NZB mice increases the antibody response to certain antigens, but this effect is not seen in older NZB mice who may have lost their suppressor T

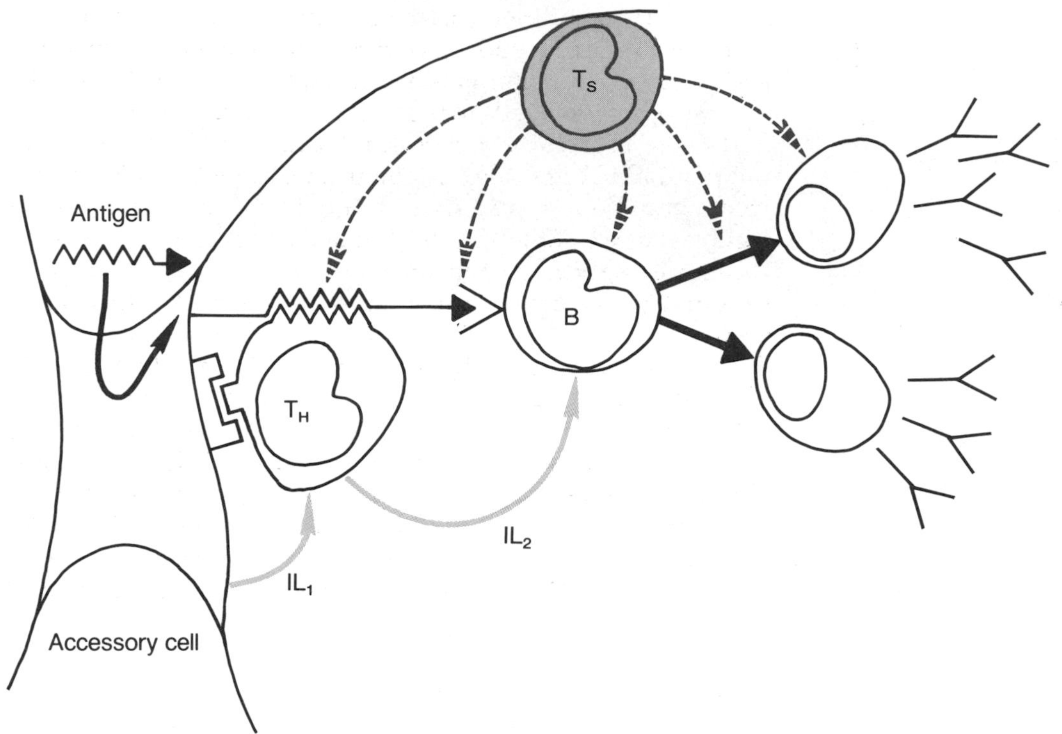

Figure 11-4. T suppressor cells and tolerance. During an immune response, T helper/inducer cells activate not only B cells but also T suppressor cells. T suppressor cells produce an antigen-specific factor that can act at the T_H or B cell level to inhibit the immune response to that antigen only.

cell population and thus become prone to development of certain "autoallergic" diseases. (4) Lymphocytes from mice with chronic suppression of a given immunoglobulin allotype suppress expression of that allotype on normal cells in vitro or upon passive transfer into a normal host. (5) Lymphocytes stimulated by certain mitogens, such as concanavalin A, inhibit the immune response of normal cells. (6) Removal of the bursa of Fabricius in chickens may lead to the appearance of T cells that suppress IgA- or IgG-bearing B cells. Each of these observations supports the concept that a certain population of T cells controls the response of B cells. The mechanism through which T cells suppress the response of B cells is unclear. Suppressor T cells may prevent presentation of antigen, block the function of T helper cells, inhibit proliferation of B cells, or block the differentiation of B cells to antibody-secreting plasma cells.

Suppressor T cells may also limit the activity of other T cells. The part of the T cell population that exerts a suppressor effect is probably about 10% to 20%. Certain T cells inhibit mixed lymphocyte reactions and the blastogenic response to mitogens such as phytohemagglutinin or to specific antigens. In addition, treatment of recipient rats with antithymocyte serum (ATS) may increase the severity of a graft versus host reaction produced upon transfer of thymus cells. Since the graft versus host reaction is T cell mediated, the ATS may depress suppressor T cells of the host that control the graft versus host cells. Therefore, suppressor T cells may function in the tolerant animal and may be the primary mechanism for preventing antibody production by B cells or cellular immunologic reaction by other T cells. When the suppressor T cells are specific for a given antigen, the immune response to other antigens may be normal in animals rendered tolerant by this mechanism.

In a mouse model, Ig class–specific T_S cells that act only on B cells for IgE have also been identified. After immunization with antigen in complete Freund's adjuvant, a population of T_S cells in the spleen (pass through nylon wool, killed by anti-Thy + C) inhibits the production of IgE by primed B cells, but does not affect IgG production to the same antigen. These T_S cells produce a soluble factor when exposed to specific antigen that acts only on B cells of the IgE class (Fig. 11-5). This model,

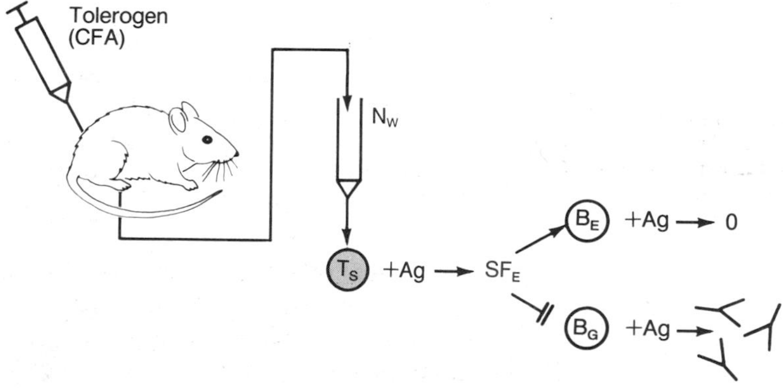

Figure 11-5. Demonstration of suppressor T cell factor specific for IgE antibody. T suppressor cells obtained by passage over nylon wool of spleen cells from animals immunized with antigen in complete Freund's adjuvant produce a suppressor factor (SF_e) that specifically inhibits B cells from making IgE antibody when the B cells are reexposed to the same antigen, but has no effect on B cells having the capacity to make IgG antibody to the same antigen.

if applicable to man, could have far-reaching implications in regard to specific immunotherapy for IgE-mediated allergic reactions.

The properties of a population of suppressor cells known as *natural* suppressor cells are listed in Table 11-2. Natural suppressor cells are active upon T cell–mediated reactions primarily to MHC alloantigens, but are not antigen specific. Such cells could be responsible for both neonatal tolerance and tolerance in immunosuppressed adults. These cells are null cells in the large granular lymphocyte population. In irradiated adults, there seems to be a short-lived reappearance of natural

Table 11-2. Properties of Natural Suppressor Cells

Found in fetal and neonatal animals
Disappear a few days after birth
Activity demonstrable in irradiated adults
Not induced by antigen
Not antigen specific
Suppress:
Mixed lymphocyte reactions
Generation of T_K cells
Graft versus host reactions
Have neither T nor B markers
Are large granular lymphocytes
Do not suppress B cells

suppressor cells and, later, the presence of an antigen-specific T suppressor cell that can be induced upon exposure to antigen shortly after irradiation. This latter T suppressor cell may be important in prolonging suppression to host (recipient) tissue and modifying graft versus host disease if allogeneic cells such as bone marrow cells are transferred to an adult after irradiation.

Blocking Antibody

Earlier, it was pointed out that specific antibody may act through a feedback mechanism to limit the production of specific antibody and to control the extent of an immune response. During the induction of tolerance, a phase of antibody production sometimes occurs prior to the establishment of the tolerant state. It is tenuous to postulate that such blocking antibody can induce tolerance, as it is impossible to induce adoptive tolerance by passive transfer with antiserum.

However, the extent of an immune response might be limited by feedback inhibition of antibody production (see Chapter 10). Conflicting evidence exists regarding whether this inhibition acts on accessory macrophages, T cells, B cells, or some interaction step (Fig. 11-6). It has been suggested that the immunological activities of T cells can be blocked by antigen–antibody complexes. Although there is little concrete evidence to support this, it is possible that antigen–antibody complexes could bind to the surface receptors of helper T cells in such a way as to block reaction with free antigen and prevent helper function. Such blocking effects of antibody–antigen complexes have been postulated as preventing tumor and tissue graft rejection.

Idiotype Network

Each antibody variable region itself might be the antigen recognized by a series of autoantibodies that suppress the specific immune response (auto-anti-idiotype network) (Fig. 11-7). T cells as well as specific antibodies may have idiotypic determinants and may be subject to regulation by anti-idiotypes. Anti-idiotype sera are able to block T cell functions in some

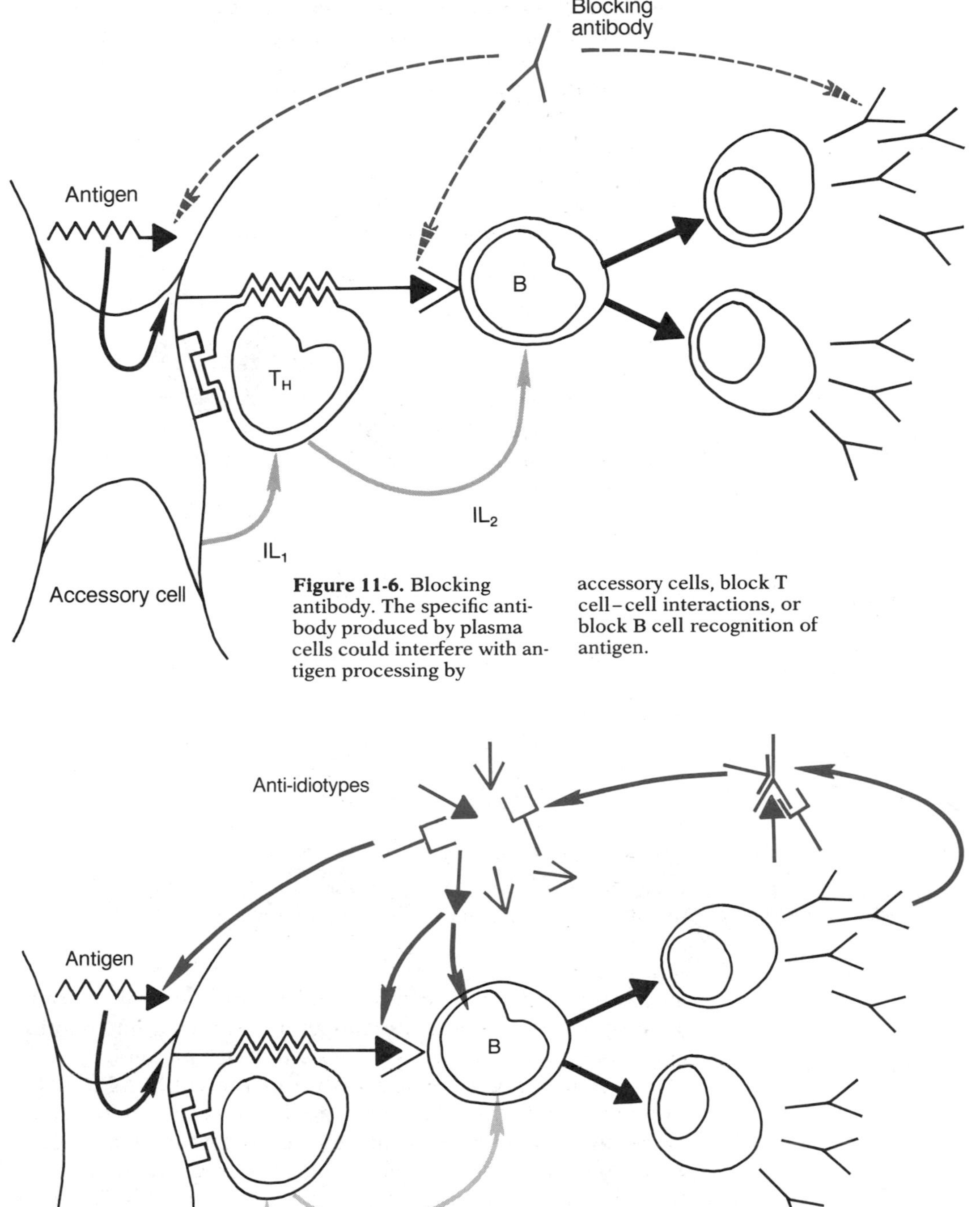

Figure 11-6. Blocking antibody. The specific antibody produced by plasma cells could interfere with antigen processing by accessory cells, block T cell–cell interactions, or block B cell recognition of antigen.

Figure 11-7. Anti-idiotypes and tolerance. The production of anti-idiotypic antibody to the antibody may block antigen processing, T helper–T cell–B cell cooperation, or B cell response to the antigen.

experimental systems. It is postulated that the presence of small amounts of such anti-idiotypes (undetectable by most techniques) is responsible for maintenance of self tolerance in some systems. (See also Chapter 10.)

Antigen Catabolism

The tolerant state may be established because of the inability of the affected animal to metabolize the antigen properly for antigen presentation, so that the stimulation necessary for a specific immune response is not made available (Fig. 11-8). Such

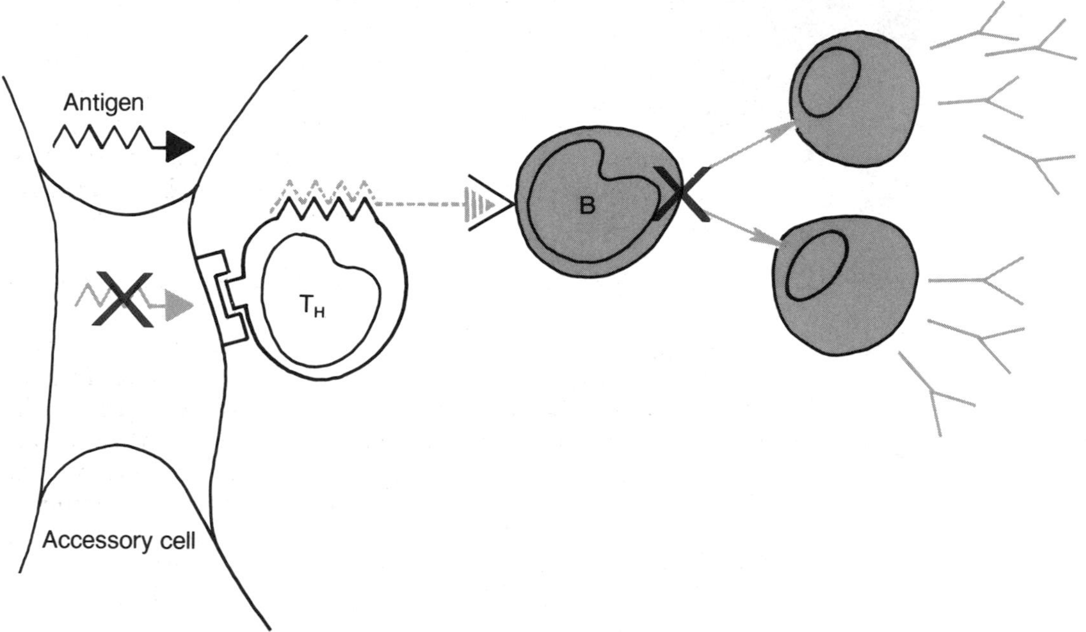

Figure 11-8. The tolerogenic effect of unprocessed antigen. If B cells or T cells are exposed directly to unprocessed antigens in the absence of antigen-presenting cells, class II MHC, or IL1, they may not respond to the specific antigens. Tolerance could be broken when the antigen processing mechanism is mature.

ineffective antigen processing could be due to a failure of the macrophage to process the antigen to immunogenic peptides expressed in association with class II MHC markers.

Tolerance may be a function of the cell type that first contacts the antigen. According to this concept, the induction of an immune response requires the processing of antigen by macrophages, which prepares the antigen for recognition by specific immunologically reactive T and/or B cells. Direct interaction of the unprocessed antigen with the specific reactive cells may result in the loss of the ability of these cells to be immunologically stimulated (tolerance). The processing of immunogen by macrophages is an immunologically nonspecific event, but the loss of recognition by specifically reactive lymphocytes results in antigen-specific tolerance.

Summary

There is no single explanation for all of the natural and experimental phenomena that are grouped under the umbrella of tolerance. Different mechanisms may explain different phenomena, or more than one mechanism may be operative in a given situation. Different cells with the capacity to respond to a specific antigen (immunologically competent cells) may undergo induction upon contact with the antigen: this may result in immunity (antibody-producing plasma cells or sensitized lymphocytes), immune memory, or tolerance. The outcome depends on the dose and type of antigen and on the state of the potentially responding individual. It is also possible that some reactive cells are killed by reaction with tolerogen or that an immunogen may be presented in a nonimmunogenic manner, causing tolerance. However, tolerance is best considered as an active process involving the production of tolerant cells that cannot respond to an immunogen, suppressor cells, or antibodies that inhibit potentially responding cells.

Split Tolerance and Immune Deviation

Split tolerance refers to the lack of response to an antigen as measured by one type of effector mechanism, while another effector arm is quite active. In some human infectious diseases, individuals may demonstrate high antibody titers but little or no cellular immunity (and vice versa) to the antigens of the infecting agent. In leprosy and chronic mucocutaneous candidiasis, good cellular response with low or no antibody responses is associated with effective protective immunity, whereas high antibody titers and low cellular responses are associated with progressive infection.

Immune deviation refers to the changing of one type of immune response to another. Effective therapy for leprosy is associated with a change from hormonal to cellular immunity. Therapy for IgE-mediated allergic reactions may be effected by changing the predominant antibody response from one immunoglobulin class (IgE) to another (IgG) by repeated antigenic challenge.

Immune Paralysis

An effect similar to tolerance may be induced by injection of moderate amounts of nondegradable antigen (Felton's immunological paralysis) (Fig. 11-9). In such cases, antibody-producing cells may be identified if they are removed from the animal, but secreted antibody is rapidly bound to the circulating antigen. Usually antigens bound to antibody (complexes) are taken up by macrophages (phagocytosis), and both antigen and antibody are degraded. With an undegradable antigen, only the antibody is destroyed and the antigen is released so that it may again combine with antibody. Thus, any antibody formed is removed rapidly by antigen so that circulating antibody is not detectable. This "paralysis" of antibody by antigen has been likened to a treadmill.

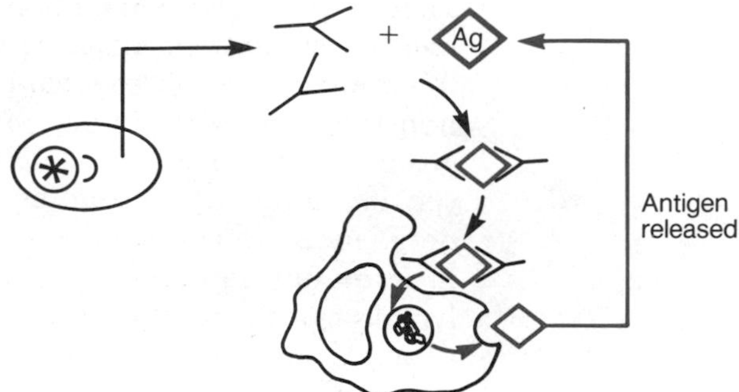

Figure 11-9. Immune paralysis. Immune paralysis refers to the consumption of antibody by poorly degradable antigens. The antibodies produced after injection of such an antigen react with the antigen to form antibody–antigen complexes. These complexes are taken up by the reticuloendothelial system (macrophages), where the antibody is catabolized but the antigen is released into the circulation system. In this manner, the antigen continues to react with and remove antibody so that titers of circulating antibody may not be demonstrable.

Desensitization

Therapeutic "hyposensitization" may involve tolerance, immune deviation, or *desensitization.* Desensitization is a temporary state of unresponsiveness in an already immunized animal, induced by relatively large doses of degradable antigen administered in such a way as to be relatively innocuous. Desensitization occurs as a result of combination between antigen and antibody; the specific antibody or sensitized cells are exhausted by reaction with the specific antigen. This is similar to the effect observed in immunological paralysis. However, since the antigen is degradable, resynthesis of antibody or re-formation of sensitized cells will result in the desensitized state being overcome, usually in a few days, with restoration of the immune state of the treated individual. The duration of the desensitized state depends on the rate at which the desensitized individual is producing the specific antibody or specifically sensitized cells and on the amount of antigen used for desensitization. Desensitization must be differentiated from clinical hyposensitization, which most likely is dependent upon a different mechanism.

Tolerance and Immunity

Immune tolerance may be a more common or more natural state than immune reactivity. An individual is likely to be presented with small amounts of antigen (everyday contact with nonpathogenic organisms) or very high and continued doses of antigen (an individual's own serum proteins), in a manner more conducive to the production of tolerance than to the production of active immunity. The immunologist has worked most often in dose ranges likely to result in active immunity and commonly uses nonspecific adjuvants to enhance immune responses. These adjuvants generally have the effect of mobilizing lymphoid cells and concentrating reactive cells at the site of antigen deposition; a similar effect would occur in the case of an infection with an organism capable of producing an inflammatory response. The role of tolerance or lack of tolerance is important in the understanding of autoimmune diseases and transplantation.

Autoimmunity

Specific immune tolerant states provide mechanisms whereby an immune response to self antigens, *autoimmunity,* is prevented. Thus, establishment of tolerance to self antigens could be considered the natural state for self antigens. Autoimmunity may then be defined as a loss of tolerance to self antigens. With recognition of the destructive power of the immune system when directed to specific antigens, it becomes obvious that an immune response to one's own antigens could be disastrous. At the end of the last century Paul Ehrlich coined the term *horror autotoxicus* for such circumstances. However, we now know that autoimmune responses are in fact quite common. Autoantibodies can be found in many normal individuals and increase in frequency with aging. In the 1960s Pierre Grabar hypothesized that autoantibodies might be important for reacting with and causing the elimination of defective or denatured molecules. Antibody-excess immune complexes are cleared rapidly by the reticuloendothelial system (see Chapter 12). Thus autoantibodies could act as carrier molecules to clear the body of effete molecules.

The reality of the situation actually lies somewhere between horror autotoxicus and garbage collection. We now know that many diseases are attributable to an autoimmune response, whereas, on the other hand, many otherwise healthy individuals may have detectable autoantibodies in their blood. The ability to induce tolerance is related to two major factors: the degree of complexity of the antigen and the amount of antigen present (see Table 11-1). The relationship of concentration of serum proteins to the incidence of autoantibodies (B cells) or autoreactive T cells to these proteins as seen by William Weigle is illustrated in Figure 11-10. As shown, autoreactivity to some determinants such as IgG idiotypes occurs naturally and may be physiological. Autoantibodies are found to a variety of other serum proteins less frequently. Autoreactive T cells occur much less frequently and may be associated with tissue lesions (thyroglobulin — thyroiditis; myelin basic protein — encephalomyelitis). Polyclonal activation of B cells may result in a number of autoantibodies. In most instances, these are of low avidity and are not associated with tissue lesions (see below).

Autoantibodies and Autoallergic Disease

A number of antibodies to tissue or serum antigens have been observed in the sera of human patients with certain diseases (Table 11-3).

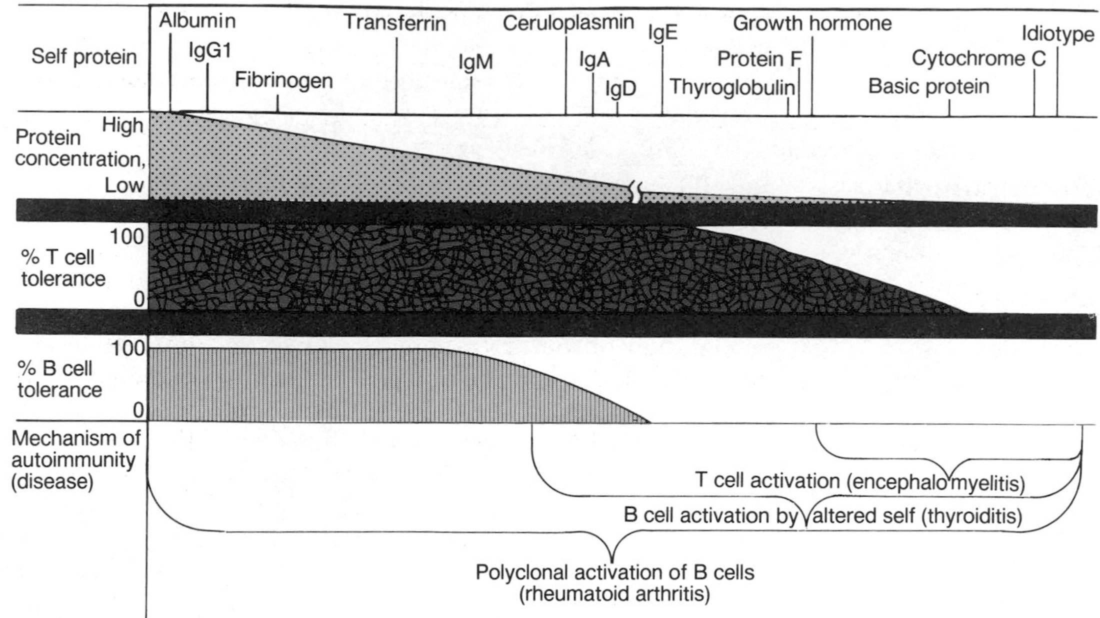

Figure 11-10. Theoretical relationship between serum protein concentration and degree of T and B cell tolerance.

Autoantibodies to cardiac muscle may be demonstrated in some patients following myocardial infarction. The induction of these antibodies may be due to alteration of myocardial antigens secondary to necrosis; the antibodies found react (? cross-react) with normal myocardial antigens. It is not likely that these antibodies play a role in the original infarction, but they have been implicated in the postinfarction syndrome, and autoantibodies to the conductive tissue of the heart (Purkinje's fibers) may be responsible for chronic heart block. Henry Kaplan has shown that there are antigens of group A streptococci that cross-react with cardiac tissue. The occurrence of this type of antibody suggests that an appropriate streptococcal infection may break tolerance to normal cardiac tissue antigens (see Fig. 11-2), with the resulting autoallergic reaction and production of rheumatic fever. Autoantibodies are also found after cardiopulmonary bypass perfusion or massive blood transfusion.

The significance of most autoantibodies is unknown. In some cases, but certainly not all, a pathogenic function has been convincingly demonstrated. Antinuclear antibody in lupus erythematosus, rheumatoid factor in rheumatoid arthritis, antiacetylcholine receptor in myasthenia gravis, anti-

Table 11-3. Some Human Diseases in Which Serum Antibodies to Serum or Tissue Antigens Have Been Found by Various Methods

Disease	Antigen	Method of Antibody Detection
Addison's disease, idiopathic	Adrenal	CF, F
Dermatitis, chronic	Dermis	F, A
Glomerulonephritis, poststreptococcal	Kidney	CF, F, H, A
Other kidney diseases	Kidney	F, A
Viral hepatitis	Liver, spleen, smooth muscle	CF, F, H, A, P
Cirrhosis of liver	Liver, spleen, kidney	CF, F, H, A
Lung diseases (emphysema, asthma, tuberculosis)	Lung	CF, GC, P
Lupus erythematosus	Liver, spleen, kidney, muscle, platelets, blood cells, nucleoprotein, RNA, DNA, histone	CF, F, A
Multiple sclerosis	Brain or white matter	CF, tissue culture demyelination
Carcinomatous neuropathy	Neurons	F, CF (gray, white)
Other CNS diseases (cerebrovascular accident)	Brain	CF
Myasthenia gravis	Muscle, thymus, thyroid	CF, F, H, GC
Myocardial infarction	Heart	H, P
Orchitis, infertility	Sperm	A
Pancreatitis, chronic cystic fibrosis	Pancreas glandular epithelium	P, H
Pernicious anemia	Intrinsic factor, parietal cell microsomes	CF, F, inhibition
Atrophic gastritis	Gastric mucosa	
Rheumatic fever	Heart, muscle, joint	CF, F, H, GC
		P, H, A
Rheumatoid arthritis	Heart, muscle, joint, subcutaneous nodules, aggregated γ-globulin	
Scleroderma, dermatomyositis	Kidney, muscle, joint, cell nuclei	F
Sjögren's syndrome	Salivary gland, liver, kidney, thyroid cell nuclei	CF, P, F, H
Syphilis	Wassermann antigen	CF, A
Thyroiditis, myxedema, thyrotoxicosis	Thyroglobulin, globular epithelium, gastric mucosa cell nuclei	P, CF, H, F
Ulcerative colitis	Mucosal glands, mucus	CF, F, H, P
Uveal injury	Uveal pigment	CF

A, agglutination of other antigen-coated particles; CF, complement fixation; CNS, central nervous system; F, fluorescent antibody fixation; GC, antiglobulin consumption; H, hemagglutination, passive; P, precipitation.

(Modified from Waksman, BH: Medicine, 41:93, 1963. Copyright 1962, The Williams & Wilkins Co.)

erythrocyte antibody in autoallergic hemolytic anemia, and antiheart antibody in rheumatic fever are almost certainly significant in the etiology of these autoallergic diseases. Other autoantibodies are characteristic of a specific disease entity and are useful diagnostic aids but are without obvious roles in causation of the disease. Antibodies that bind to hepatocytic mitochrondria may be detected by the fluorescent antibody technique in the sera of patients with primary biliary cirrhosis and chronic active hepatitis, but not in the sera of patients with other forms of cirrhosis or extrahepatic biliary obstruction. One is left with the explanation that many autoantibodies are more likely to be the result than the cause of tissue alteration or breakdown.

Criteria for Identification of Autoimmunity

There are certain characteristics, ideally identifiable in all immune responses, that should be sought in diseases of suspected autoimmune etiology. These include (1) a well-defined immunizing event (infection, immunization, vaccination), (2) a latent period (usually 6–14 days), (3) a secondary response (a more rapid and more intense reaction on second exposure to the antigen), (4) an ability to transfer the sensitive state with cells or serum from an affected individual to a normal individual, (5) a specific depression of the sensitive state by large amounts of antigen (desensitization), (6) identification and isolation of the antigen in a pure form, and (7) chemical characterization of the antigen. All, or even a few, of these criteria can rarely, if ever, be established for human diseases. The criteria are most closely approximated in certain blood dyscrasias such as autoimmune hemolytic anemia. However, these criteria can be met in experimental models that mimic human diseases.

Presumptive findings consistent with, but not strong evidence for, an allergic mechanism in disease states include (1) a morphologic picture consistent with known allergic reactions; (2) demonstration of specific antibody or of a positive delayed skin reaction; (3) depression of complement during some stage of the disease; (4) beneficial effect of agents known to inhibit some portion of an allergic reaction (steroids, radiation, cyclosporine); (5) identification of a reasonable experimental model in animals that mimics the human disease; (6) association with other possible autoallergic diseases; and (7) increased familial susceptibility to the same disease or other autoallergic diseases.

Theories of Autoimmunization

1. The tissues involved in autoallergic diseases are derived from ectoderm or endoderm and are regarded as foreign by the immune apparatus, which is mesodermal. These autoantigens are substances that are absent or sequestered during

the immune neutral period of development and, therefore, fail to induce tolerance like other body antigens. Blood–tissue barriers normally prevent these antigens from reaching the circulation and the immune apparatus. When viral infection, injury, or other episodes cause breakdown of blood–tissue barriers and release of these sequestered antigens into circulation, an allergic reaction may occur.

2. Viral infections or other events cause alteration of tissue substances not normally antigenic, so that they are recognized as antigen by the immune system. This hypothesis has received experimental support. William Weigle has been able to break tolerance using chemically modified antigens. By immunizing animals with aqueous homologous thyroglobulin to which arsenilic or sulfanilic acid haptens had been coupled, he was able to induce experimental autoallergic inflammation of the thyroid; the supposition is that tolerance to autologous proteins can be broken by antigenically modified proteins of the same class.
3. T helper cells may be stimulated to activate previously inactivated B cells (cross-reactive autoimmunity).
4. The function of suppressor cells may be lost. Suppressor cells may prevent other immunologically competent cells from responding to self antigens. Presentation of the antigen in a particular manner may circumvent suppressor cell activity. Suppressor cells are short-lived and may become less numerous with aging, permitting other cells to respond to self antigens. The incidence of autoallergic diseases and autoantibodies increases with age, presumably because atrophy of the thymus with aging results in a failure in the ability of the thymus to produce new T suppressor cells.
5. B cells may be nonspecifically activated by B cell mitogens that lead to *polyclonal activation,* that is, a nonspecific increase in immunoglobulin molecules of different specificities or IgG classes. Some of the immunoglobulins produced may react with self antigens. In this manner polyclonal activation may result in autoantibody production.
6. According to the clonal selection theory of Burnet (see above) an alteration, not in the tissue in which the lesion appears but in the cells of the immune system, leads to autoimmunity. Because of an unknown mechanism, some immunologically competent cells, which do not normally react against tissues of the same animal, go out of control and recognize normal tissue substances as antigens.
7. The effects of blocking antibodies or the idiotype network may be lost. These effects appear to be cyclic. Thus the extent of an immune response may be held at a low level by the idiotype network. However, an antigenic exposure may affect one or some of the members of the anti-idiotypic reac-

tants in the network, permitting an autoimmune response to become manifested. Wavering of control is a possible explanation for the frequent cyclic remissions and relapses that are common occurrences in diseases caused by autoimmunity.

8. A recently suggested mechanism is the induction of class II MHC expression on cells normally not expressing class II MHC, permitting antigen presentation and induction of an immune response.

A summary of B cell control mechanisms in autoantibody responses and B cell proliferation responses that could progress to lymphoma is given in Figure 11-11.

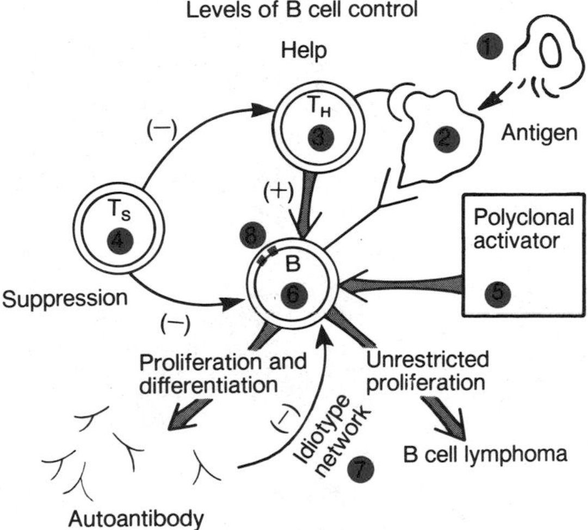

Figure 11-11. Control of B cells: autoantibody production and B cell lymphoma. Loss of control of B cells may occur at a number of possible sites: (1) Sequestered antigens may be released into the circulation and become available for immunization. (2) Alteration of self antigens or unusual antigen presentation (i.e., associated with viral infections) may lead to stimulation of B cells and breaking of tolerance to self antigens. (3) Increased T_H (helper) activity may occur, resulting in inappropriate stimulation of normal B cells. (4) A loss of suppressor activity (T_S) could result in increased T_H activity or B cell proliferation. (5) Polyclonal activators (bacterial endotoxins, etc.) may bypass control mechanisms and activate B cells directly to produce antibodies nonspecifically. (6) An inherent (somatic) change may occur in a B cell, resulting in loss of tolerance due to production of a new reactive clone. (7) Fluctuations in idiotype network antibodies may permit greater production of previously suppressed autoantibodies. (8) Expression of class II MHC (IA) on cells not normally expressing class II MHC, leading to antigen presentation and induction of an immune response.

Summary

Immune tolerance is the specific loss of the ability to produce an immune response to a given antigen; normal responses to other antigens remain intact. Some possible mechanisms of tolerance are:

1. Clonal elimination/anergy: elimination or inactivation in

the tolerant animal of the cells responsible for recognizing and responding to the given antigen.

2. Suppressor cells: active inhibition of reactive cells present in the animal by specific suppressor cells.
3. Blocking antibody: reaction of potentially responding cells blocked by specific antibody or antibody–antigen complexes.
4. Network theory: anti-idiotype antibodies that act on the surface of cells are boosted by rising levels of idiotype-containing antibodies.
5. Immunogen processing: Immunogen reaches the potentially responding cells in an unprocessed form, rendering them nonreactive. Unprocessed antigen may induce suppressor cells.

Normally an individual develops tolerance to his own antigens during development (natural tolerance). A loss of natural tolerance is believed to be responsible for autoimmune diseases. However, many normal individuals have demonstrable autoantibodies without evidence of disease. Breaking of tolerance to self antigens may have a normal function or may cause disease.

References

Tolerance

Neonatal

Auerbach R, Clark S: Immunological tolerance: transmission from mother to offspring. Science 189:84, 1975.

Billingham RE, Brent L: Acquired tolerance of foreign cells in newborn animals. Proc R Soc B 146:28, 1956.

Boyden SV: Natural antibodies and the immune response. Adv Immunol 5:1, 1965.

Burnet FM, Fenner F: The Production of Antibodies. Melbourne, Macmillan, 1949.

Hasek M, Langerova A, Hraba T: Transplantation immunity and tolerance. Adv Immunol 1:1, 1961.

Howard JC, Michie D: Induction of transplantation immunity in newborn mice. Transplant Bull 29:91, 1962.

Hraba T: Mechanisms and role of immunological tolerance. *In* Kallos P, Goodman HC, Hasek M, Inderbitzen T (eds): Monographs in Allergy. Basel, Karger, 1968.

Medawar PB: Actively acquired tolerance of foreign cells. Nature 172:603, 1953.

Moller G (ed): Transplantation Tolerance. Immunol Rev 46, 1979.

Owen RD: Immunogenetic consequence of vascular anastomoses between bovine twins. Science 102:400, 1945.

Streilein JW: Neonatal tolerancc: towards an immunogenetic definition of self. Immunol Rev 46:125, 1979.

Triplett EL: On the mechanism of immunologic self recognition. J Immunol 89:505, 1962.

Weigle WO: Immunological unresponsiveness. Adv Immunol 16:61, 1973.

Clonal Elimination/Anergy

Basten A, Miller JFAP, Sprent J, Cheers C: Cell-to-cell interaction in the immune response. X. T cell-dependent suppression in tolerant mice. J Exp Med 140:199, 1974.

Benjamin DC: Neonatally induced tolerance to HcG: duration in B cells and absence of specific suppressor cells. J Immunol 119:311, 1977.

Burnet FM: The Clonal Selection Theory of Acquired Immunity. London, Cambridge University Press, 1959.

Burnet FM: The Integrity of the Body: A Discussion of Modern Immunological Ideas. Cambridge, Harvard University Press, 1962.

Chiller JM, Habicht GS, Weigle WO: Cellular sites of immunologic unresponsiveness. Proc Nat Acad Sci USA 65:551, 1970.

Chiller JM, Rombard CG, Weigle WO: Induction of immunological tolerance in neonatal and adult rabbits. Cell Immunol 8:28, 1973.

Dresser DW, Mitchison NA: The mechanism of immunological paralysis. Adv Immunol 8:128, 1968.

Mitchison NA: Induction of immunological paralysis with two zones of dosage. Proc R Soc Land [Biol] 161:275, 1966.

Moller G (ed): Mechanism of B cell tolerance. Immunol Rev 43, 1979.

Nossal GJV: Cellular mechanisms of immunological tolerance. Ann Rev Immunol 1:33, 1983.

Nossal GJV, Pike BL: Evidence for the clonal abortion theory of B lymphocyte tolerance. J Exp Med 141:904, 1975.

Parks E, Weigle WO: Current perspectives on the cellular mechanisms of tolerance induction. Clin Exp Immunol 39:257, 1980.

Scibienski RJ, et al: Active and inactive states of immunologic unresponsiveness. J Immunol 113:45, 1974.

Weigle WO: Termination of acquired immunological tolerance to protein antigens following immunization with altered protein antigens. J Exp Med 116:913, 1962.

Suppressor Cells

Argyris BF: Adoptive tolerance: transfer of the tolerant state. J Immunol 90:29, 1963.

Argyris BF: Adoptive tolerance transferred by bone marrow, spleen, lymph node or thymus cells. J Immunol 96:273, 1966.

Baker PJ, Stashak PW, Ambsbaugh DF, Prescott B: Regulation of the antibody response to type III pneumococcal polysaccharide. II. Mode of action of thymic-derived suppressor cells. J Immunol 112:404, 1974.

Baker PJ, Stashak PW, Ambsbaugh DR, Prescott B, Barth RF: Evidence for the existence of two functionally distinct types of cells which regulate the antibody response to type III pneumococcal polysaccharide. J Immunol 105:1581, 1970.

Benjamin DC: Evidence for specific suppression in the maintenance of immunologic tolerance. J Exp Med 141:635, 1975.

Cantor H, Asofsky R: Paradoxical effect of anti-thymocyte serum on the thymus. Nature 243:39, 1973.

Dorf ME, Benacerraf B: Suppressor cells and immunoregulation. Annu Rev Immunol 2:126, 1984.

Dutton RW: Inhibitory and stimulatory effects of Concanavalin A on the response of mouse spleen cell suspensions to antigen. II. Evidence for separate stimulatory and inhibitory cells. J Exp Med 138:1496, 1973.

Gershon R, Cohan P, Hencin R, Liebhaber SA: Suppressor T cells. J Immunol 108:586, 1972.

Gershon R, Kondo K: Cell interactions in the induction of tolerance: the role of thymic lymphocytes. Immunology 18:723, 1970.

Gershon R, Kondo K: Infectious immunological tolerance. Immunology 21:903, 1971.

Green DR, Flood PM, Gershon R: Immunoregulatory T-cell pathways. Annu Rev Immunol 1:439, 1983.

Ha T-Y, Waksman BH, Treffers HP: The thymic suppressor cell. I. Separation of subpopulations with suppressor activity. J Exp Med 139:13–23, 1974.

Kerbel RS, Eidinger D: Enhanced immune responsiveness to a thymus-independent antigen early after adult thymectomy: evidence for short-lived inhibitory thymus-derived cells. Eur J Immunol 2:114–118, 1972.

Moller G (ed): Unresponsiveness to Haptenionated Self Molecules. Immunol Rev 50, 1980.

Okumura K, Tada T: Regulation of homocytotropic antibody formation in the rat. VI. Inhibitory effect of thymocytes on the homocytotropic antibody response. J Immunol 107:1682–1689, 1971.

Scibienski RS: Active and inactive states of immunologic unresponsiveness. J Immunol 113:45, 1974.

Strober S: Natural suppressor cells, neonatal tolerance and total lymphoid irradiation: exploring obscure relationships. Annu Rev Immunol 2:219, 1984.

Weber G, Kolsch E: Transfer of low zone tolerance to normal syngeneic mice by θ positive cells. Eur J Immunol 3:767, 1973.

Blocking Antibody

Bansal SC, et al: Cell-mediated immunity and blocking serum activity to tolerated allografts in rats. J Exp Med 137:590, 1973.

Brent L, et al.: Attempts to demonstrate an in vivo role for serum blocking factors in tolerant mice. Transplantation 14:382, 1972.

Gorczynski R, Kontiainen S, Mitchison NA, Tigelar RE: Antigen–antibody complexes as blocking factors on the T lymphocyte surface. *In* Edelman GM (ed): Cellular Selection and Regulation in the Immune Response. New York, Raven Press, 1974, p143.

Hasek M, et al: Attempts to compare the effectiveness of blocking factors and enhancing antibodies in vivo and vitro. Transplantation 20:95, 1975.

Hellstrom I, Hellstrom KE, Allison AC: Neonatally induced tolerance may be mediated by serum borne factors. Nature 230:49, 1971.

Moller G (ed): Regulation of the immune response by antibodies against the immunogen. Immunol Rev 49:1980.

Voisin GA: Immunologic facilitation: a broadening of the concept of the enhancement phenomenon. Prog Allergy 5:328, 1971.

Wright PW, et al: In vitro reactivity in allograft tolerance. Persistence of cell mediated cytotoxicity and serum blocking activity in highly tolerant rats. Transplantation 19:437, 1975.

Idiotype Network

Cazenave PA: Idiotype–antiidiotype regulation of antibody synthesis in rabbits. Proc Nat Acad Sci USA 74:5122, 1977.

Cerny J, Kelsoe G: Priority of the anti-idiotypic response after antigen administration: artifact or integrating network mechanism. Immunol Today 5:61, 1984.

Herzenberg LA, Tokuhisa K, Hayakawa K: Epitope-specific regulation. Annu Rev Immunol 1:609, 1983.

Hoffman GW: A theory of regulation and self–nonself discrimination. Eur J Immunol 5:638, 1975.

Jerne NK: Towards a network theory of the immune system. Ann Immunol (Inst Pasteur) Ser C125:373, 1974.

Jerne NK: The immune system: a web of V domains. Harvey Lect 70:93, 1975.

Kelsoe G, Reth M, Rajewsky K: Control of idiotype expression by monoclonal antiidiotope bearing antibody. Immunol Rev 52:75, 1980.

Kohler H, Muller S, Bona C: Internal antigen and immune network. Proc Soc Exp Biol Med 178:189, 1985.

Moller G (ed): Idiotype Networks. Immunol Rev 79, 1984.

Moller G (ed): Idiotypes on T Cells and B Cells. Immunol Rev 27, 1975.

Nisonoff A, Bangasser SA: Immunological suppression of idiotypic specificities. Transplant Rev 27:100, 1975.

Paul WE, Bona C: Regulatory idiotopes and immune networks. A hypothesis. Immunol Today 3:9, 1982.

Rajewsky K: Symmetry and asymmetry in idiotypic interactions. Ann Immunol (Inst Pasteur) 1340:133, 1983.

Rajewsky K, Takemori T: Genetics expression and function of idiotypes. Annu Rev Immunol 1:569, 1983.

Rodkey LS: Studies of idiotypic antibodies: production and characterization of auto-antiidiotypic antisera. J Exp Med 139:712, 1974.

Antigen Processing

Ada GL, Nossal GJV, Pye J: Antigens in immunity. XI. The uptake of antigen in animals previously rendered immunologically tolerant. Aust J Exp Biol Med Sci 43:337, 1965.

Ada GL, Parish CR: Low zone tolerance to bacterial flagellin in adult rats. A possible role for antigen localized in lymphoid follicles. Proc Nat Acad Sci USA 61:556, 1968.

Aldo-Benson M, Borel Y: The tolerant cell: direct evidence for receptor blockade by tolerogen. J Immunol 112:1793, 1974.

Garvey J, Eitzman DV, Smith RI: The distribution of S^{35} labeled bovine serum albumin in newborn and immunologically tolerant adult rats. J Exp Med 112:533, 1960.

Humphrey JH: The fate of antigen. Proc R Soc Lond [Biol] 146:34, 1956.

Kripke ML: Immunological unresponsiveness induced by ultraviolet irradiation. Immunol Rev 80:87, 1984.

Moller G (ed): Role of macrophages in the immune response. Immunol Rev 40, 1978.

Schwartz RS, Ryder RJW, Gottlieb BAA: Macrophages and antibody synthesis. Prog Allergy 14:81, 1970.

Unanue ER: The regulatory role of macrophages in antigenic stimulation. Part two. Symbiotic relationship between lymphocytes and macrophages. Adv Immunol 31:1, 1981.

Split Tolerance

Ishizaka K: Cellular events in the IgE antibody response. Adv Immunol 23:1, 1976.

Ishizaka K: Regulation of IgE synthesis. Annu Rev Immunol 2:259, 1984.

Ishizaka K, Ishizaka T: Mechanisms of reaginic hypersensitivity and IgE antibody response. Immunol Rev 41:109, 1978.

Katz DH: The allergic phenotype: manifestation of "allergic breakthrough" and imbalance in normal "damping" of IgE antibody production. Immunol Rev 41:77, 1978.

Lee WY, Sehon AN: Suppression of reaginic antibodies. Immunol Rev 41:200, 1978.

Rogers TJ, Balish E: Immunity to candida albicans. Microbiol Rev 44:660, 1980.

Turk JL, Bryceson ADM: Immunological phenomena in leprosy and related diseases. Adv Immunol 13:209, 1971.

Immune Paralysis

Felton LD: The significance of antigen in animal tissue. J Immunol 61:107, 1949.

Halliday WJ: Immunological paralysis of mice with pneumococcal polysaccharide antigens. Bacteriol Rev 35:267, 1971.

Autoimmunity

Battisto JR, Claman HN (eds): Immunological Tolerance to Self and Not-self. Ann NY Acad Sci 392, 1982.

Grabar D: Autoantibodies and the physiologic role of immunoglobulin. Immunol Today 4:337, 1983.

Moller G (ed): Autoimmunity and Self–Nonself Discrimination. Immunol Rev 31:1976.

Smith HR, Steinberg AD: Autoimmunity: a perspective. Annu Rev Immunol 1:175, 1983.

12 | Inflammation

Inflammation is the primary process through which the body repairs tissue damage and defends itself against infection (see Chapter 1). Inflammation may be initiated by either immune or nonimmune pathways, but both pathways employ similar effector mechanisms. Activation of immune pathways is initiated by a specific reaction of immunoglobulin antibody or sensitized T lymphocytes with antigen. The in vivo effects of immune activation are determined by amplification mechanisms that are also components of nonimmune inflammatory processes. These amplification mechanisms, rather than the specific immune reaction alone, are largely responsible for the tissue lesions actually observed. Nonimmune inflammation is initiated by release of bacterial products or components of dying tissue cells.

The function of inflammation is to deliver plasma and cellular components of the blood to extravascular tissues. The extravasation of plasma fluid into tissue (edema) causes dilution of toxic materials and increases lymphatic flow. Phagocytic blood cells infiltrate inflamed tissue and destroy bacteria. At late stages, fibrosis walls off foci of infection. As a physiological response to injury, inflammation clears and restores damaged tissue; as a pathologic process, inflammation produces tissue damage (lesions).

The Process of Inflammation

The phases of inflammation are given in Table 12-1. The following sequence of events occurs during an inflammatory response: (1) increased blood flow (vasodilation) preceded by transient vasoconstriction, (2) increased vascular permeability leading to edema (vasopermeability), (3) infiltration by poly-

Table 12-1. Phases of Inflammation: Neurologic, Vascular, Cellular

Initiating event	→	Acute vascular response (minutes)	→	Acute cellular response (hours)	→	Chronic cellular response (days)	→	Scarring or resolution (weeks)
Trauma, necrosis, infection	→	Vasodilation, increased vasopermeability (hyperemia, edema)	→	Neutrophil infiltrate (pus)	→	Mononuclear cell infiltrate[a]	→	Fibrosis or clearing

[a] Lymphocytes, macrophages, and plasma cells.

morphonuclear neutrophils, (4) infiltration by lymphocytes and macrophages (chronic inflammation), leading to (5) resolution (restoration of normal structure) or (6) scarring (filling in of areas of tissue destruction by fibroblasts and collagen) (see Fig. 12-1). The first three events are considered *acute* inflammation; the latter three stages, *chronic* inflammation.

Inflammation is initiated by trauma, tissue necrosis (death), infection, or immune reactions. The immediate response is a temporary vasoconstriction causing blanching of the skin. The mechanism for this is not well understood, but is believed to be mediated by the sympathetic nervous system. Vasoconstriction is followed within seconds by the acute vascular response resulting in increased blood flow (hyperemia) and edema. If there has been only mild injury, such as is caused by stroking the skin, the inflammatory process may be limited to this phase only. However, if there is sufficient cell death or infection the acute cellular phase will follow. Changes in blood flow lead to margination of neutrophils next to endothelial cells, followed by emigration of neutrophils into the adjacent tissue. Contraction of endothelial cells causes leakage (diapedesis) of red blood cells, which progresses to hemorrhage if necrosis of endothelial cells occurs. Exposure of fibrinogen and fibronectin provides sites for platelet aggregation and activation. Alterations in the viscosity of the blood and the electrostatic charge of plasma may aggregate red cells into stacks like pancakes (rouleau formation) as the normal negative repelling charge of the erythrocytes is lost. Depending on the degree of injury or infection, the acute cellular phase may be sufficient to clear the tissue. However, it is usually necessary for the chronic cellular infiltrate of lymphocytes and macrophages to effect removal of tissue debris or dead bacteria. The macrophage is the major player in this process. If damage is sufficient to result in loss of normal tissue, fibroblastic proliferation and scarring will occur.

The gross manifestations of the acute vascular response (the *triple response*) may be evoked by scratching the skin. The triple response proceeds as follows:

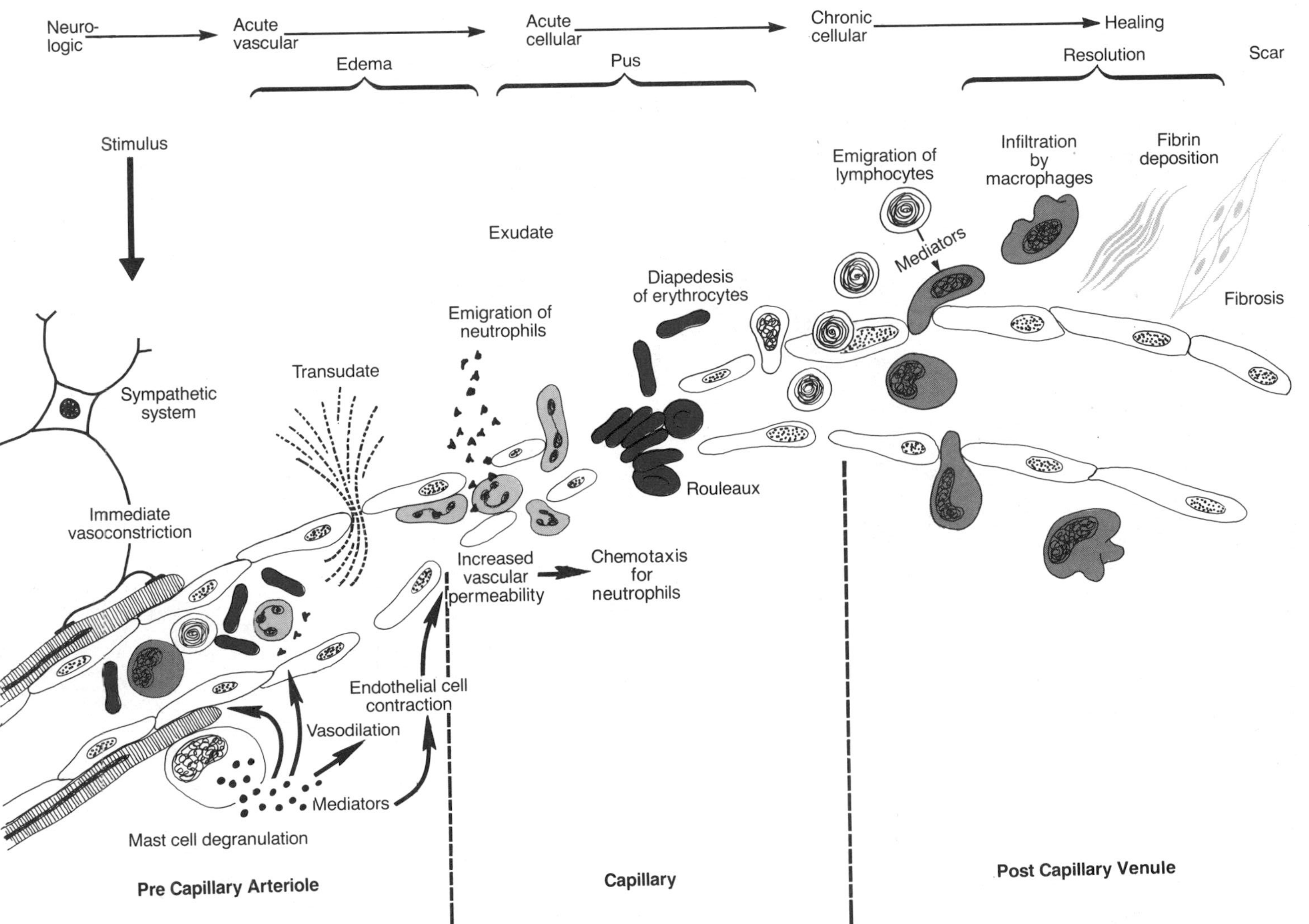

Figure 12-1. The sequence of events in the process of inflammation.

1. 3–50 seconds: thin red line (vasodilation of capillaries)
2. 30–60 seconds: flush (vasodilation of arterioles)
3. 1–5 minutes: wheal (increased vascular permeability, edema)

The term *wheal* refers to pale, soft, swollen areas on the skin caused by leakage of fluid from capillaries. Some individuals react to skin stroking by marked wheal formation, such that words may actually be written on the skin by whealing (dermatographism).

The ancient Greeks, who recognized the four classic cardinal signs of inflammation (Fig. 12-2), considered inflammation

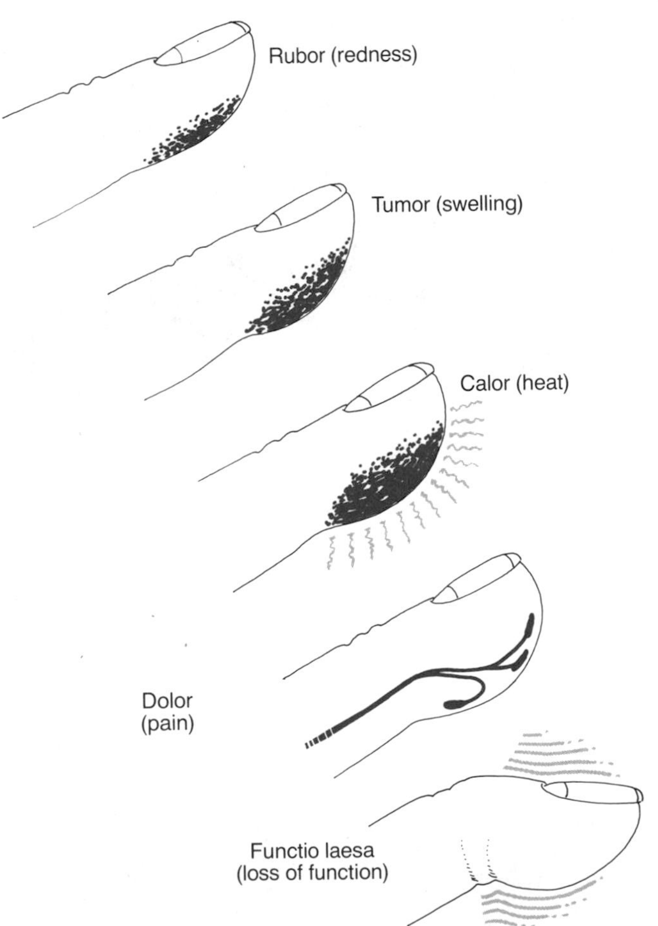

Figure 12-2. The five cardinal signs of inflammation.

to be a disease. Later the fifth sign, loss of function, was added by the great German pathologist Rudolf Virchow. Increased blood flow is manifested grossly by redness (*rubor*) and increased local temperature (*calor*). The increased blood flow delivers serum factors and blood cells to the tissue. The increase in vascular permeability permits exudation of plasma from the capillaries or postcapillary venules into the tissue, causing edema and increase in tissue mass (*tumor*). Tissue swelling and chemical mediators act on nerve endings to produce pain (*dolor*). Swelling and pain lead to loss of function (*functio laesa*).

Chemical mediators are signaling molecules that act on smooth muscle cells, endothelial cells, or white blood cells to induce, maintain, or limit inflammation. The agents that act first in the sequence affect smooth muscle cells of precapillary arterioles to produce dilation and increased blood flow. Increased vascular permeability occurs in two phases: early (within minutes) and late (6–12 hours). The early phase is mediated by histamine and serotonin, whereas several other mediators contribute to the later phase. Late-phase mediators are derived from a variety of sources including arachidonic acid metabolites, breakdown products of the coagulation system (fibrin split products), peptides formed from blood or tissue proteins (bradykinin), and activated complement components, as well as factors released from bacteria, necrotic tissue, neutrophils (inflammatory peptides), lymphocytes (lymphokines), and monocytes (monokines). The generation of these factors and their effects will be presented in more detail below.

Histologically, the essential feature of acute inflammation is infiltration of the tissue by neutrophils. Neutrophils are believed to pass through gaps in capillary endothelium and are attracted to sites of inflammation by chemotactic factors. Tissue necrosis is caused by release of proteolytic enzymes into the tissue from the lysosomes of the neutrophils. Neutrophilic infiltrate is followed by infiltration by mononuclear (round) cells (i.e., lymphocytes and macrophages). Macrophages, although they move less rapidly than neutrophils, are also attracted by chemotactic mediators and are activated to phagocytose and digest necrotic tissue or inflammatory products, including effete neutrophils that have become damaged in the inflammatory process. If tissue damage is not extensive, the inflammation will be limited by controlling factors such as enzyme inhibitors and oxygen scavengers. Macrophages will then clear the inflamed area, and the tissue will return to normal (*resolution*). However, if tissue damage is extensive or the initiating stimulus persists, then mediators of chronic inflammation are activated. If tissue damage is significant or the organ has limited ability to regenerate, resolution cannot be achieved and the damaged tissue will be replaced by fibroblastic proliferation and collagen deposition (*fibrous scar*). If extensive, fibrous scarring may lead to a compromise in normal function. The fibrotic process may include proliferation of both fibroblasts and endothelial cells (capillaries), which forms granulation tissue, so named because grossly it has the appearance of small granules like sand. If the inflamed tissue contains material that is difficult for macrophages to digest (such as silica or complex lipids), a particular form of chronic inflammation, *granulomatous* (like granulation tissue), takes place. The process of inflammation is modified by infection, immune products, tissue death (necrosis), and foreign bodies. Examples of the lesions of different stages of inflammation in different tissue are given later in this chapter.

Some terms used to describe various manifestations of the inflammatory process are listed in Table 12-2. The manifestations of inflammation depend upon the severity and location of the reaction as well as the nature of the inflammatory stimulus. Systemic effects of inflammation include fever and increased numbers of white blood cells (leukocytosis). Fever is caused by increase in the metabolic rate of muscular tissue secondary to effects of *pyrogens* released from damaged tissue that act on the hypothalamus. Leukocytosis is caused by increased production and release of white cells from the bone marrow.

Table 12-2. Definitions of Terms Used to Describe Manifestations of Inflammation

Hyperemia: increased blood in tissue, caused by vasodilation.

Edema: excess fluid in tissues, caused by increased vascular permeability.

Transudate: physiologic, low-protein-concentration edema fluid, containing albumin; specific gravity less than 1.012; cleared by lymphatics.

Exudate: pathologic, high protein edema fluid containing immunoglobulins and macroglobulin; specific gravity greater than 1.02.

Pus: exudate rich in white cells and necrotic debris, caused by emigration of neutrophils and release of enzymes.

Fibrinoid necrosis: enzymatic digestion of tissue resulting in an appearance like fibrin; example: fibrinoid necrosis of vessels in vasculitis.

TYPES OF EXUDATE

Serous: thin fluid (like transudate).

Fibrinous: stringy, containing fibrin.

Suppurative: pus (neutrophils and necrotic debris).

Hemorrhagic: bloody (vascular necrosis).

Fibrous: healed exudate, scar, adhesions.

TYPES OF LESIONS

Ulcer: surface erosion.

Abscess: cavity filled with pus.

Cellulitis: diffuse inflammatory infiltrate in tissue.

Pseudomembrane: fibrinous or necrotic layer on epithelial surface.

Catarrhal: excess mucus production.

The Cells of Acute Inflammation

The cellular players in the process of acute inflammation include mast cells, neutrophils, platelets and eosinophils, which act in sequence. They are activated by a variety of chemical processes and, in turn, produce and release a number of chemical mediators. Most of the manifestations of the acute vascular response are the result of chemical mediators released from mast cells.

Mast Cells

Mast cells contain granules with a variety of biologically active agents (Table 12-3), which, when released extracellularly (de-

Table 12-3. Mast Cell Mediators

Mediator	Structure/Chemistry	Source	Effects
Histamine	β-Imidazolylethylamine	Mast cells, basophils	Vasodilation; increase vascular permeability (venules), mucus production
Serotonin	5-Hydroxytryptamine	Mast cells (rodent), platelets, cells of enterochromaffin system	Vasodilation; increase vascular permeability (venules)
Neutrophil chemotactic factor	MW > 750,000	Mast cells	Chemotaxis of neutrophils
Eosinophil chemotactic factor A	Tetrapeptide	Mast cells	Chemotaxis of eosinophils
Vasoactive intestinal peptide	28-Amino-acid peptide	Mast cells, neutrophils, cutaneous nerves	Vasodilation; potentiate edema produced by bradykinin and C5a des-Arg
Thromboxane A_2	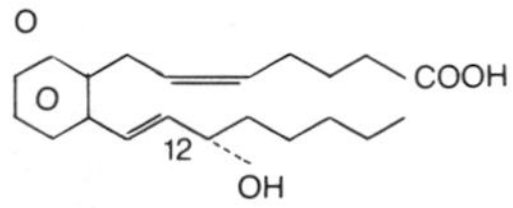 O, O, COOH, 12, OH	Arachidonic acid (cyclooxygenase pathway)	Vasoconstriction, bronchoconstriction, platelet aggregation
Prostaglandin E_2 (or D_2)	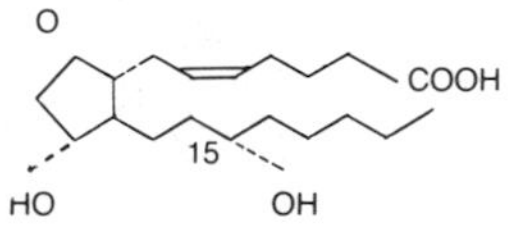 O, COOH, 15, HO, OH	Arachidonic acid (cyclooxygenase pathway)	Vasodilation; potentiate permeability effects of histamine and bradykinin; increase permeability when acting with leukotactic agent; potentiate leukotriene effect; hyperalgesia
Leukotriene B_4	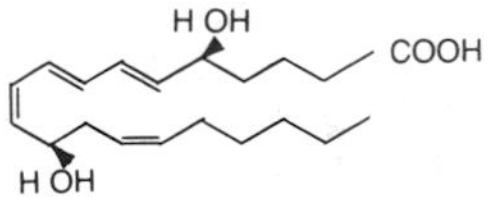 H OH, COOH, H OH	Arachidonic acid (lipoxygenase pathway)	Chemotaxis of neutrophils; increase vascular permeability in the presence of PGE_2
Leukotriene D_4	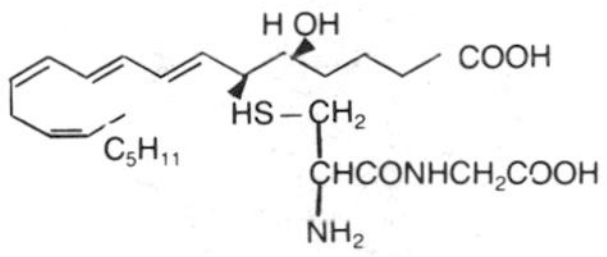 H OH, COOH, $HS-CH_2$, C_5H_{11}, $CHCONHCH_2COOH$, NH_2	Arachidonic acid (lipoxygenase pathway)	Increase vascular permeability
Platelet-activating factor	Acetylated glycerol ether phosphocholine	Basophils, neutrophils, monocytes, macrophages	Release of mediators from platelets, neutrophil aggregation, neutrophil secretion, superoxide production by neutrophils; increase vascular permeability

granulation), cause contraction of endothelial cells, thus opening up vessel walls to permit egress of antibodies, complement, or inflammatory cells into tissue spaces. Mast cells were observed by early histologists to be filled with cellular material (the granules). The term *mast cell* was applied to indicate that these cells appeared to be stuffed as if by overeating (German *Mast*, "forced fattening"). The cellular granules contain biologically active agents produced by the mast cell, which are released upon activation of the cells. Mast cells are usually located adjacent to small arterioles and in submucosal tissues where released vasoactive mediators would be expected to be most active in causing relaxation of smooth muscle cells and dilatation of arterioles. In classic anaphylactic reactions, mast cells are degranulated by reaction of antigen with IgE antibody that adheres to the surface of mast cells because of a specific configuration of the Fc part of the antibody molecules. Mast cells have receptors for IgE that are composed of two chains, α and β. The α chain (MW 50,000) extends from the cell surface and is believed to combine with IgE. Upon reaction of antigen with IgE antibody on the surface of the mast cells, a complex cellular activation mechanism causes the mast cells to release the pharmacologically active agents contained in cytoplasmic granules (Fig. 12-3).

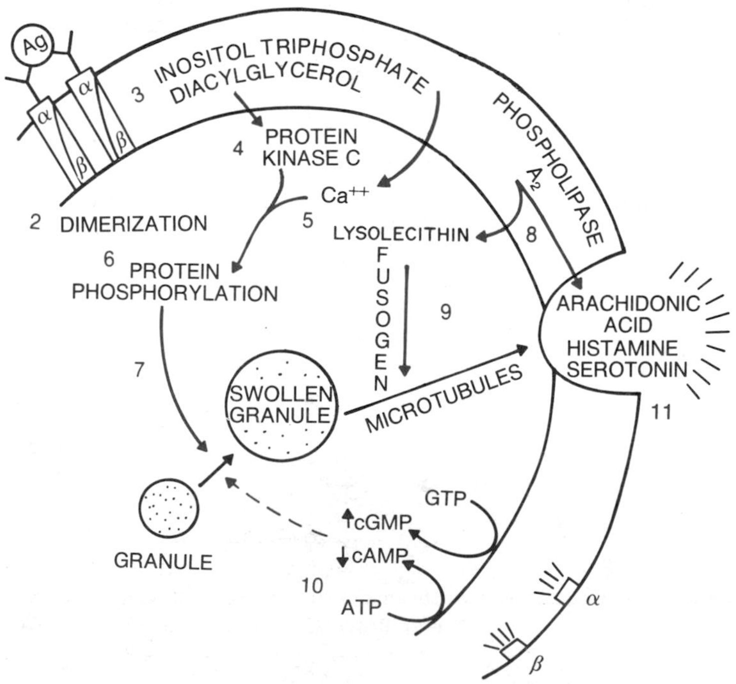

Figure 12-3. Postulated steps in mast cell degranulation. (1) Binding of antigen (allergen), crosslinking two IgE molecules on mast cell surface. (2) Dimerization of IgE receptors: α, MW 50,000, attached to IgE; β, MW 30,000. (3) Activation of phospholipase C; action of phospholipase C on membrane phosphatidylinositol-4,5-biphosphate to form inositoltriphosphate and diacylglycerol. (4) Activation of protein kinase C. (5) Mobilization of intracellular Ca^{++}. (7) Enlargement of granules by protein kinases. (8) Activation of phospholipase A_2 with formation of lysolecithin and arachidonic acid. (9) Lysolecithin acts as "fusogen" causing granule to fuse with membrane and release contents. (10) Activation of granules dependent on levels of cAMP and cGMP, which in turn are regulated by α and β adrenergic receptors. (11) Release of histamine and membrane phospholipids (arachidonic acid).

The pharmacologically active agents of mast cells are the chemical mediators of atopic or anaphylactic hypersensitivity. The effects of their release are described in more detail in Chapter 17. The major effects of mast cell mediators are listed in Figure 12-4. The major early events in inflammation—vasodilation and increased vascular permeability—are mediated by the immediate degranulation of mast cells and the release of histamine and serotonin. Later vascular events, occurring 6–12 hours after initiation of inflammation, are mediated by prostaglandins and leukotrienes produced as a result of metabolism of phospholipids from membrane-like material released from mast cell granules (see below). Chemotaxis of neutrophils and eosinophils is affected by leukotrienes as well as by platelet-activating factor. Enzymes activated by solubilization of granular material may also contribute to tissue damage and/or repair.

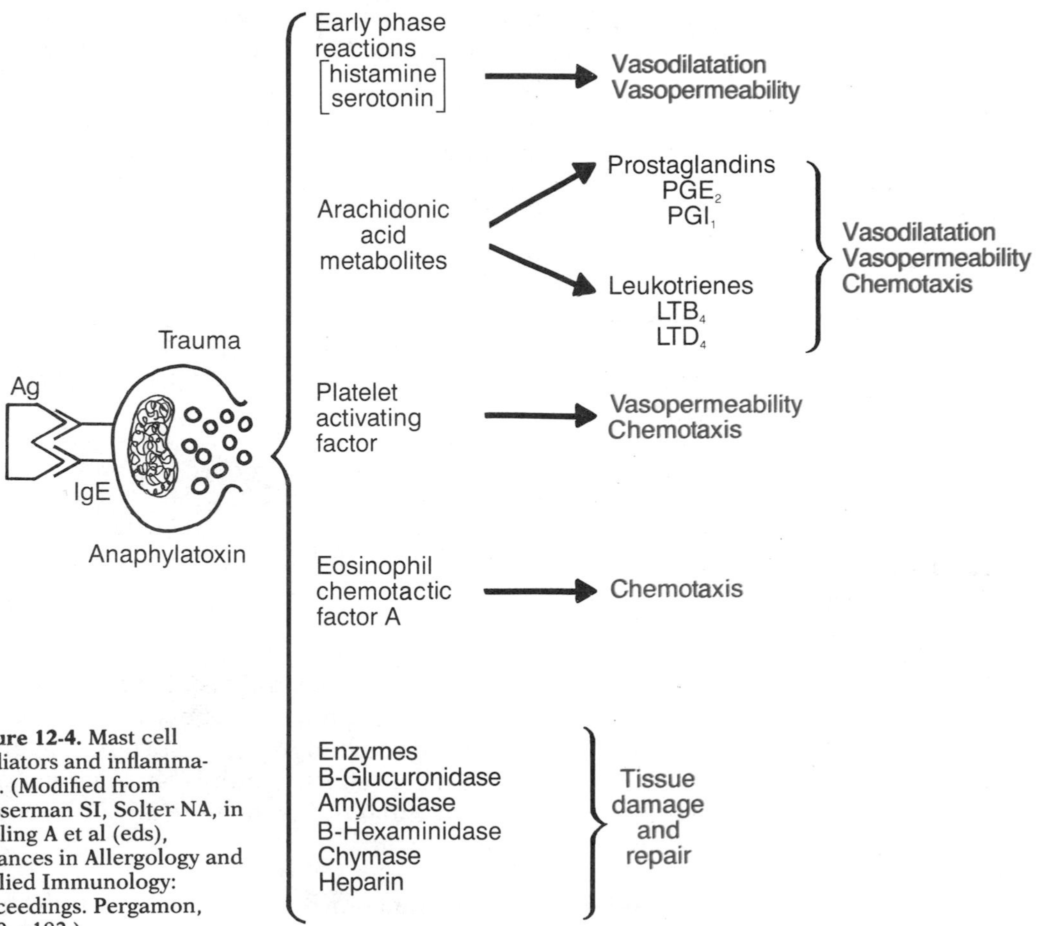

Figure 12-4. Mast cell mediators and inflammation. (Modified from Wasserman SI, Solter NA, in Oehling A et al (eds), Advances in Allergology and Applied Immunology: Proceedings. Pergamon, 1980, p192.)

Histamine

Histamine is the major preformed mast cell mediator. Injection of histamine into the skin produces the typical wheal and flare reaction of the immediate acute vascular response. Histamine causes endothelial cell contraction and vasodilation leading to edema (wheal) and redness (flare). Histamine is formed from the amino acid L-histidine by the action of the enzyme L-histidine decarboxylase, found in the cytoplasm of mast cells and basophils. The biologic effects of histamine are mediated by two distinct sets of receptors, H_1 and H_2 (Table 12-4). Effects

Table 12-4. H_1- and H_2-Dependent Actions of Histamine

H_1 Receptor–Mediated	H_2 Receptor–Mediated	H_1 and H_2
Increased cGMP	Increased cAMP	Vasodilation (hypotension)
Smooth-muscle constriction (bronchi)	Smooth muscle dilation (vascular)	Flush
Increased vascular permeability	Gastric-acid secretion	Headache
Pruritus	Mucous secretion	
Prostaglandin generation	Inhibition of basophil histamine release	
	Inhibition of lymphokine release	
	Inhibition of neutrophil enzyme release	
	Inhibition of eosinophil migration	
	Inhibition of T-lymphocyte–mediated cytotoxicity	
Antagonized by "classical" antihistamines	Antagonized by cimetidine	

Modified from Metcalfe DD, Kaliner M: Mast cells and basophils, in Oppenheim JJ, Rosenstreich DL, Potter M (eds), Cellular Functions in Immunity and Inflammation. New York, Elsevier, 1981.

mediated through H_1 receptors are the classic acute vascular inflammatory events. Anti-inflammatory effects, as well as vasodilation, are mediated through H_2 receptors. Thus, histamine may activate acute vascular effects, yet inhibit acute cellular inflammation. Acute cellular inflammation is mediated by products of arachidonic acid.

Arachidonic Acid Metabolites

Major mediators of inflammation are the metabolic derivatives of arachidonic acid. Arachidonic acid is derived from membrane phospholipids that are broken down by phospholipases. In the human, membrane phospholipids are released from mast cells during the early phase of acute inflammation but may also be derived from other cell membranes. The metabolism of arachidonic acid is believed to occur mainly in macrophages, but metabolites may also be synthesized by most, if not all, cells that take part in an inflammatory response, including the mast cell. Metabolism of arachidonic acid occurs via two major pathways: the cyclooxygenase pathway and the lipoxygenase pathway (Fig. 12-5). The cyclooxygenase pathway gives rise to prostaglandins; the lipoxygenase pathway to leukotrienes.

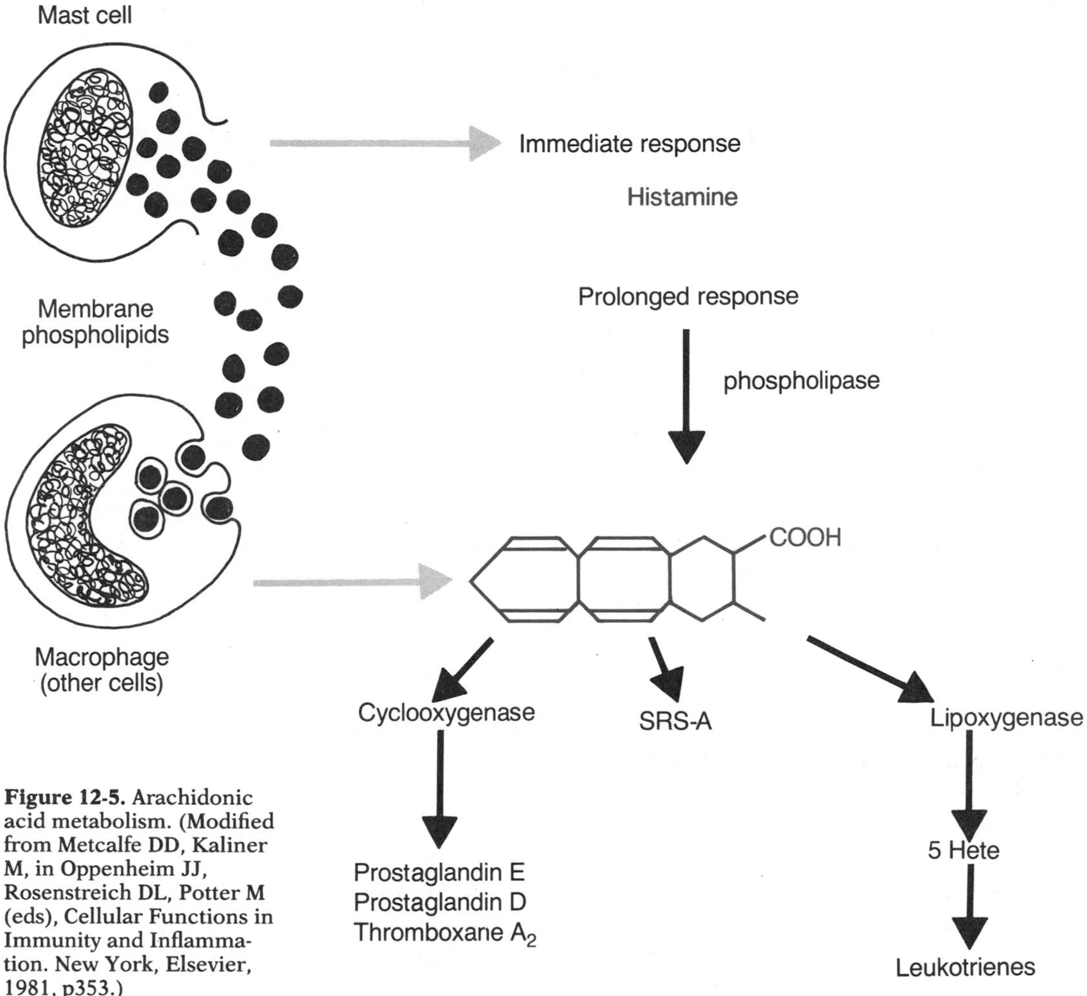

Figure 12-5. Arachidonic acid metabolism. (Modified from Metcalfe DD, Kaliner M, in Oppenheim JJ, Rosenstreich DL, Potter M (eds), Cellular Functions in Immunity and Inflammation. New York, Elsevier, 1981, p353.)

Prostaglandins. The prostaglandins are derived by oxidation of prostanoic acid (cyclooxygenation).

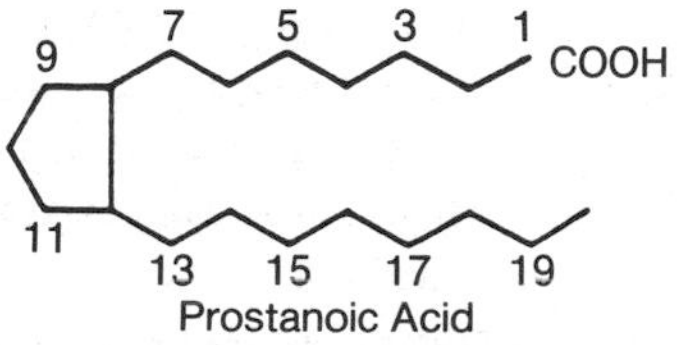

9 7 5 3 1 COOH
11 13 15 17 19
Prostanoic Acid

The numerical subscript in each prostaglandin (PG) refers to the number of unsaturated bonds. PGE_1 has one unsaturated bond at the 13 – 14 position; PGE_2 has two unsaturated bonds, at the 5–6 and at the 13–14 positions. The letter designations refer to the position of bonds in the ring structure:

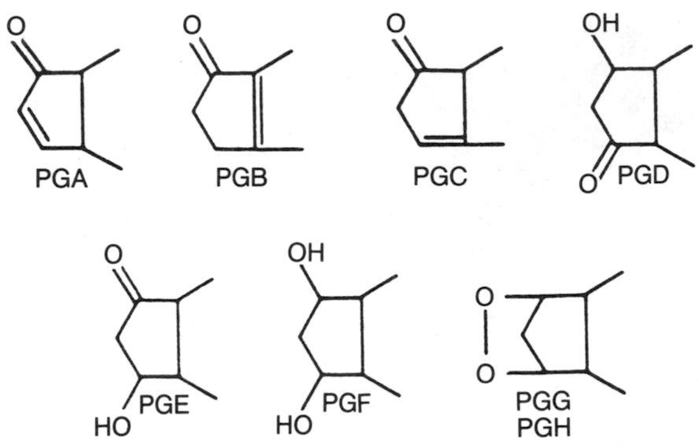

PGA PGB PGC PGD

PGE PGF PGG PGH

Prostaglandins were originally identified in seminal fluid and were believed to be produced by the prostate. It is now known that other tissue cells, particularly mast cells, are the major source of prostaglandins. Prostaglandins are prominent in anaphylactic reactions. The most active components are PGE_2 and PGD_2, which produce vasodilation, increase vascular permeability, and cause hyperalgesia (increased sensitivity to pain). The primary source for thromboxane A_2 is the platelet. Thromboxane A_2 is also produced by the cyclooxygenase pathway and is active in vasoconstriction, bronchoconstriction, and platelet aggregation. These metabolites are rapidly metabolized to inactive forms (PGE_1, PGD_1, and thromboxane B_2) by further oxygenation. The nonsteroidal anti-inflammatory drugs (NSAID), such as aspirin, act to inhibit cyclooxygenase and block formation of these inflammatory mediators.

Leukotrienes. The products of the lipoxygenase pathway are called leukotrienes. They are generated by leukocytes and mast cells. Again the subscript denotes the number of double bonds. The activity of leukotrienes C_4, D_4, and E_4 is believed to be responsible for a factor previously called *slow reacting substance of anaphylaxis* (SRS-A); that of leukotriene B_4 is chemotactic for eosinophils (*eosinophilic chemotactic factor of anaphylaxis,* ECFA) and neutrophils. Although prostaglandins are responsible for some of the late vascular effects of anaphylaxis, they may also modulate anaphylaxis by increasing cyclic nucleotide levels of mast cells and inhibiting histamine release.

Polymorphonuclear Neutrophils

Neutrophilic polymorphonuclear leukocytes are the major cellular component of the acute inflammatory reaction. Neutrophils are characterized by numerous cytoplasmic granules that contain highly destructive hydrolytic enzymes (Table 12-5). At

Table 12-5. Antimicrobial Systems in Neutrophils

Oxygen Dependent	Oxygen Independent
Myeloperoxidase	Lysozyme
Superoxide anion (O_2^-)	Lactoferrin
Hydroxyl radical (OH^-)	Cationic proteins
Singlet oxygen ($^1O_2$)	Neutral proteases
Hydrogen peroxide	Acid hydrolases

least three cytoplasmic granules are identifiable: specific granules (lactoferrin, etc.), azurophilic granules (lysosomes containing acid hydrolases and other enzymes), and a third granule compartment containing gelatinase. Neutrophils may be attracted to sites of inflammation by a number of chemotactic factors (Table 12-6). Neutrophils have cell surface receptors for

Table 12-6. Chemotactic Factors for Neutrophils

Complement
C_5a
C_5a des-Arg
Kallikrein
Fibrinopeptide B
f-Met tripeptides
Collagen peptides
Transfer factor (lymphokine)
Neutrophil chemotactic factors of:
Fibroblasts
Macrophages (interleukin 1)
Lymphocytes
Platelet-activating factor
Leukotriene B_4

some of these factors, such as activated fragments of complement (see below) and formylmethionyl tripeptides. Acute inflammatory reactions need not be initiated by immune mechanisms and are frequently associated with bacterial infections (such as staphylococcal and streptococcal infections) or traumatic tissue injury. In these situations neutrophils are attracted into sites of inflammation by chemotactic factors released by the infecting organism (f-Met peptides) or by products of damaged tissue, such as fibronectin, fibrin or collagen degradation products, or factors produced by other inflammatory cells. In immune complex reactions, neutrophils are attracted by formation of activated complement components (see below) following antibody–antigen reaction in tissues. Upon attraction to sites of inflammation, neutrophils attempt to engulf and digest complexes consisting of bacteria coated with antibody and complement. However, phagocytosis by neutrophils is usually accompanied by release of the lysosomal enzymes from these cells into the tissue spaces, particularly if the antigen is difficult for the polymorphonuclear neutrophil to ingest. The lysosomal acid hydrolases cause local tissue digestion at the site of the reactions. The characteristic lesion is fibrinoid necrosis —areas of acellular digested tissue that look like fibrin but lack any fibrillar appearance. Reactive oxygen metabolites (Table 12-5), primarily involved in bacterial killing, may also damage infiltrating neutrophils and adjacent tissues, resulting in the formation of pus.

Complement

The complement system consists of a set of up to 20 serum proteins that form a controlled sequence for production of activated molecules (Table 12-7). The complete activation sequence occurs on the surface of cells and involves a series of molecular interactions during which fragments as well as new multimolecular complexes with biologic activity are formed. Activation of the complement system via the classic sequence is initiated by antibody–antigen reactions, whereas an alternate pathway may be activated by certain bacterial products. Activated components mediate a variety of tissue responses, including cell lysis, chemotaxis of neutrophils and monocytes, enhancement of phagocytosis, and increased vascular permeability. These activated components also interact with other accessory systems, including the coagulation and fibrinolytic systems, to amplify and/or limit the acute inflammatory reaction. The major functions of activated complement fragments are to open blood vessels and to attract and activate polymorphonuclear neutrophils.

Classical Pathway

A simplified diagrammatic representation of the *classical pathway* for complement activation is shown in Figure 12-6, and the sequence described in detail in Table 12-8. The first component of complement, C1, has the capacity to bind and be activated by antibody molecules that have been altered in their Fc region by reaction with antigen. The Ig classes that are active in fixing complement are IgG and IgM. One molecule of IgM is capable of activating C1, whereas two molecules of IgG reacting close together are required. Activation of C1 may take place in a fluid phase, as when antibody reacts with soluble antigens in the bloodstream; or activation may occur on the surface of cells, as is the case when antierythrocyte antibody reacts with a red cell. In order for two IgG molecules to achieve close enough apposition on a red cell to activate C1, approximately 600 to 1000 molecules must bind to the cell, whereas only one IgM molecule is required.

The components of the classical pathway leading to cell lysis are C1 through C9. In the activation sequence occurring at the cell surface, C1 functions as a recognition unit, C2–C4 as an activation unit, and C5–C9 as a membrane attack unit. When C1 attaches to antibody, it becomes activated as an enzyme (C1 esterase), which cleaves C4 and C2 into two fragments each

Table 12-7. Complement Components

Component	Function	Molecular Weight	Number of Polypeptide Chains	Serum Concentration ($\mu g/ml$)	Site of Synthesis
CLASSICAL PATHWAY					
C1q	Recognition	400,000	18	200	Small intestine epithelium
C1r	Enzyme	160,000	2	—	Small intestine epithelium
C1s	Enzyme	80,000	1	120	Small intestine epithelium
C2	Activation	115,000	1	30	Macrophages
C3	Activation	180,000	2	1,200	Macrophages
C4	Activation	210,000	3	400	Liver epithelium
C5	Attack	180,000	2	75	Macrophages
C6	Attack	128,000	1	60	Liver
C7	Attack	150,000	3	60	—
C8	Attack	150,000	3	15	—
C9	Attack	75,000	1	Trace	Liver
ALTERNATE PATHWAY					
Properdin		190,000	4	20	Macrophages
Factor B	C3 Activator	100,000	1	225	Macrophages
Factor D	C3 Coactivator	25,000	4	Trace	Macrophages
C3	Activation	210,000	3	400	Macrophages

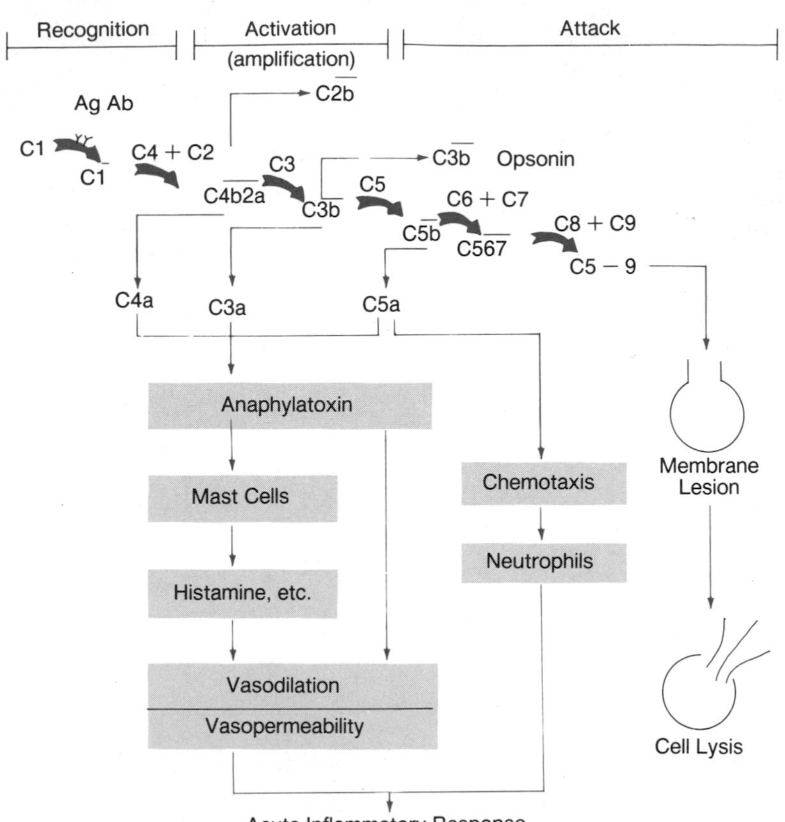

Figure 12-6. Classical pathway of complement activation. Following reaction of antibody with antigen, a cascade reaction of complement components is activated. C1 functions as a recognition unit for the altered Fc of two IgG or one IgM molecule(s); C2 and C4, as an activation unit leading to cleavage of C3. C3 fragments have a number of biological activities: C3a anaphylatoxin, and C3b is recognized by receptors on macrophages (opsonin). C3b also joins with fragments of C4 and C2 to form C3 convertase, which cleaves C5. C5 then reacts with C6 through C9 to form a membrane attack unit that produces a lesion in cell membranes, through which intracellular components may escape (lysis).

(C4a and C4b, C2a and C2b). One of the fragments of C4 (C4b) and one of the C2 fragments (C2a) join together and bind to new sites on the cell surface. Other fragments, C4a and C2b, are released into the fluid phase. C4a has weak anaphylatoxic activity, whereas C2b is converted by plasmin into a C2b kinin-like molecule believed to be responsible for the lesions of hereditary angioedema (see below). The complex of C4b2a forms an enzyme, C3 convertase, which binds and cleaves C3 into C3a and C3b. C3b binds to new sites on the cell surface. As activated C1 can cleave many molecules of C4 and C2 and the C4b2a complex can cleave many molecules of C3, these serve as amplification steps. C3a is released into the fluid phase, where it functions as anaphylatoxin. Phagocytic cells have receptors for C3b; C3b serves as an opsonin (enhances phagocytosis). In addition C3b forms a trimolecular complex with C4b2a (C4b2a3b) that is able to cleave C5 into C5a and C5b (C5 convertase). C5a is released into the fluid phase and C5b binds to the cell surface. C5a is a polypeptide of MW 15,000 with the most potent chemotactic and anaphylatoxic activity of any chemical mediator. C4a and C3a do not have chemotactic activity. In tissues C5a is rapidly broken down to C5a des-Arg by

Table 12-8. Sequence and Mechanism of Immune Hemolysis

Reaction	Biochemical Event
E + A → EA	Reaction of erythrocyte and antierythrocyte antibody.
EA + C1 → EAC1q*	C1q attaches to antibody at a site on Fc portion of Ig antibody bound to the cell.
C1r → $\overline{\text{C1r}}$	Bound C1q* converts C1r to active form by cleavage of C1r.
C1s → $\overline{\text{C1s}}$	$\overline{\text{C1r}}$ activates C1s by cleavage of C1s.
C4 → $\overline{\text{C4a}}$ + C4b* C2 → C2a* + $\overline{\text{C2b}}$	$\overline{\text{C1s}}$ cleaves C4 into $\overline{\text{C4a}}$ and C4b* and C2 into C2a* and $\overline{\text{C2b}}$; plasmin acts on C_2b to produce C_2b kinin; $\overline{\text{C4a}}$ has weak anaphylatoxin activity.
C4b* + C2a* → $\overline{\text{C4b2a}}$	C4b* and C2a* combine to form C3 convertase.
C3 → $\overline{\text{C3a}}$ + C3b*	$\overline{\text{C4b2a}}$ cleaves C3 into $\overline{\text{C3a}}$ and C3b*; $\overline{\text{C3a}}$ (anaphylatoxin) causes smooth muscle contraction and degranulation of mast cells.
C3b* + C4b2a → $\overline{\text{C4b2a3b}}$	C3b* binds to activated bimolecular complex of $\overline{\text{C4b2a}}$ to form a trimolecular complex, C5 convertase, that is a specific enzyme for C5. Macrophages have receptors for C3b, so that C3b acts as opsonin.
C5 → $\overline{\text{C5a}}$ + C5b*	C5 is cleaved into $\overline{\text{C5a}}$ and C5b* by C5 convertase; $\overline{\text{C5a}}$ has anaphylactic and strong chemotactic activity for polymorphonuclear neutrophils.
$\overline{\text{C5b*}}$ + C6789 → $\overline{\text{C5b.9}}$	C5b* reacts with other complement components to produce a macromolecular complex that has the ability to alter cell membrane permeability. $\overline{\text{C8}}$ is most likely the active component, with $\overline{\text{C9}}$ increasing efficiency of $\overline{\text{C8}}$ and producing maximal cell lysis.

E, erythrocyte; A, antibody to erythrocyte.
$\overline{\text{C1}}$, $\overline{\text{C4}}$, etc.: a line above the C number indicates the activated form of the component.
C4a, C4b, etc.: the lower-case letters indicate cleavage products of the parent complement molecule.
C4b*, C2a*: the asterisk indicates a cleavage product that contains an active binding site for other complement components.

cleavage of the amino-terminal arginine. C5 des-Arg is inactive as anaphylatoxin but retains potent chemotactic activity for neutrophils in the presence of whole serum. Anaphylatoxins C5a and C3a (and, weakly, C4a) produce direct contraction of smooth muscle. Addition of these complement fragments will produce contraction of intestine, uterine, tracheal, or other smooth muscle in vitro (Schultz–Dale test), followed by a refractory period termed *tachyphylaxis* that is specific for C3a or C5a (i.e., C3a desensitizes the muscle to further stimulation by C3a but not by C5a). This suggests separate, distinct receptors for C3a and C5a on smooth muscle. In addition, anaphylactic complement fragments induce the release of histamine from mast cells via receptors for C3a and C5a on the mast cell. C5a induces acute inflammation if activated in tissue by soluble antibody–antigen complexes (toxic complex reactions). C5b binds to the cell surface, where it reacts with the remaining complement components, C6–C9, to produce a multimolecular complex that is capable of inserting itself into the cell membrane, forming a channel that permits release of the cytoplasm (lysis).

Alternate Pathway

The complement cascade may be activated by another set of proteins similar to C4, C2, C1, and C3; this is called the *alternate pathway*. A more detailed schematic representation of both the classical and alternate pathways of complement activation is shown in Figure 12-7. The alternate pathway is activated by

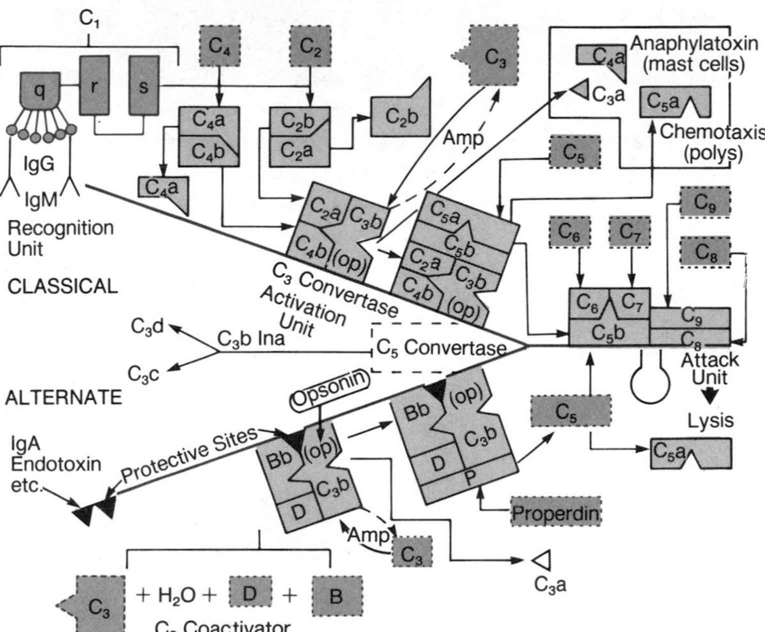

Figure 12-7. Details of the classical and alternate pathways of complement activation. For description, see text.

materials such as bacterial lipopolysaccharide (endotoxin), yeasts (zymosan), or IgA antibody. Three factors—initiating factor, factor B, and factor D—interact in a manner similar to that of the first three complement components of the classical pathway, producing a complex of activated B (Bb) and D that functions as a C3 convertase. A trimolecular complex of Bb, D, and C3b is then formed that is stabilized by the addition of another component, properdin. This complex functions as C5 convertase in activation of C5 and the remaining components of the attack unit.

Regulation and Amplification Mechanisms in the Complement System

Regulation of the complement system is accomplished by a set of inactivators. Complement activation occurs at low levels normally at all times as well as at high levels during inflammation. If left uncontrolled, the cascade of activation could result in serious damage to normal tissue. A number of inactivators of complement have been identified, which act on different stages of complement activation (Table 12-9). Included are C1q inhibitor, C1 esterase inhibitor, the C3 esterase inhibitor system, a membrane activation complex (MAC) inhibitor that competes with cell membrane sites for C5–9, and serum carboxypepti-

Table 12-9. Regulatory Components of the Complement System

C1q inhibitor	Inactivates C1q binding
C1 esterase inhibitor	Inactivates esterase activity
C3 convertase inhibitor system	Inactivates C3 convertase
MAC inhibitor	Competes with cell surface for C5–9
Serum carboxypeptidase N	Inactivates anaphylatoxin

dase N, which inactivates anaphylatoxin (C5a). A deficiency of the C1 esterase inhibitor is found in hereditary angioedema. These patients exhibit massive acute transient swelling of areas of the skin, the bronchi, or the gastrointestinal tract, associated with depressed serum levels of C4 and C2 because of an inability to inactivate C1 esterase. This reaction results in the continued formation of C4 and C2 fragments, particularly C2b; C2b is converted by plasmin to a molecule with kinin-like activity. The C2b–kinin causes contraction of endothelial cells and edema. The reaction continues for approximately 24 hours, which is essentially the biological life of C1 esterase in the absence of C1 esterase inhibitor.

The C3 esterase inhibitor system consists of at least six different components (Table 12-10). The major inactivator is

Table 12-10. Regulatory Proteins of Complement C3 Convertase

Regulator	Properties	Function	Deficiency State
CR1 (C3b/C4b receptor)	MW 160,000–250,000 Cell membrane of neutrophils, macrophages, and erythrocytes	Binds C3b and C4b; promotes phagocytosis and degranulation; cofactor for C3b inactivator; increases decay of C4b2a and C3bBb (C3 convertases)	Hemolytic anemias, chronic granulomatous disease
Factor H	MW 150,000–160,000 Serum glycoprotein	Cofactor for C3b INH; binds C3b, increases decay of C3bBb in the alternative pathway	Low C3, recurrent infections, C3 detectable on erythrocytes
C4-binding protein	MW 540,000–590,000 Serum protein	Binds C4b; cofactor for C3b INH; increases decay of C4b2a	
Decay-activating factor (DAF)	MW 70,000 Cell membrane glycoprotein	Binds C3bBb or C4b2a; increases decay of C3 convertase of both classical and alternative pathway	Paroxysmal nocturnal hemoglobulinuria (lysis of RBC)
JP45-70	MW 45,000–70,000 Membrane	Binds C3b; inactivates C3 convertase (preferential for classical pathway)	
C3b inactivator (C3b INII)	Serine protease endopeptidase	Inactivates C3b by cleavage of α chain; requires cofactors	Low C3, recurrent infections, angioedema

C3b inactivator (C3b INH). C3b INH is an enzyme that cleaves the α chain of C3b to C3bi, then further cleaves C3bi to C3c and C3d. A number of cofactors are involved for the classical and alternate pathways of formation of C3 convertase. CR1, C4bp, and DAF displace C2a from C4b, whereas CR1, factor H, and DAF displace Bb from C3b. This displacement results in decay of C3 convertase and permits cleavage of the C3b by C3b INH. CR1, C4bp, and factor H are closely linked genetically, but are not linked to the MHC complex. Two other complement receptors are CR2 and CR3. CR2 is the binding site for C3d on B cells. The function of this receptor is not known, but it also functions as the binding site for Epstein–Barr virus on B cells. CR3 is a receptor for C3bi on phagocytic cells. Individuals with decreased CR3 receptors have defects in neutrophil functions and increased bacterial infections.

Activation of complement components is an essential feature of cytotoxic and immune complex reactions and may play a role in initiating some delayed cellular reactions, as well. The fixation of complement to a cell surface by action of antibody or via the alternate pathway is responsible for cytolytic reactions. Opsonization is activated because of coating by C3b (or C4b), and lysis of cells by formation of the membrane attack complex C5–9. The chemotactic effect of C5a attracts polymorphonuclear leukocytes and is largely responsible for the participation of these cells in immune complex reactions. The anaphylatoxic effects of C3a and C5a cause separation of endothelial cells. This serves to open vascular barriers to inflammatory cells so that neutrophils, lymphocytes, and macrophages may emigrate from the blood and induce inflammation in tissues.

Platelets

The role of platelets in inflammation is not well understood. Platelets contain heparin and serotonin, so that release of these mediators may contribute to the acute vascular phase of inflammation. Platelets also produce oxygen radicals, which may cause tissue damage. However, the major role of platelets is to block damaged vessel walls and prevent hemorrhage.

Platelets react at sites of vascular damage via a receptor for a triplet peptide, arginine-glycine-asparagine (Arg-Gly-Asp), present in fibrin, fibronectin, and vitronectin. At sites of vascular damage the extracellular matrix proteins fibronectin and vitronectin are exposed, and fibrin is formed through activation of the clotting system (see below). Platelets bind to these molecules, forming clumps of platelets that plug up leaks in the vascular system.

The Coagulation System

Any significant inflammation will result in activation of the coagulation system; several components of this system may serve as inflammatory mediators (Fig. 12-8). The coagulation

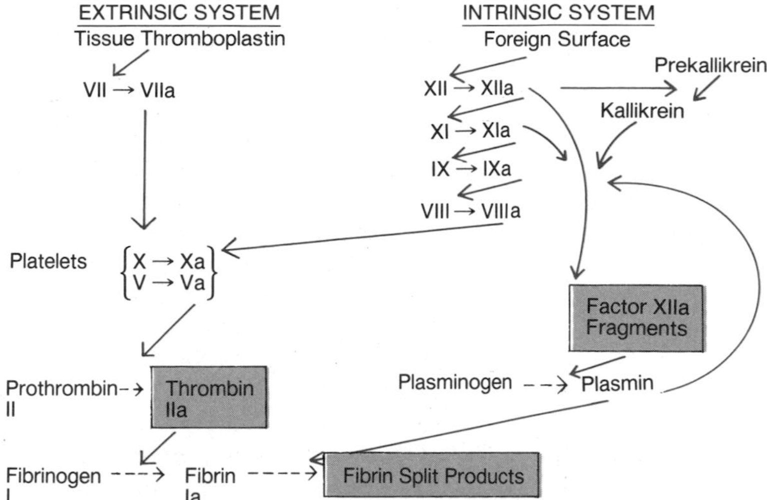

Figure 12-8. The coagulation system and inflammation.

system responds to various stimuli by the formation of platelet plugs and insoluble protein aggregates (fibrin) formed from soluble precursors. Fibrin forms clots that serve to stop bleeding following injury to blood vessels. The fibrinolytic system is activated soon after clot formation in order to limit the extent of fibrin deposition and to initiate dissolution of fibrin so that circulation can be restored to injured tissues. Fibrin may also act as a scaffold for the ingrowth of fibroblasts and capillaries to initiate repair. If fibrin formed intravascularly is not cleared, multiple areas of tissue necrosis (infarcts) may occur. This is known as disseminated intravascular coagulation (see Shwartzman Reaction below). The kinin system increases vascular permeability in areas of inflammation and may be activated by intermediate products of the coagulation cascade.

Roman numerals designate the major components of the coagulation system; a Roman numeral followed by the letter *a* indicates the active fragment of that factor. Coagulation products active in inflammation are fragments of Hageman factor (XIIa) and of thrombin (IIa), and fibrin split products. The coagulation system consists of three major parts: the extrinsic system, the intrinsic system, and the common thrombin–fibrin pathway. The extrinsic system is activated by the action of tissue thromboplastin on factor VII. The intrinsic system involves activation of a series of components beginning with factor XII (Hageman factor). The common pathway is the activation of factors X and V on platelets with the subsequent formation of thrombin and fibrin. Kallikrein, activated factor XI, and plasmin can all act to cleave activated factor XII to produce fragments that initiate fibrinolysis and kinin release, as well as generate a plasma factor that enhances vascular permeability. Activated factor XII converts prekallikrein to kallikrein (see The Kinin System below), so that activation of the intrinsic coagulation system also generates inflammatory mediators.

The Kinin System

Peptides that are active as mediators of inflammation may be generated from a number of cells and tissue products. Of these the most active is the kinin system. The components of this system are generated by the cleavage of plasma proteins into active peptides by proteolytic enzymes of the kallikrein system or trypsin. Kallikreins are small proteolytic enzymes found in tissues (particularly glandular organs) and in plasma, that act on large molecules such as kininogens to produce active peptides. Kallikreins are activated from prekallikreins by the action of activated factor XII (Hageman factor) of the intrinsic coagulation system.

Prekallikrein in plasma exists as a single polypeptide chain with an intrachain disulfide bond. There is also a tissue form, which is slightly different. Activated factor XII (XIIa) cleaves polypeptide chain to form an active two-chain disulfide-linked kallikrein molecule.

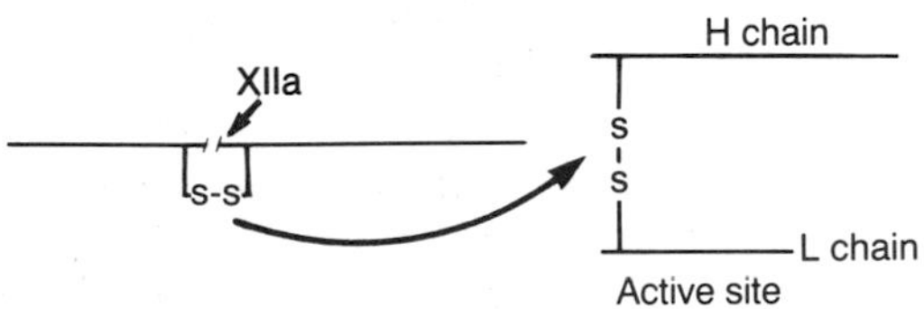

Kallikrein, factor XIIa, factor XI, and trypsin act on kininogens to produce biologically active fragments (see Fig. 12-9). The active peptides are kallidin and bradykinin. Kallidin is a

Activated Hageman Factor (XIIa)

Prekallikrein → Kallikrein or Trypsin

Kininogens → (plasma or tissue) Kallidin → (Amino-peptidase) Bradykinin → (Kininase) Inactive Peptides

H-Arg.Pro.Pro.Gly.Phe.Ser.Pro.Phe.Arg.OH

H-Lys.Arg.Pro.Pro.Gly.Phe.Ser.Pro.Phe.Arg.OH

Figure 12-9. The kinin system.

decapeptide and bradykinin is a nanopeptide formed by cleavage of the amino-terminal lysine from kallidin. These mediators, particularly bradykinin, are highly active in stimulating vasodilation and increased vascular permeability but are rapidly catabolized by kininases into inactive peptides.

Eosinophils

Polymorphonuclear eosinophils are distinguished by the affinity of their cytoplasmic granules for acidic dyes such as eosin, resulting in an intense red staining. This staining is primarily due to the presence of a major basic protein (MBP) that binds acid dyes. Eosinophils are found predominantly in two types of inflammation: allergy and parasitic worm infections. Some chemotactic factors for eosinophils are listed in Table 12-11. These factors are derived from inflammatory cells, complement, or worm extracts. Eosinophils contain many of the same lysosomal enzymes as neutrophils, but appear to function quite differently by limiting or controlling the extent of inflammation. Injection of eosinophils into sites of inflammation induced by histamine, serotonin, or bradykinin effectively diminishes the inflammation. Antibody–antigen complexes are phagocytosed and deactivated by eosinophils. The major basic protein appears to inhibit the action of heparin. These products are uniquely equipped to inactivate inflammatory mediators of mast cells (Table 12-12). In addition, eosinophils are cytotoxic to schistosome larvae through an antibody-dependent cell-mediated mechanism.

Table 12-11. Chemotactic Factors for Eosinophils

Factor	Origin
Histamine	Mast cells
Eosinophilic chemotactic factor A	Mast cells
Neutrophil peptides	Neutrophils
Eosinophil stimulator promoter	Lymphocytes
C5a	Complement
Worm extracts	*Ascaris*

Table 12-12. Eosinophil Modulating Factors for Mast Cell Products

Mast Cell Product	Eosinophil Product
Histamine	Histaminase
SRS-A (leukotrienes)	Arylsulfatase
Heparin	MBP
(Chemotactic factors)	Esterase

Interrelationships of Inflammatory Cells and Systems in Acute Inflammation

A composite of inflammatory mechanisms and interrelationships is illustrated in Figure 12-10. The complement, kinin, coagulation, and mast cell systems as well as bacterial products contribute to vasodilation, increased vascular permeability, and chemotaxis of the primary cellular mediator of acute inflammation, the neutrophil. The neutrophil and its lysosomal enzymes are responsible for killing microorganisms, on the one hand, or causing tissue necrosis, on the other hand.

Products of the complement, kinin, coagulation, and mast cell systems produce vasoactive and chemotactic mediators of acute inflammation. The major mediators are highlighted by boxes in Figure 12-10.

The anaphylactic peptides C3a and C5a are the major inflammatory mediators derived from complement. Cells de-

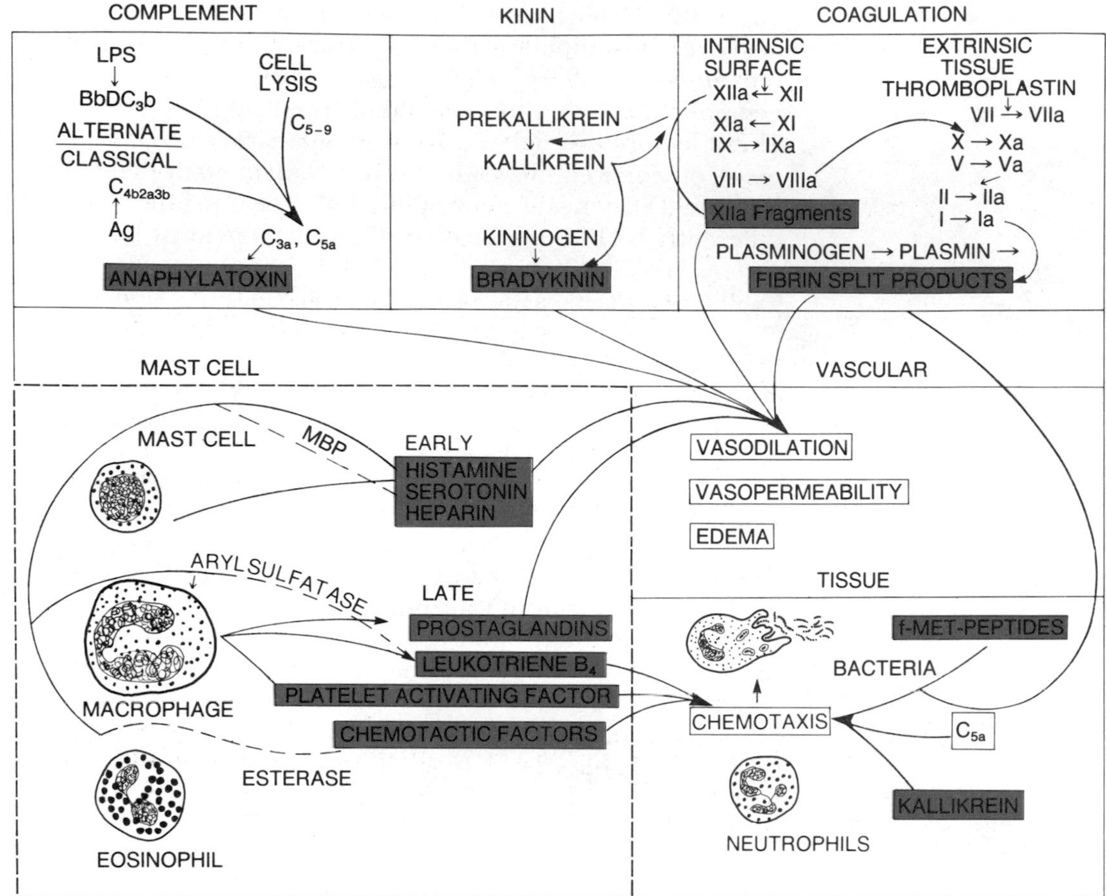

Figure 12-10. Interrelationships of inflammatory cells and systems in acute inflammation.

stroyed by the activation of complement may contribute indirectly through release of intracellular contents that may cause further tissue destruction (enzymes) or activate the extrinsic coagulation system. Activation of the intrinsic coagulation system produces a series of active fragments. Activated factor XII (Hageman factor) contributes to generation of three inflammatory mediators: bradykinin, Hageman factor fragments, and fibrin split products. Mast cells contribute directly by release of mediators such as histamine and serotonin and indirectly by providing arachidonic acid precursors for generation of leukotrienes, prostaglandins, and other factors. These systems act to increase blood flow and vascular permeability, leading to edema, in addition to attracting polymorphonuclear neutrophils and eosinophils to sites of inflammation. Neutrophils destroy infecting organisms by phagocytosis and digestion but also release lysosomal enzymes that may produce tissue damage. Eosinophils are believed to modulate inflammatory reactions by deactivating mast cell mediators.

Adult Respiratory Distress Syndrome

The adult respiratory distress syndrome (ARDS) is the result of diffuse damage to the alveolar epithelium and capillary endothelium of the lung (alveolar wall). This causes increased capillary permeability, interstitial and intraalveolar edema, fibrin exudation, and hyaline membrane formation. ARDS is an increasingly frequent cause of death in patients with diffuse respiratory infections, burns, oxygen toxicity, or narcotic overdose or who undergo open cardiac surgery.

The etiology of ARDS is not precisely defined but is thought to involve shock, oxygen toxicity, complement activation, bacterial products, or a combination of these. In oxygen toxicity associated with artificially assisted respiration, free radicals injure endothelium, causing increased permeability, and epithelium, inducing alveolar edema. Complement activation generates C5a, which induces leukocyte aggregation and activation in the lung. Alveolar cell injury causes loss of surfactant and collapse of air spaces. The role of the different acute inflammatory mechanisms in ARDS is not clear at this time, but most likely involves multiple mediators and may be potentiated by a failure of inactivation mechanisms.

The Cells of Chronic Inflammation

The cells of chronic inflammation are lymphocytes, macrophages, and plasma cells. To contrast these with the cells of acute inflammation (*polymorphonuclear* cells), the cells of chronic inflammation collectively are termed *mononuclear* cells. The function of lymphocytes and macrophages in chronic inflammation is presented here; plasma cells are also present in many forms of chronic inflammation and represent antibody producing cells resulting from stimulation of B cells by antigens.

Lymphocytes

Lymphocytes are prominent in chronic inflammation and are the immune-specific effector cells of delayed hypersensitivity. In immune-specific inflammation, lymphocytes are activated by specific reaction with antigen to release lymphokines responsible for delayed hypersensitivity. In nonimmune chronic inflammation, it is not clear what attracts lymphocytes to sites of inflammation. Lymphocytes do not respond chemotactically to factors that attract other white blood cells. Lymphocytes activated by antigen secrete a number of biologically active inflammatory mediators (Table 12-13). The major function of these mediators appears to be the attraction and activation of macrophages, but other functions such as increasing vascular permeability, killing target cells, and controlling lymphocyte proliferation have been attributed to lymphokines.

Table 12-13. Lymphokines

Factor	MW	Produced by	Effect
Migration inhibitory factor	15,000–70,000	Activated TD cells	Inhibits migration of macrophages
Macrophage activating factor	35,000–55,000	Activated TD cells	Increases lysosomes in macrophages; increases phagocytic activity
Macrophage chemotactic factor	12,500	1. Activated TD cells 2. Lysates of PMNs 3. Ag-Ab complexes (complement)	Attracts macrophages; gradient chemotaxis
Lymphotoxin	Multiple (10,000–200,000)	Activated TK or NK cells	Causes lysis of target cells
Lymphocyte stimulating factor	85,000	Activated TD cells	Stimulates proliferation of lymphocytes
Proliferation inhibitory factor	70,000	Activated TD cells	Inhibits proliferation of lymphocytes
Aggregation factor		Activated TD cells	Causes lymphocytes and macrophages to adhere together
Interferon	20,000–25,000	Activated TD cells	Inhibits growth of viruses; activates NK cells
Lymphocyte-permeability Factor	12,000	Lymph node cells	Increases vascular permeability
Transfer factor	10,000	Activated TD cells	Induces antigen-specific delayed hypersensitivity after passive transfer
Skin reactive factor	10,000	Activated TD cells	Induces inflammation upon injection into skin
Cytophilic antibody	160,000	Plasma cells	Binds to macrophages; stimulates phagocytosis of specific antigen
Leukocyte inhibitory factor	68,000	Activated T cells	Inhibits neutrophil mobility
Osteoclast activating factor	17,000	T and B cells	Stimulates osteoclasts to absorb bone

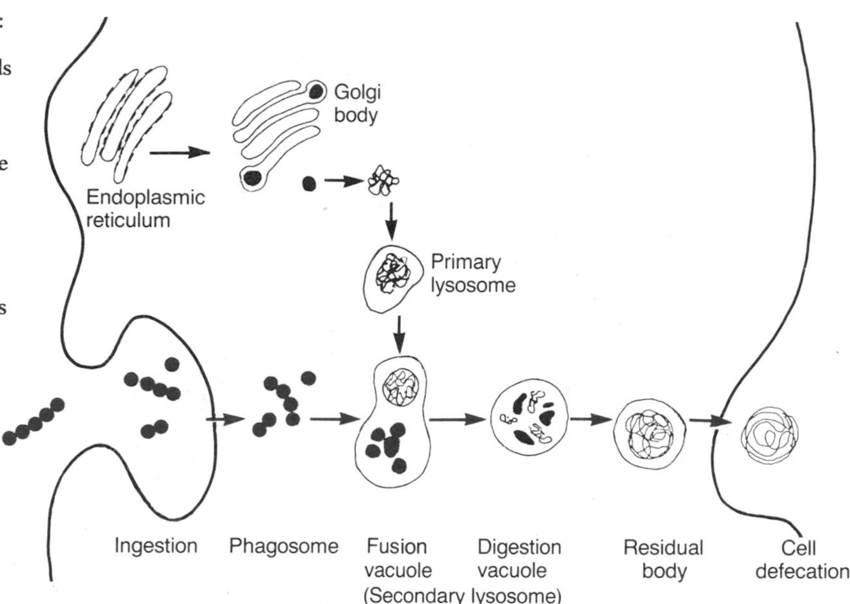

Figure 12-11. Phagocytosis: stages of intracellular digestion and different kinds of lysosomes. Foreign material is ingested into a phagosome. Phagosome fuses with primary lysosome (formed by Golgi body), which contains enzymes to digest ingested material. Resulting fusion vacuole is termed a secondary lysosome. When digestion is ended, some material may remain in residual body, or be eliminated from cell by cell defecation.

Macrophages

Macrophages (see Chapter 2) play an important role in chronic inflammation in general, and in delayed hypersensitivity reactions in particular. Macrophages usually infiltrate sites of inflammation several hours after polymorphonuclear cells. The main function of macrophages is to phagocytose damaged tissue components, microorganisms, or other cells (Fig. 12-11). In this manner, by the action of potent macrophage lysosomal enzymes, the macrophage clears the tissue of the products of inflammation and sets the stage for resolution of the inflammatory process. In delayed hypersensitivity reactions, macrophages are attracted and activated by *lymphokines* produced by reaction of antigen with specifically sensitized lymphocytes (T_D cells) (see Table 12-13).

Phagocytosis

The stages of phagocytosis are illustrated in Figure 12-12. Coating of bacteria by complement or antibody enhances phagocytosis, although phagocytosis certainly occurs in the absence of antibody and complement. Cell surface aggregation of receptors precedes invagination of the cell membrane. Ingestion of material is accompanied by ion fluxes (positive ions entering cell) and superoxide formation. After formation of a phagocytic vacuole, fusion with enzyme containing lysosomes (phagolysosome) and digestion of phagocytosed material occurs.

Products of Macrophages

The products of macrophages that are important for consideration in inflammation are (1) the cytoplasmic constituents re-

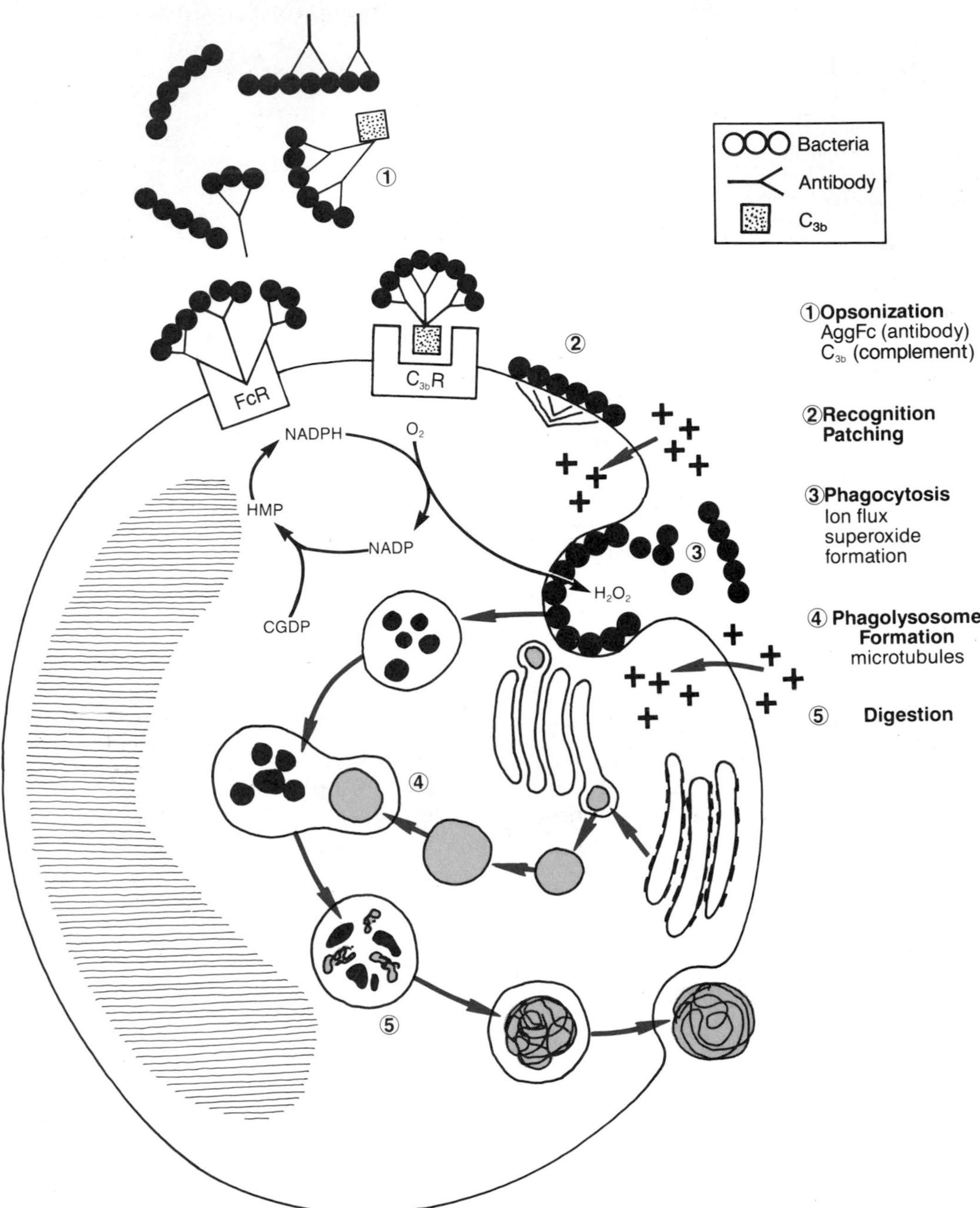

Figure 12-12. Schematic drawing of steps in phagocytosis: (1) opsonization —aggregated Fc of antibody, formation of C3b; (2) recognition through receptors and patching; (3) ingestion—cation influx stimulates transduction of hexose monophosphate shunt and conversion of O_2 to H_2O_2; (4) fusion of lysosome and phagosome to form phagolysosome involving microtubules; (5) digestion of bacteria in phagolysosome.

Table 12-14. Cellular, Cell Surface, and Secreted Products of Macrophages

I. CELLULAR	
Peroxidase (RER) 5′ nucleotidase	Aminopeptidase Alkaline phosphatase
II. CELL SURFACE RECEPTORS	
Fc receptor I (IgG_2a) Fc receptor II (IgG_2b) IgM C3b Lymphokines Protein aggregates (nonspecific) Fibronectin	High-density lipoprotein Lactoferrin Insulin Fibrinogen Asialoglycoprotein f-Met-Leu-Phe
III. SECRETED BIOLOGICALLY ACTIVE PRODUCTS OF MACROPHAGES	

Hydrolytic enzymes
  Lysosomal hydrolases
  Neutral proteases
  Collagenase
  Plasminogen activator
  Elastase
  Lysozyme
  Arginase
	Cell stimulatory proteins
	  Colony-stimulating factor
	  Interleukin 1
	  Interferon
	  Tumor necrosis factor
	  Osteoclast activating factor
	Others
	  Complement components
	    (C2, C3, C4, C5, factor B)
	  Oxygen intermediates
	  α_2 macroglobulin
	  Prostaglandins

sponsible for cellular metabolism and the degradation of phagocytosed material, (2) the cell surface receptors that contribute to phagocytosis, and (3) the secreted products that may cause tissue damage (Table 12-14). Depending on the nature of the inflammatory stimulus, the macrophage functions to clear necrotic tissue and to eradicate invading organisms, leading to resolution of the acute inflammatory response or, if the organism persists, to initiate a chronic or prolonged defensive reaction, granulomatous inflammation. Macrophages may also release products to stimulate specific immune functions to aid in the defense against persistent microorganisms.

The importance of macrophages in inflammation was emphasized by Eli Metchnikoff almost 100 years ago. Macrophages are attracted to sites of inflammation by a number of chemotactic factors (see Table 12-15). The most potent are those derived from activated lymphocytes (lymphokines), but factors may also be derived from other cell types. In addition, macrophages are attracted by C5a and by f-Met peptides. Thus macrophages are attracted to sites of acute inflammation both by products of immune specific activation of lymphocytes and by products of nonimmune cells. In addition, lymphocytes activated by non-

Table 12-15. Growth-Stimulating, Chemotactic, and Activation Factors Acting on Macrophages

Substance	Physicochemical Characteristics (MW)	Source	Functional Properties
Macrophage colony-stimulating factor (CSF)	70,000	Fibroblasts	Macrophage colony formation from bone marrow cells. Also induces macrophage secretion
Macrophage growth factor (MGF)	Same as CSF	Fibroblasts, activated T lymphocytes	Acts on promonocytes
Factor inducing monocytosis (FIM)	18,000–23,000	Unknown	Increases macrophages in blood
Leukocyte-derived chemotactic factor (LDCF)	12,000	Activated T lymphocytes	Chemotactic for macrophages
Plasminogen activator inducer (IPA)		Activated T lymphocytes	Stimulates plasminogen activator secretion
Macrophage stimulatory protein (MSP)	100,000	Unknown	Increases spreading and phagocytosis
Factor Bb	65,000	Alternate complement pathway	Increases spreading and phagocytosis; inhibits migration
Macrophage activating factor (MAF)	50,000–60,000	Activated T lymphocytes	Increases macrophage tumoricidal and microbicidal function
Migration inhibitory factor (MIF)	25,000–60,000	Activated T lymphocytes	Inhibits migration
Soluble immune response suppressor (SIRS)	Similar to MIF	Activated T lymphocytes	
Interferon	Several MW species	Fibroblasts, activated T lymphocytes	Both Types I and II activate macrophages
Macrophage aggregating factor	>100,000	Activated T lymphocytes	Distinct from MIF. Causes clumping of macrophages in vivo and in vitro; may be fibronectin
C5a	15,000	Complement activation	Chemotactic
f-Met peptides	Tripeptides	Bacteria	Chemotactic
Phorbol esters		Tumor promotors	Activate macrophage secretion
LPS (endotoxin)		Bacteria	Activates macrophages

Modified from Rosenstreich DL: The macrophage, in Oppenheim JJ, Rosenstreich DL, Potter M (eds), Cellular Functions in Immunity and Inflammation. New York, Elsevier, 1981, p 140.

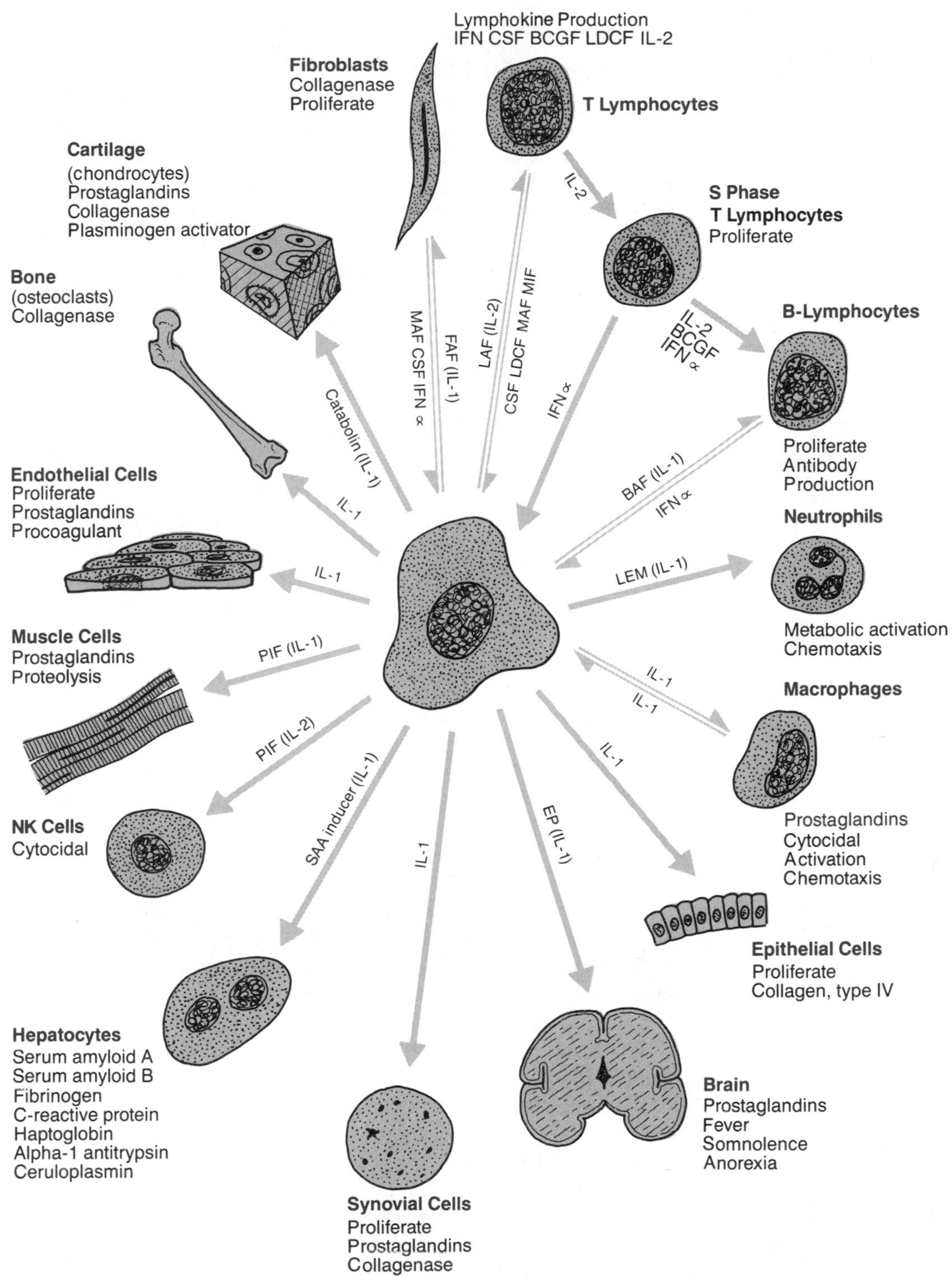

Figure 12-13. Effects of IL1 on target cells and tissues. The diagram shows bidirectional interactions between macrophages and lymphoid cells or fibroblasts mediated by IL1 and other cytokines, and the activities of target cells known to be augmented by IL1. IFN, interferon; CSF, colony stimulating factor; BCGF, B cell growth factor; LDCF, lymphocyte-derived chemotactic factor; SAA, serum amyloid A; PIF, proteolysis-inducing factor; EP, endogenous pyrogen.

immune specific mitogens, such as endotoxin (lipopolysaccharide, LPS) or other bacterial products, will produce lymphokines active on macrophages. Activated macrophages have an increased capacity for phagocytosis and an increased capacity to digest phagocytosed objects and, in addition, secrete factors (monokines) active in inflammation and immune reactions (see Table 12-14). Activated macrophages have changes in lysosomal enzyme content: a decrease in 5′ nucleotidase and an increase in aminopeptidase and alkaline phosphatase as well as an increase in adenosine triphosphate and in production of superoxide anion and hydrogen peroxide. There is also an increase in activity of cell surface receptors on macrophages, in particular for Fc of immunoglobulin and for C3b.

Interleukin 1

A major macrophage mediator (monokine) is interleukin 1 (IL1). This mediator has a large number of biological effects (Fig. 12-13). Active investigation has led to the conclusion that the activities attributed to interleukin 1 may, in fact, be caused by more than one mediator.

Origin and Development of Macrophages

Macrophages are derived from bone marrow cells and are stimulated to mature to activated effector cells by a number of factors. These factors are listed in Table 12-15, and the stages of action of the factors given in Figure 12-14.

Phagocytic Deficiencies

In some cases, either because of the nature of the phagocytosed material or because of an insufficiency in lysosomal hydrolases, ingested particles or organisms are not killed and digested. Some organisms (e.g., *Histoplasma capsulatum*) have the ability to survive phagocytosis and reproduce within phagocytes. Infection with such an agent may result in the presence of large numbers of viable organisms in the cytoplasm of phagocytic cells. Some inorganic particles (e.g., silica) cannot be digested, remain in phagocytic cells, and eventually cause destruction of the phagocyte (phagocytic suicide), tissue damage and fibrosis, and increased susceptibility to certain infections. Certain human diseases are characterized by abnormalities in phagocytosis (phagocytic dysfunction). Such phagocytic deficiencies are usually associated with susceptibility to infections. These diseases are presented in more detail in Chapter 24.

Activated Macrophages

An acquired cellular resistance to microbial infection may be observed in an infected host whose mononuclear phagocytes have an increased capacity for destroying infected organisms (i.e., the host has activated macrophages). Macrophage activation may occur by increasing the number of lysosomes per cell, by increasing the amount of hydrolytic enzymes in each lysosome, or by increasing the number of phagocytes available. Once such an increased capacity has been established, it is

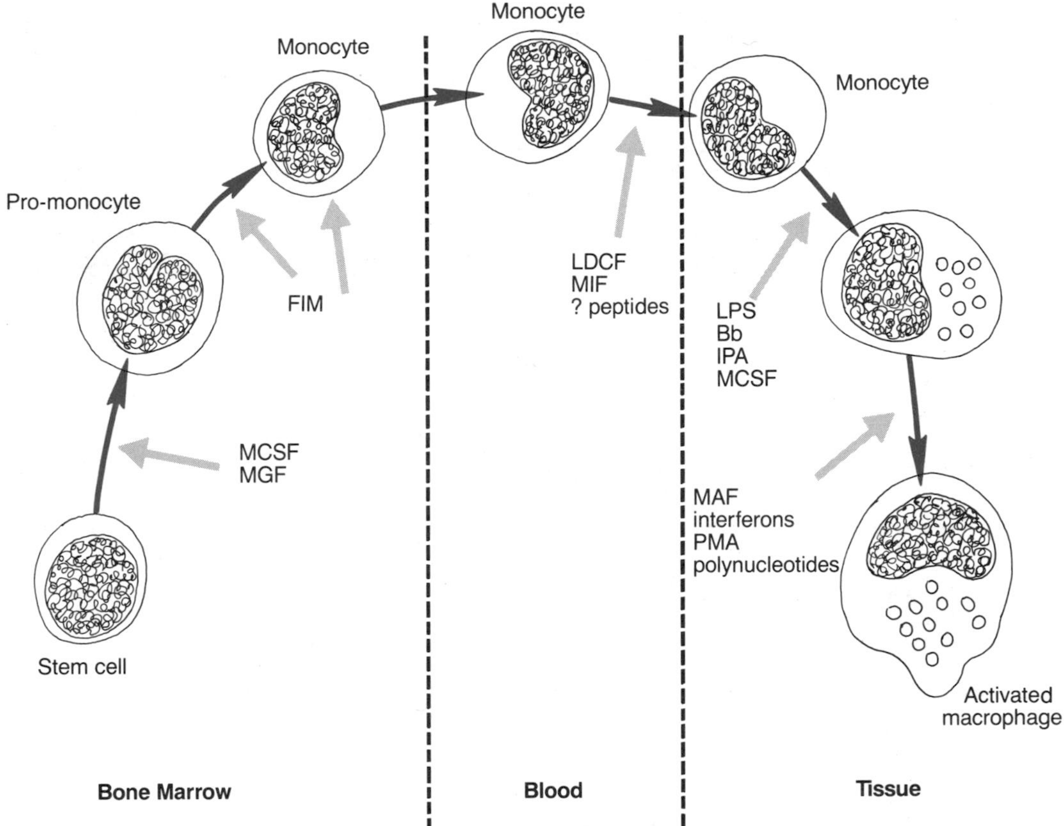

Figure 12-14. Postulated stages in development and activation of macrophages. The proliferation and differentiation of monocytes are stimulated by factors that act on bone marrow precursors. Monocytes are released into the peripheral blood and are attracted to sites of inflammation by inflammatory mediators, where they are stimulated by other factors to become activated for increased phagocytosis and secretion.

active against infections caused by unrelated organisms. A number of agents have been found that cause activation of macrophages. These include bacillus Calmette-Guérin (BCG), *Listeria monocytogenes,* toxoplasma, endotoxin, levamisole, and polynucleotides (Fig. 12-15). A considerable interest in the role of this phenomenon in enhancing tumor immunity has developed because of the possibility of limiting tumor growth with activated macrophages. This type of cellular immunity has been termed *immune phagocytosis,* even though this "immunity" is nonspecific.

The Reticuloendothelial System

The reticuloendothelial system (RES) is a multiorgan collection of cells whose primary common functional capacity is phagocytosis. Two general types of phagocytes are recognized —wandering and fixed. The wandering cells are the monocytes of the peripheral blood. These cells may be found in other

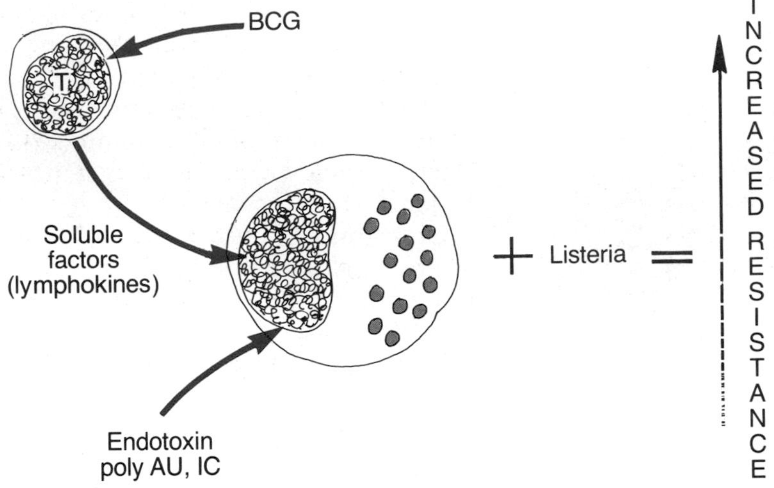

Figure 12-15. Nonspecific macrophage activation. Macrophages may acquire an increased capacity to destroy infective organisms or target cells after treatment with a variety of agents. Bacillus Calmette-Guérin acts upon T cells, which produce a soluble factor that affects macrophages. Endotoxins and polynucleotides act directly on macrophages. The mechanism of action of these agents is not understood, but as a result of macrophage activation, an experimental animal will resist a normally infectious challenge dose of an infectious agent. The chart (bottom) indicates that the dose of *Listeria monocytogenes* required to kill an experimental animal is significantly higher after treatment of the animals with BCG.

organs, for example in the sinusoids of lymphoid organs or the connective tissue (stroma) of many organs, where they may be only temporary residents. The fixed cells (histiocytes) are permanent residents in these tissue locations. Histiocytes may be found in liver (Kupffer cells or sinusoid-lining cells), spleen (sinusoid-lining cells, reticular cells, dendritic macrophages), lymph nodes, connective tissue, brain (microglia), bone marrow, adrenals, thymus, and lungs (alveolar macrophages). If particles such as carbon or vital dyes are injected into the blood, the Kupffer cells of the liver and the phagocytic cells of the spleen ingest most of them; if the particles are inhaled, the pulmonary alveolar macrophages ingest them; if they are injected into connective tissue, the local phagocytes ingest them; if the particles are injected into the brain, the microglia destroy them. All these cells have in common the ability to ingest foreign materials.

Phagocytic Index

Measurement of the phagocytic capacity of an animal may be accomplished by determining the rate of disappearance of stable, inert, uniform particles such as gelatin-stabilized carbon particles. Upon intravenous injection of such particles, about 90% are taken up by the liver, most of the remainder by the spleen. Carbon clearance is measured after saturation of the clearing mechanism, because a dose of particles lower than the saturation dose is cleared during the first few passages of the blood through the liver. Determination of carbon clearance under these conditions primarily measures liver blood flow. If a dose large enough to saturate the reticuloendothelial system is given, a two-stage elimination occurs: (1) a rapid clearance as the particle-laden blood first passes through the liver and spleen, and (2) a slower clearance, which occurs upon recirculation through the previously saturated reticuloendothelial system. The slope of this second curve is the *phagocytic index.* It measures regeneration of phagocytic capacity after saturation.

The clearance of particles from the blood by the reticuloendothelial system follows first-order reaction kinetics:

reactant → product

or

particles in blood → ingestion by RES

The change in concentration of the particles in the blood over a given time is related to the concentration at the start of the experiment, as follows:

$$dC/dt + KC_0.$$

This becomes:

$$C_t = C_0 10^{-Kt}$$

where

C_t = concentration at time t,
C_0 = initial concentration,
t = time,
K = constant (phagocytic index).

Solving for K:

$$K = \frac{\log C_1 - \log C_2}{t_2 - t_1}$$

After injection of a dose of carbon particles sufficient to saturate the reticuloendothelial system, the concentration of carbon in the blood at a given time is determined (C_1, t_1). After a period of several hours, the animal is bled and the concentration of carbon again determined (C_2, t_2). K, the phagocytic index, can then be determined from the formula given above.

Stimulation of the Reticuloendothelial System

A number of agents may affect the phagocytic index. Products of microorganisms, such as the cell wall of yeast (zymosan), bacterial endotoxins, extracts of *Mycobacterium tuberculosis,* living and killed organisms, simple lipids such as triglycerides, and hormones such as estrogen, have all been shown to increase carbon clearance. The ability of some organisms such as *Salmonella typhimurium* to increase phagocytic activity results in increased resistance of the host to other infecting microorganisms (see Activated Macrophages, above). Antibody to a given organism or particle may increase the capacity of the host to phagocytose antibody-coated particles (opsonin). The mechanisms of action of agents that stimulate phagocytic clearance are not clear.

Blockade of the Reticuloendothelial System

Phagocytic clearance may be depressed by overloading the reticuloendothelial system. Thus, a saturating dose of carbon may decrease the clearance of a second dose of carbon. Blockade of the reticuloendothelial system with fibrin results in a decreased clearance of fibrin formed after blockade (see above). Agents that blockade the system have similar properties. Colloidal carbon blockades the system for a second dose of carbon or for similar agents but does not affect the clearance of chromic phosphate. This suggests different phagocytic receptors for different particles.

Shwartzman Reaction

The Shwartzman reaction is not an immune reaction but an alteration in factors affecting intravascular coagulation and reticuloendothelial clearance.

Local Shwartzman Reaction

The local Shwartzman reaction is a lesion confined to a prepared tissue site (usually skin) and is a two-stage reaction. The tissue site is prepared by the local injection of an agent (gram-negative endotoxin) that causes accumulation of polymorphonuclear leukocytes. It is believed that the granulocytes then condition the site by releasing lysosomal acid hydrolases that damage small vessels, setting up the site for reaction to a provoking agent. A mild inflammatory reaction may serve as a preparative event. Provocation is accomplished by injection into the prepared site of agents that initiate intravascular coagulation (gram-negative endotoxins, antigen–antibody complexes, starch). The lesion is caused by intravascular clotting with localization of platelets, granulocytes, and fibrin at the site of preparation, forming white cell thrombi that lead to necrosis of vessel walls and hemorrhage. The administration of nitrogen mustard (decreased granulocytes) or vasodilators inhibits the reaction, whereas agents that block the reticuloendothelial system (e.g., carbon) increase the intensity of the reaction. Specific immunization is not necessary. Although immune reactions may serve as either a preparatory or provocative event, nonimmune reactions are also effective.

Generalized Shwartzman Reaction (Disseminated Intravascular Coagulation)

The classic generalized Shwartzman reaction is elicited by giving a young rabbit two intravascular injections of endotoxin 24 hours apart (Fig. 12-16). After the first injection, a few fibrin thrombi are found in vessels of liver, lungs, kidney, and spleen capillaries. Following the second injection, many more thrombi are found. Bilateral renal cortical necrosis and splenic hemorrhage and necrosis are prominent. The fibrin thrombi do

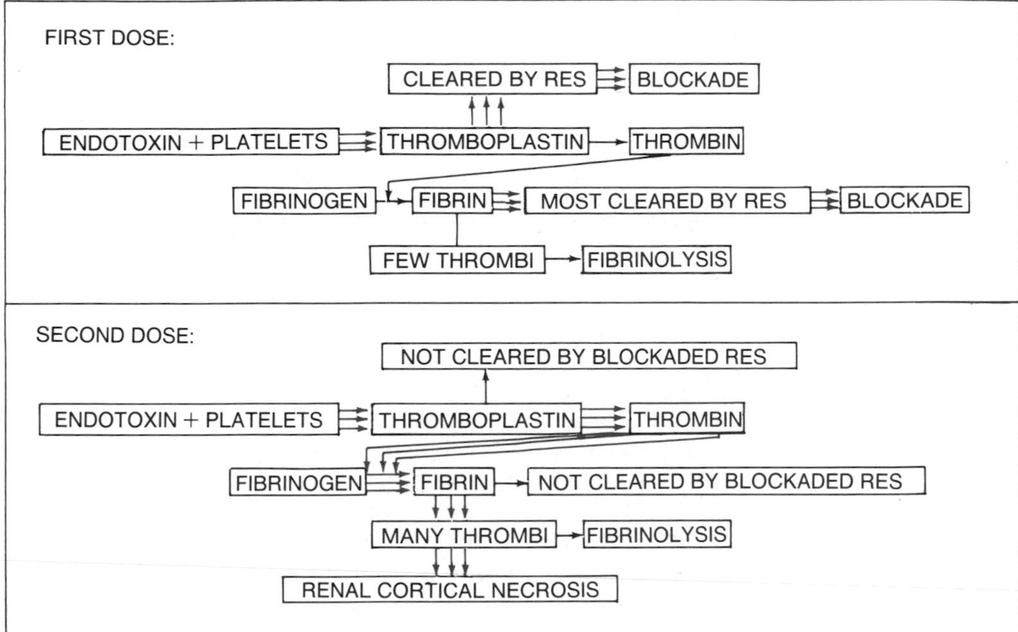

Figure 12-16. Mechanism of generalized Shwartzman reaction induced by endotoxin. Classic generalized Shwartzman reaction is elicited by giving rabbits two doses of endotoxin 24 hours apart. Primary effect of first (preparatory) dose of endotoxin is to cause release of platelet thromboplastin. Most of this thromboplastin is cleared by reticuloendothelial system (RES). Some thrombin triggers conversion of fibrinogen to fibrin, but again most of this fibrin is cleared by reticuloendothelial system. If an animal is examined after one dose of endotoxin (preparative dose), a few fibrin thrombi are found in vessels of liver, lungs, and spleen. These thrombi appear to be quickly removed by fibrinolysis, with no damage to treated rabbit. However, because of action of reticuloendothelial system in clearing thromboplastin and fibrin, blockade of reticuloendothelial system occurs. This blockade permits second dose of endotoxin to produce severe intravascular coagulation. Second dose (provocative dose) initiates same release of platelet thromboplastin as first dose, but with reticuloendothelial system blockaded, this thromboplastin is not cleared; most goes on to form thrombin and initiate conversion of fibrinogen to fibrin. This fibrin cannot be cleared by the blockaded reticuloendothelial system and most becomes lodged in capillaries, capillaries of renal glomeruli in particular. Fibrinolytic system is not capable of overcoming large amounts of fibrin formed in a short period of time. End result may be fatal renal cortical necrosis.

not contain clumps of platelets or leukocytes. In human disease, the generalized Shwartzman reaction develops as an acute and frequently fatal complication of an underlying disease, such as infection. This is called disseminated intravascular coagulation. It is triggered by one or more episodes of intravascular clotting leading to the formation of multiple fibrin or fibrin-like thrombi that lodge in small vessels. Such thrombi are prominent in the kidney or adrenal glands and cause necrosis and/or hemorrhage. Three steps appear to be necessary:

1. Intravascular clotting with fibrin formation.
2. Deposition of fibrin in small vessels. In order for this to happen, at least one, and usually all, of the following condi-

tions must apply: depression of reticuloendothelial clearance of altered fibrinogen; decrease in blood flow through affected organs; liberation of enzymes by granulocytes, which help precipitate fibrin.

3. Once deposited, the fibrin is not removed by fibrinolysis.

Agents that cause blockade of reticuloendothelial clearance (thorotrast, carbon, endotoxin, cortisone) serve as priming agents, and agents that activate intravascular clotting (endotoxin, antigen–antibody complexes, synthetic acid polysaccharides) serve as provoking agents.

Endotoxin Shock

Endotoxin shock is different from the Shwartzman reaction in that no preparative injection is necessary; shock can be induced in any species (the Shwartzman reaction occurs only in man and rabbit); shock occurs with equal intensity at any age (young rabbits are much more sensitive than old rabbits to the Shwartzman reaction); thrombi are not prominent in endotoxic shock, which features hemorrhage and necrosis, and cortisone enhances the Shwartzman reaction but does not affect endotoxic shock. Endotoxin may function by activation of complement components causing vasodilation and increased vascular permeability.

The Shwartzman Reaction and Pregnancy

A single injection of endotoxin in pregnant rabbits produces a generalized Shwartzman reaction. Bilateral renal cortical necrosis has been reported in septicemia following induced abortion in humans. Clinical evidence indicates that bilateral renal cortical necrosis in this circumstance represents a human equivalent of the generalized Shwartzman reaction due to endotoxemia during pregnancy. Pregnancy serves as the preparative step, because fibrinolytic activity and reticuloendothelial clearance are decreased during pregnancy. The occurrence of gram-negative septicemia during delivery or abortion serves as the provocative step, leading to hypotension and intravascular clotting. In addition, intravascular dissemination of amniotic fluid during delivery may activate fibrin formation. This may be followed by thrombocytopenia and hemorrhage or a typical generalized Shwartzman reaction with bilateral renal cortical necrosis. Fibrin occurs within glomerular capillary loops within 48 hours of the provocation. Hemorrhagic necrosis of the adrenals and/or renal cortical necrosis may occur 60 hours to 40 days later. However, most episodes of pregnancy-associated Shwartzman reaction do not progress to fatal renal cortical necrosis.

Review of Inflammatory Mediators

A summary of the role of different mediators at different stages of the inflammatory process is given in Figure 12-17. The early vascular stages are largely caused by mast cell mediators. In some instances products of the coagulation, kinin, and comple-

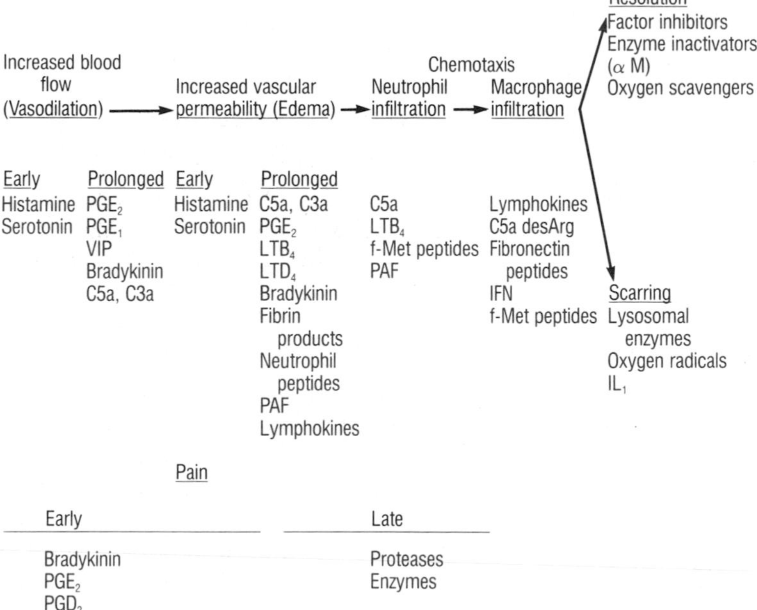

Figure 12-17. Summary of the role of mediators in the process of inflammation. PGE, prostaglandin E; PGD, prostaglandin D; C, complement components; VIP, vasoactive intestinal polypeptide; LTB, leukotriene B; LTD, leukotriene D; PAF, platelet-activating factor; IFN, interferon; IL1, interleukin 1.

ment systems may be active. The acute cellular stage is mediated by complement, leukotrienes, or bacterial or tissue products. The chronic cellular stage is influenced mainly by lymphokines. The outcome of the inflammatory process depends largely on the degree of injury and is effected mainly by macrophages, which either clear the inflamed tissue or set the stage for fibroblast proliferation and scarring. Because of the difficulty in studying this complex process, which can really only be duplicated in vivo, the precise action of the various mediators is not well understood.

Manifestations of Inflammation in Tissues

Examples of morphologic manifestations of different stages of inflammation in tissues include four different organs in which inflammation is initiated by different etiologies: (1) vessels—vasculitis induced by antigen–antibody reaction or inflammatory mediators; (2) lung—pneumonia induced by infection; (3) heart—myocardial infarction induced by blockage of blood flow (coronary thrombus), and (4) kidney—glomerulonephritis induced by antibody–antigen reaction and activation of complement (Table 12-16).

The initiating event is different, but the subsequent sequence of events is similar. Acute inflammation is first manifested in vessels by increased blood flow (congestion) and increased vascular permeability (edema). Chemotactic factors attract and activate polymorphonuclear neutrophils. If enzyme release from neutrophils occurs in the vessel walls, fibrinoid (fibrin-resembling) necrosis is seen. This is followed by lymphocyte and macrophage infiltration. If resolution does not

Table 12-16. Manifestations of Inflammation in Tissue

Organ	Etiology	Inciting Event	Stages of Inflammation: Acute	Subacute	Chronic
Vessel (vasculitis)	Multiple	Multiple; cell injury, infection	Increased blood flow and vasopermeability (edema) →		Resolution
			Poly infiltrate (pus)—Mononuclear cells →		Resolution / Scarring
			Necrosis—Hemorrhage →		Scarring
Lung (pneumonia)	Infection	Release of bacterial products	Edema, congestion →		Resolution
			Poly infiltrate—Macrophages →		Resolution / Scarring
			Hemorrhage—*Necrosis*—Fibroblast proliferation →		Scarring
Heart (infarct)	Disturbance of flow	Necrosis of myocardial cells	Edema, congestion Poly infiltrate—Macrophage— Fibroblast proliferation →		Scarring
Kidney (glomerulonephritis)	Immune inflammation	Deposition of Ag-Ab complexes, activation of complement	Increased glomerular permeability (proteinuria) →		Resolution
			Poly infiltrate—mononuclear infiltrate *Necrosis*—Hematuria—Epithelial proliferation →		Scarring (uremia)

occur, subendothelial fibroblastic proliferation leads to narrowing of the vessel wall (endarteritis) and eventually to infarction of tissue. In the lung, congestion and edema due to increased blood flow and vascular permeability are followed by polymorphonuclear infiltration, and then macrophage infiltration, fibroblast proliferation, and scarring (organizing pneumonia). In myocardial infarction, necrosis of myocardial cells is seen first. Release of cytoplasm from necrotic cells produces vasodilation and endothelial cell contraction (increased vascular permeability — edema), and chemotaxis for polymorphonuclear cells. This is followed by macrophage infiltration, fibroblast and capillary proliferation (granulation tissue), and scarring. In the renal glomerulus the sequence of events is initiated by activation of complement following deposition of antibody–antigen complexes in the basement membrane. This produces changes in the endothelial cells and basement membrane that result in leakage of protein in the urine (proteinuria, the equivalent of edema in other organs) and chemotaxis of polymorphonuclear neutrophils. Enzymes released by polymorphonuclear cells cause destruction of the basement membrane, and red cells pass into the urine (hematuria, the equivalent of hemorrhage in other tissues). Subacute glomerular inflammation is manifested by proliferation of epithelial cells and continued thickening of the basement membrane (membranoproliferative glomerulonephritis). The major consequence of the inflammatory process changes from increased glomerular permeability (proteinuria, hematuria) to decreased filtration as the basement membrane becomes thickened (uremia). As in other organs, chronic inflammation is manifested by fibrosis and scarring. Thus, in each organ the process of inflammation is essentially the same, leading to resolution or scarring through similar stages.

Summary

Inflammation is the process of delivery of proteins and cells to sites of tissue damage or infection and their activation at these sites. The process proceeds from acute, subacute, and chronic stages to resolution or scarring. Tissue lesions and extent of reaction are determined by inflammatory mechanisms mediated by serum protein or cellular systems. The serum protein systems include complement, coagulation, fibrinolysis, and kinin; the cellular systems include polymorphonuclear leukocytes, mast cells (or basophils), platelets, eosinophils, lymphocytes, macrophages, and the reticuloendothelial system. Each of these systems has a homeostatic function and is controlled by interrelated feedback mechanisms. Excessive or inadequate activation of these systems may have serious effects. Manifestions of the stages of inflammation in different tissues are similar even though the inflammatory process is initiated by different events (infections, tissue necrosis, antibody–antigen reaction).

References

General

Braunsteiner R, Zuker-Franklin D (eds): The Physiology and Pathology of Leukocytes. New York, Grune & Stratton, 1962.

Florey HW (ed): General Pathology, 4th ed. Philadelphia, Saunders, 1970.

Hunter J: A Treatise on the Blood, Inflammation and Gun Shot Wounds, Vol I. London, G. Nicoll, 1974.

Larsen CL, Henson PM: Mediators of inflammation. Annu Rev Immunol 1:335, 1983.

Lepow IH, Ward PA (eds): Inflammation: Mechanisms and Control. New York, Academic Press, 1972.

Movat HZ (ed): Inflammation, Immunity and Hypersensitivity. New York, Harper & Row, 1971.

McCutcheon M: Chemotaxis in leukocytes. Physiol Rev 26:319, 1946.

Oppenheim JJ, Rosenstreich DL, Potter M: Cellular Functions in Immunity and Inflammation. New York, Elsevier, 1981.

Spector WG, Willoughby DA: The inflammatory response. Bacteriol Rev 27:117, 1963.

Suter E, Ramseier H: Cellular reactions in infection. Adv Immunol 4:117, 1964.

Thomas L, Uhr JW, Grant L (eds): International Symposium on Injury, Inflammation and Immunity. Baltimore, Williams & Wilkins, 1964.

Zweifach BW, Grant L, McClusky RT (eds): The Inflammatory Response, Vol 3. New York, Academic Press, 1974.

Van Arman CG (ed): White Cells in Inflammation. Springfield, Ill., Thomas, 1974.

Mast Cells

Anderson P, Slorach SA, Uvnas B: Sequential exocytosis of storage granules during antigen-induced histamine release from sensitized rat mast cells in vitro. An electron microscopic study. Acta Physiol Scand 88:359, 1973.

Austen KF, Orange RP: Bronchial asthma: the possible role of the chemical mediators of immediate hypersensitivity in the pathogenesis of subacute and chronic disease. Annu Rev Resp Dis 112:423, 1975.

Bach MK: Mediators of anaphylaxis and inflammation. Annu Rev Microbiol 36:371, 1982.

Benditt BR, Lagunoff D: The mast cell: its structure and function. Prog Allergy 8:195, 1964.

Bennich H, Johansson SGO: Structure and function of human immunoglobulin E. Adv Immunol 13:1, 1971.

Berridge MJ: The molecular basis of communication within the cell. Sci Am 253:142, 1985.

Chakrin L, Bailey D: Leukotrienes. Orlando, Fla., Academic Press, 1984.

Davis P, Bailey PJ, Goldenberg MM, Ford-Hutchinson AW: The role of arachidonic acid oxygenation products in pain and inflammation. Annu Rev Immunol 2:335, 1983.

Dvorak HF, Dvorak AM: Basophils, mast cells, and cellular immunity in animals and man. Hum Pathol 3:454, 1972.

Ishizaka K, Ishizaka T, Hornbrook MH: Physico-chemical properties of human reaginic antibody. IV. Presence of a unique immunoglobulin as a cause of reaginic activity. J Immunol 97:75, 1966.

Metcalf DD, Kaliner M, Donlon MA: The mast cell. CRC Crit Rev Immunol 3:24, 1981.

Mota I: Mast cells and anaphylaxis. Ann NY Acad Sci 103:264, 1963.

Paton WDM: The release of histamine. Prog Allergy 5:79, 1958.

Uvnas B: Mechanism of histamine release in mast cells. Ann NY Acad Sci 103:278, 1963.

Wasserman SI: The human lung mast cell. Environ Health Perspect 55:259, 1984.

Neutrophils

Becker EL: Enzyme activation and the mechanism of neutrophil chemotaxis. Antibiot Chemother 19:409, 1974.

Boyden S: The chemotactic effect of mixtures of antibody and antigen on polymorphonuclear leucocytes. J Exp Med 115:453, 1962.

Cochrane CG: Immunologic tissue injury mediated by neutrophilic leukocytes. Adv Immunol 9:97, 1968.

Fantone JC, Ward PA: Role of oxygen-derived free radicals and metabolites and leukocyte-dependent inflammatory reactions. Am J Pathol 107:397, 1982.

Goldstein IM: Polymorphonuclear leukocyte lysosomes and immune tissue injury. Prog Allergy 20:301, 1976.

Naccache PH, Shaafi RI: Granulocyte activation: biochemical events associated with the mobilization of calcium. Surv Immunol Res 3:288, 1984.

Schiffmann E, Corcoran BA, Wahl SA: N-formylmethyl peptides as chemoattractants for leukocytes. Proc Nat Acad Sci USA 72:1059, 1975.

Spicer SS, Hardin JH: Ultrastructure, cytochemistry, and function of neutrophil leukocyte granules. Lab Invest 20:488, 1969.

Zigmond SH: Chemotaxis by polymorphonuclear leukocytes. J Cell Biol 77:269, 1978.

Complement

Cochrane CG, Ward PA: The role of complement in lesions induced by immunologic reactions. *In* Grabar P, Miesher P (eds): Immunology, Vol IV. Basel, Schwabe, 1966.

Cohen S: The requirement for the association of two adjacent rabbit γ-G antibody molecules in the fixation of complement by immune complexes. J Immunol 100:407, 1968.

Gewurz H, Shin HJ, Mergenhagen SE: Interactions of the complement system with endotoxic lipopolysaccharide: consumption of each of the six terminal complement components. J Exp Med 128:1049, 1968.

Gotze O, Muller-Eberhard HJ: Lysis of erythrocytes by complement in the absence of antibody. J Exp Med 132:898, 1970.

Gotze O, Muller-Eberhard HJ: The alternative pathway of complement activation. Adv Immunol 24:11, 1976.

Hirsch RL: The complement system. Its importance in the host response to viral infection. Microbiol Rev 46:71, 1982.

Hugli TE: Structure and functions of the anaphylatoxins. Springer Semin Immunopathol 7:93, 1984.

Humphrey JH, Dourmashkin RR: The lesions in cell membranes caused by complement. Adv Immunol 11: 75, 1969.

Johnson BJ: Complement: a host defense mechanism ready for pharmacological manipulation. J Pharmacol Sci 66:1367, 1977.

May JE, Frank MM: A new complement-mediated cytolytic mechanism—the C1 bypass activation pathway. Proc Nat Acad Sci USA 70:649, 1973.

Mayer MA: Membrane damage by complement. Johns Hopkins Med J 148:243, 1981.

Muller-Eberhard HJ: Chemistry and reaction mechanisms of complement. Adv Immunol 8:1, 1968.

Muller-Eberhard HJ: Complement. Annu Rev Biochem 38:389, 1969.

Pangburn MK, Muller-Eberhard HJ: The alternative pathway of complement activation. Springer Semin Immunopathol 7:163, 1984.

Rapp HJ, Borsos T: Complement research: fundamental and applied. JAMA 198:1347, 1966.

Reid KBM: Application of molecular cloning to studies on the complement system. Immunology 55:185, 1985.

Rosenberg LT: Complement. Annu Rev Microbiol 19:285, 1965.

Seeman P: Ultrastructure of membrane lesions in immune lysis, osmotic lysis and drug induced lysis. Fed Proc 33:2116, 1974.

Verroust PJ, Wilson CB, Cooper NR, Edgington TS, Dixon FJ: Glomerular complement components in human glomerulonephritis. J Clin Invest 53:77, 1974.

Wurz L: Properdin system and immunity. II. Interaction of the properdin system with polysaccharides. Science 122:545, 1955.

Coagulation

Pensky J, Kinz CF, Todd EW, Wedgwood RJ, Boyer JT, Lepow IH: Properties of highly purified human endotoxin. J Immunol 100:142, 1968.

Ratnoff O: The interrelationship of clotting factors and immunologic mechanisms. *In* Good RA, Fisher DW (eds): Immunology. Stanford, Sinauer, 1971, p 35.

Rodriguez-Erdmann F: Bleeding due to increased intravascular blood coagulation. N Engl J Med 273: 1370, 1966.

Sundsmo JS, Fair DS: Relationship among the complement, kinin, coagulation and fibrinolytic systems in the inflammatory reaction. Clin Physiol Biochem 1:225, 1983.

Kinin

Kaplan AP, Ghebrehiwet B, Silverberg M, Sealey JE: The intrinsic coagulation–kinin pathway, complement cascades, plasma kinin–angiotensin system and their interrelationship. CRC Crit Rev Immunol 3:75, 1981.

Schachter M: Kallikreins and kinins. Physiol Rev 49: 1969.

Silva K, Rothschild HA (eds): Bradykinin and related kinins. *In* International Symposium on Vasoactive Peptides. São Paulo, Brazil, 1967.

Spragg J: Complement, coagulation and kinin generation. *In* Sirois P,

Rola-Pleszcynski M (eds): Immunopharmacology. New York, Elseiver, 1982.

Webster ME: Kinin system. *In* Movat HZ (ed): Cellular and Humoral Mechanisms in Anaphylaxis and Allergy. New York, Karger, 1969.

Eosinophils

Beeson PB, Bass DA: The Eosinophil. Philadelphia, Saunders, 1977.

Gleich GJ, Loegering DA: The immunobiology of eosinophils. Annu Rev Immunol 2:429, 1983.

Lecks HI, Kravis LP: The allergist and the eosinophil. Pediatr Clin North Am 16:125, 1969.

Litt M: Studies in experimental eosinophilia. VI. Uptake of immune complexes by eosinophils. J Cell Biol 23:355, 1964.

Ross R, Klebanoff SJ: The eosinophilic leukocyte. Fine structural studies of changes in the uterus during the estrous cycle. J Exp Med 124:653, 1966.

Sampter M: Eosinophils: nominated but not elected. N Engl J Med 303:1175, 1980.

Lymphocytes

Cohen S: The role of cell-mediated immunity in the induction of inflammatory responses. Am J Pathol 88:502, 1977.

Ford WL, Gowans JL: The traffic of lymphocytes. Semin Hematol 6:67, 1969.

Gately MK, Mayer MM: Purification and characterization of lymphokines: an approach to the study of molecular mechanisms of cell mediated immunity. Prog Allergy 25:106, 1978.

Gowans JL, McGregor DD: The immunological activities of lymphocytes. Prog Allergy 9:1, 1965.

Oppenheim JJ, Jacobs D (eds): Leukocytes and Host Defense. Progress in Leukocyte Biology, Vol 5. New York, Liss, 1986.

Waksman BH, Namba Y: On soluble mediators of immunologic regulation. Cell Immunol 21:161, 1976.

Macrophages

Adams DO, Hamilton TA: The cell biology of macrophage activation. Surv Immunol Res 2:283, 1983.

Axline SG: Functional Biochemistry of the Macrophage. Semin Hematol 7:142, 1970.

Cohn ZA: The structure and function of monocytes and macrophages. Adv Immunol 9:163, 1968.

DeDuve C, Wattiauk R: Functions of lysosomes. Annu Rev Physiol 28:435, 1966.

Gresser I: Interferons. New York, Academic Press, 1981.

Kluger MJ, Oppenheim JJ, Powanda MC (eds): The Physiologic, Metabolic and Immunologic Activities of Interleukin 1. New York, Liss, 1985.

Mackaness GB, Blanden RV: Cellular immunity. Prog Allergy 11:89, 1967.

Murahata RI, Mitchell MS: Modulation of the immune response by BCG: a review. Yale J Biol Med 49:283, 1976.

Nelson DS: Immunobiology of the Macrophage. New York, Academic Press, 1976.

Reichard S, Kojima M (eds): Macrophage Biology. New York, Liss, 1985.

Snyderman R, Pike MC: Chemoattractant receptors on phagocytic cells. Annu Rev Immunol 2:257, 1984.

Van Furth R (ed): Mononuclear Phagocytes. Oxford, Blackwell, 1970.

Van Oss, CJ: Phagocytosis as a surface phenomenon. Annu Rev Microbiol 32:19, 1978.

Virelizier JL, Arenzanaseisdedos F: Immunological functions of macrophages and their regulation by interferons. Med Biol 63:149–159, 1985.

Reticuloendothelial System

Heller JH, Gordon AS: The reticuloendothelial system. Ann NY Acad Sci 88, 1960.

Stiffel C, Mouton D, Biozzl G: Kinetics of the phagocytic function of reticuloendothelial macrophages in vivo. *In* Van Furth R (ed): Mononuclear Phagocytes. Oxford, Blackwell, 1970, p335.

Stuart AE: The Reticuloendothelial System. Edinburgh, Livingston, 1970.

Shwartzman Reaction

Apitz KA: Study of the generalized Shwartzman phenomena. J Immunol 29:255, 1935.

Colman R, Robboy SJ, Minna JD: Disseminated intravascular coagulation: a reappraisal. Annu Rev Med 30:359, 1979.

Gilbert VE, Braude AI: Reduction of serum complement in rabbits after injection of endotoxin. J Exp Med 116:477, 1962.

Hjort PF, Rapaport SI: The Shwartzman reaction: pathologic mechanisms and clinical manifestations. Annu Rev Med 16:135, 1965.

Mori W: The Shwartzman reaction: a review including clinical manifestations and proposal for a universal or single organ third type. Histopathology 5:113, 1981.

Muller-Berghaus G: Pathophysiology of generalized intravascular coagulation. Serum Thromb Hemostasis 3:209, 1977.

Shwartzman G: Phenomena of Local Tissue Reactivity. New York, Hoeber, 1937.

13 Immune-Mediated Inflammation

Immune Effector Mechanisms

The specificity of antibody and specifically sensitized T effector lymphocytes provides a means of directing the defensive force of inflammation directly to infecting foreign organisms. The immune response in this way provides immune effector mechanisms augmented by accessory inflammatory processes that protect us against specific infections. Six immune effector mechanisms are recognized: *inactivation or activation, cytotoxic, Arthus (immune complex), anaphylactic, delayed (cellular),* and *granulomatous* (Fig. 13-1). These effector mechanisms are activated by the reaction of antibody or sensitized cells with antigens in vivo (Fig. 13-2).

The first four types of immunopathologic mechanisms are mediated by immunoglobulin antibodies. The characteristics of the reactions not only are determined by the properties of the immunoglobulin molecules involved but also depend on the nature and tissue location of the antigen and on the accessory inflammatory systems that are called into play.

The last two mechanisms, delayed hypersensitivity and granulomatous reactions, are dependent not upon antibody but upon reaction of antigen with specifically sensitized cells (T_D lymphocytes). Delayed reactions are usually elicited by soluble degradable antigens, whereas granulomatous reactions are elicited by poorly degradable antigens.

Activation of T_D cells leads to production and release of soluble factors (lymphokines) whose function is to attract and activate macrophages. The major mechanism of tissue damage is phagocytosis and destruction of cells by macrophages. If macrophages, activated by antibody or by lymphocytes, are unable to digest the material they phagocytose, masses of macrophages collect in the tissues and lead to space-occupying lesions that eventually interfere with normal tissue function (granulomas). Granulomatous reactions are not separately classified in some systems, but produce tissue lesions that are

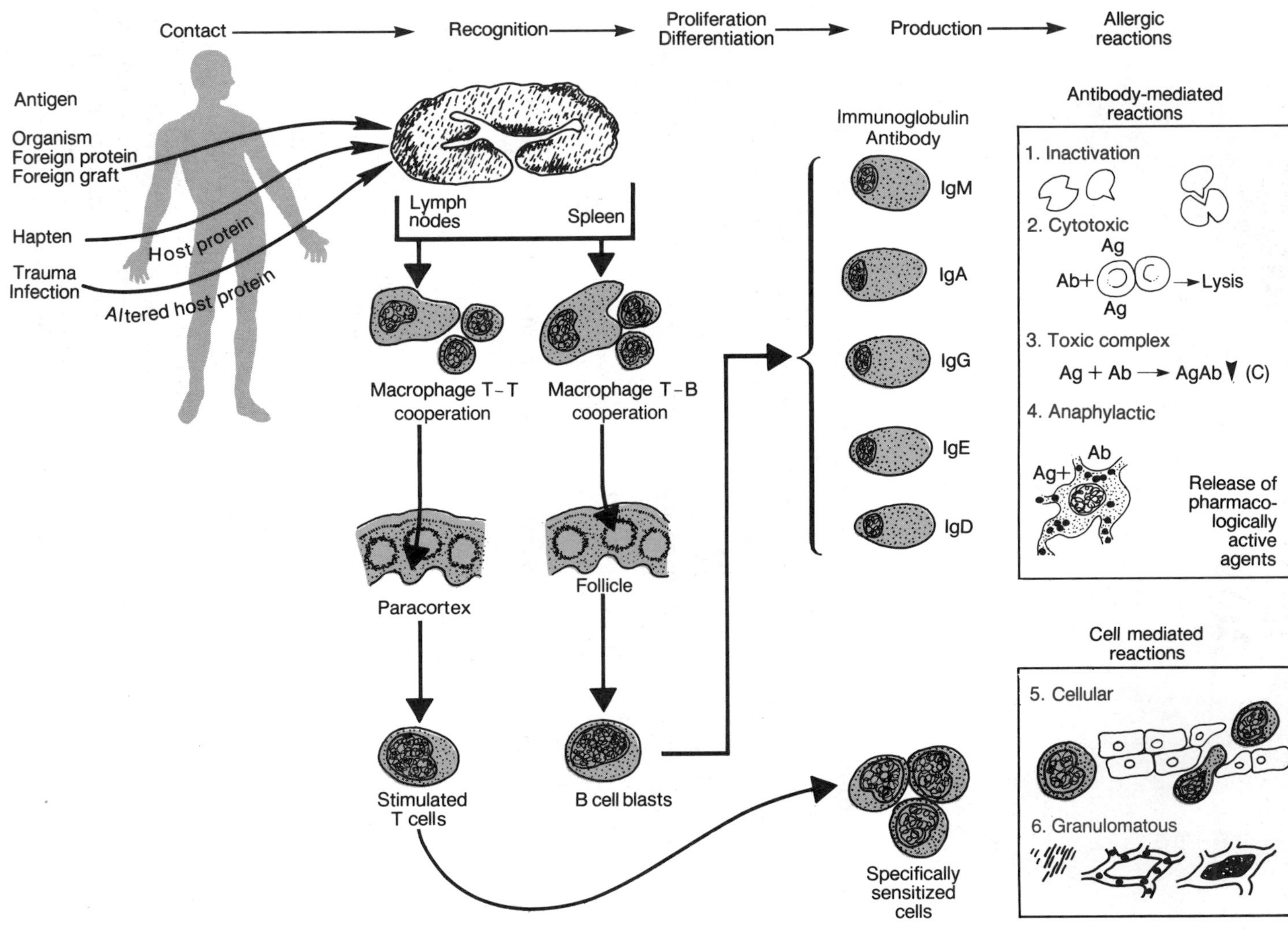
Contact
Recognition
Proliferation
Differentiation
Production
Allergic reactions
Antigen
Organism
Foreign protein
Foreign graft
Hapten
Trauma
Infection
Host protein
Altered host protein
Lymph nodes
Spleen
Macrophage T–T cooperation
Macrophage T–B cooperation
Paracortex
Follicle
Stimulated T cells
B cell blasts
Immunoglobulin
Antibody
IgM
IgA
IgG
IgE
IgD
Specifically sensitized cells
Antibody-mediated reactions
1. Inactivation
2. Cytotoxic
Ag
Ab+
Ag
Lysis
3. Toxic complex
Ag + Ab ⟶ AgAb (C)
4. Anaphylactic
Ab
Ag+
Release of pharmaco-logically active agents
Cell mediated reactions
5. Cellular
6. Granulomatous

◀ **Figure 13-1.** Immune response and immune effector mechanisms. Potential antigens (foreign material, haptens, or altered host material) induce immune reactivity. This reactivity is manifested by production of specifically reactive serum proteins (antibodies) or specifically modified cells (sensitized lymphocytes) capable of recognizing and reacting with the antigen to which the individual is exposed. As a result of this process, the following immune effector mechanisms may become manifest: (1) inactivation or activation of biologically active molecules, (2) cytotoxic or cytolytic reactions, (3) anaphylactic or atopic reactions, (4) Arthus (immune complex) reactions, (5) delayed hypersensitivity (cellular) reactions, and (6) granulomatous reactions. Also produced is a population of cells with ability to cause more rapid and more intense response to second contact with immunizing antigen (secondary response).

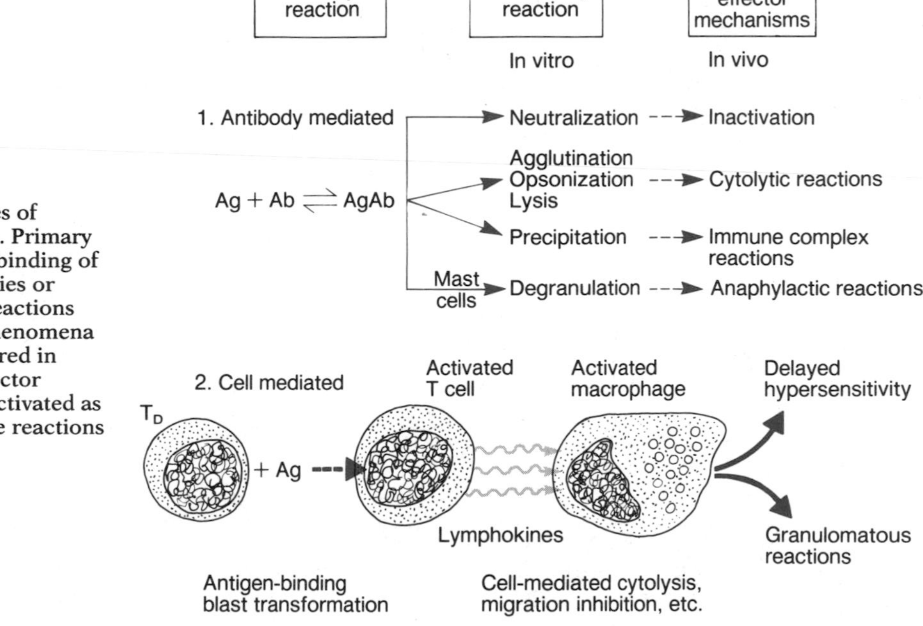

Figure 13-2. Stages of immune reactions. Primary reactions refer to binding of antigen to antibodies or cells; secondary reactions refer to various phenomena that can be measured in vitro; immune effector mechanisms are activated as a result of immune reactions in vivo.

characteristic and clearly different from delayed hypersensitivity reactions.

The first four immune reactions can be transferred with antiserum, whereas DH (delayed hypersensitivity) and granulomatous reactions are transferrable not with antiserum but with sensitized cells. When functioning properly these mechanisms deliver lethal blows to foreign agents that have invaded the body, while producing little or no damage to host tissues. However, if damage is extensive or if the immune response becomes directed to host tissue, this same mechanism may cause disease.

Until the 1960s immune reactions were not classified according to mechanism, but were presented as a bewildering list of peculiar lesions. The first working classification of four major immune mechanisms was introduced by Gell and Coombs in 1963 in their classic textbook as immune mechanisms that cause disease (immunopathologic mechanisms). The classification that we will use includes six categories (Table 13-1).

Table 13-1 Classification of Immune Mechanisms

Gell and Coombs (1963)	Roitt (1971)	Sell (1972)
—	Stimulatory	Inactivation or activation
Type II	Cytotoxic	Cytotoxic or cytolytic
Type III	Immune complex	Immune complex (Arthus)
Type I	Atopic or anaphylactic	Atopic or anaphylactic
Type IV	Delayed hypersensitivity	Delayed hypersensitivity
—	—	Granulomatous

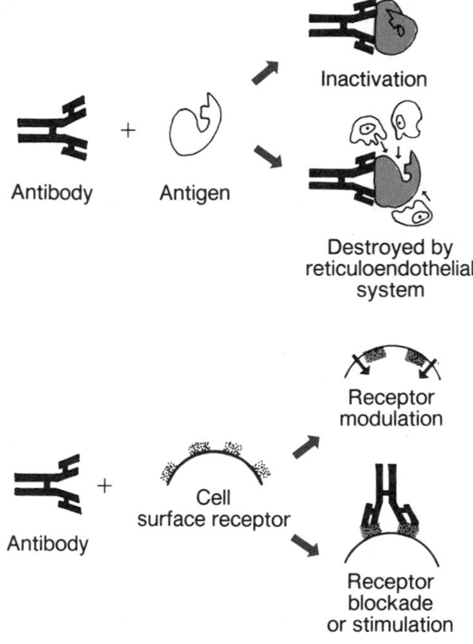

Antibody-Mediated Immune Effector Mechanisms

Inactivation or Activation

Inactivation or activation reactions occur when antibody reacts with an antigen that performs a vital function. Inactivation may occur by reaction of antibody to soluble molecules, such as bacterial toxins, or by reaction of antibody with cell surface receptors such as virus receptors. Reactions with soluble molecules produce changes in the tertiary structure of the biologically active molecule so that it no longer performs its biological function or is cleared from the circulation by the reticuloendothelial system as an immune complex. Reaction of antibody with cell surface receptors blocks or induces loss of the receptor from the cell surface by modulation.

Inactivation reactions to toxic agents, such as diphtheria or tetanus toxins, are beneficial and antibodies to virus may prevent cellular infection. In fact, this is the goal of immunization to toxoids. However, when antibody reacts with something vital for normal function, the same mechanism produces disease.

Cytotoxic or Cytolytic Reactions

Reaction of antibody with cell surface antigens results in activation of complement components and destruction of cells.

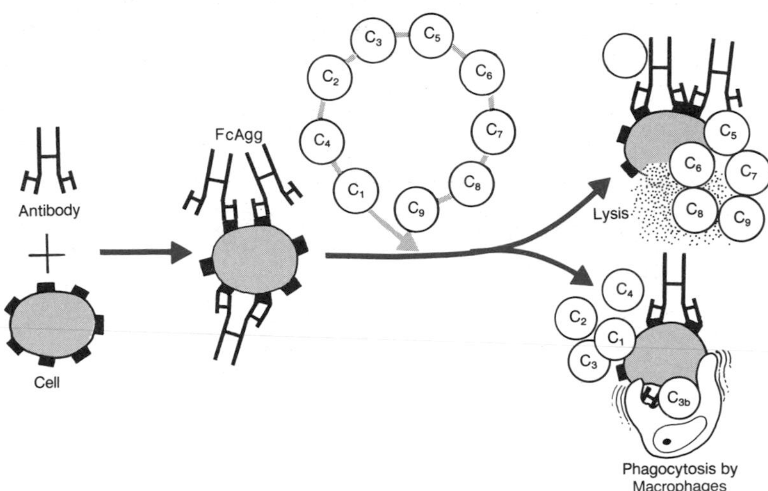

Table 13-2. Some Protective Actions of Complement

CLASSICAL COMPLEMENT PATHWAY	
Components	
C14b	Viral neutralization (e.g., herpes simplex)
C14b2a3b	Viral neutralization (e.g., Newcastle disease virus, polyoma virus)
	Adherence to lymphocytes and phagocytic cells
	Enhanced phagocytosis
	Generation of lymphokines
C14b2a3d	Adherence to lymphocytes and phagocytic cells
C1-9	Lysis of cells, bacteria, and viruses
Component fragments	
C3a	Anaphylatoxin
C3b	Enhances phagocytosis (opsonin)
	Generation of lymphokines
C3e	Leukocyte mobilization
C4a	Anaphylatoxin, weak
C5a	Chemotactic factor; anaphylatoxin, strong
ALTERNATIVE COMPLEMENT PATHWAY	
Cytolysis	
Viral neutralization	
Enhanced phagocytosis	
Macrophage activation	
Generation of anaphylatoxins (C3a, C5a)	
Generation of chemotactic factor (C5a)	

Complement components produce a realignment of membrane structures and the loss of cell membrane integrity, or the cell is coated with complement components that render the cell susceptible to phagocytosis by the reticuloendothelial system. Complement is activated by alterations in the tertiary structure of antibodies when they react with antigen. One molecule of IgM antibody reacting with a cell surface antigen is capable of activating complement and of lysing a cell, whereas two molecules of IgG antibody must react *together* to activate complement and accomplish lysis of a cell. For this reason, lytic reactions are much more effectively mediated by IgM than by IgG antibody. Other immunoglobulin classes do not fix complement and thus do not lyse cells.

Some of the protective functions of complement activation are listed in Table 13-2. Complement activation can directly inactivate viruses or bacteria and can enhance phagocytosis of infectious agents or contribute to an inflammatory response. The inflammatory activities of complement are critical for Arthus (immune complex) reactions.

Arthus (Immune Complex) Reaction

Activation of complement by reaction of antibody (usually IgG) with antigens in tissue is responsible for an inflammatory reac-

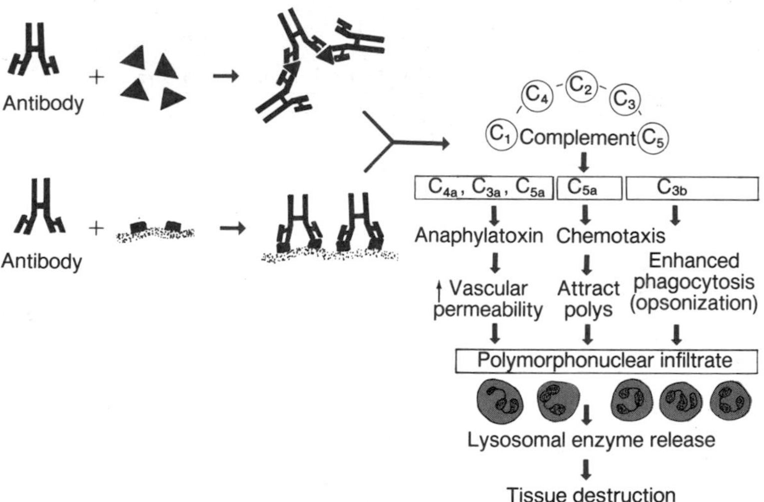

tion mediated by polymorphonuclear leukocytes. The activation of complement products C3a, C4a, and C5a can produce constriction of endothelial cells (anaphylatoxin), permitting blood components to pass into tissues. The chemotactic activity of complement fragment C5a attracts polymorphonuclear leukocytes to sites of complement activation. Damage is caused by digestion of tissue by lysosomal enzymes released from the polymorphonuclear leukocytes attracted to the tissue. Injection of antigens into the skin of animals with circulating IgG antibody results in an acute inflammatory reaction (Arthus reaction) that peaks at 6 hours and fades by 24 hours. It is characterized by perivascular necrosis and polymorphonuclear infiltration of arterioles and venules.

The protective function of immune complex reactions is to mobilize inflammatory cells at sites of acute infection. The activation of the chemotactic components of complement serves to bring polymorphonuclear cells to locations where they are needed; the released lysosomal enzymes act on infectious agents or their products, and destroy them.

Anaphylactic or Atopic Reactions

Anaphylactic or atopic reactions are initiated by pharmacologically active agents (histamine and serotonin) that are released

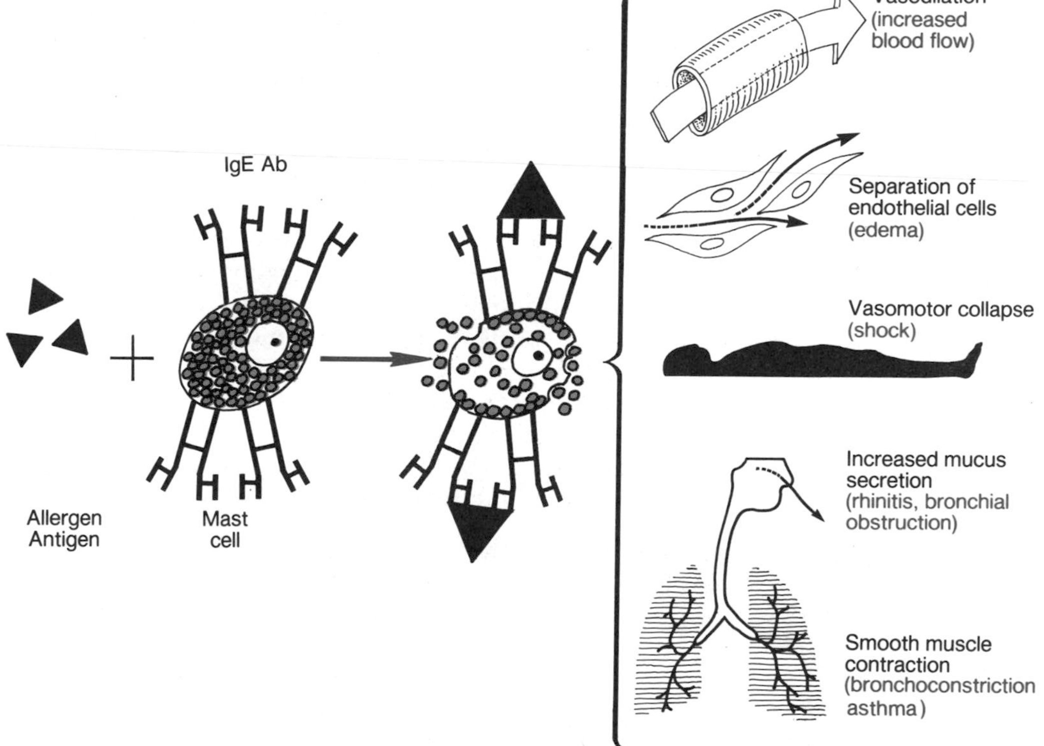

from mast cells after antibody passively bound to mast cells reacts with antigen. In addition, arachidonic acid metabolites produced by macrophages from cell membrane phospholipids released from mast cell granules contribute to later inflammatory phases of the reaction. Injection of antigen into the skin of an anaphylactically sensitive individual results in an acute reaction that peaks within 15–30 minutes and fades in 2 or 3 hours (cutaneous anaphylaxis, wheal and flare, hives). A later cellular inflammatory phase of the reaction may occur after 10–20 hours. This later phase is more evident in the biphasic bronchospastic response of the lung, where production of arachidonic metabolites by lung tissue may be more pronounced. The antibody responsible is almost always of the IgE class. Mast cells contain granules filled with pharmacological agents that act directly on smooth muscle and endothelial cells as well as cell membrane material that is metabolized to active compounds. When antigen reacts with mast cell bound IgE antibody, the cell releases the contents of its granules by a nonlytic fusion mechanism (degranulation). The released pharmacologically active agents, primarily histamine and serotonin, act on end-organ target cells to cause immediate symptoms. The membrane phospholipids are metabolized by oxidative pathways, presumably by mononuclear cells, to produce a series of biologically active compounds, leukotrienes and prostaglandins, that are responsible for later effects.

Anaphylactic or atopic reactions are elicited by reaction of antigens with IgE antibody to mast cells. The ability of IgE antibody to "fix to skin" is determined by its binding to mast cells in the skin (cytophilic antibody). The reaction can be passively transferred by injection of serum containing IgE antibody into the skin (passive cutaneous anaphylaxis). Antigen can be injected up to 45 days after injection of reaginic serum, as the antibody will remain "fixed" to mast cells in the skin. This is also referred to as the Prausnitz–Kustner reaction in honor of the authors who first described the typical reaction. Passive transfer of an Arthus reaction is demonstrable only if the antigen is injected within 24 to 48 hours after antibody, as the IgG antibody will diffuse away (it does not "fix" to mast cells).

The protective function of anaphylactic reactions is not as well understood as in other immune effector mechanisms, but several possible functions are:

Histamine and serotonin are primary mediators of increased blood flow to sites of reaction.

Anaphylactic reactions serve to open vascular endothelium, thus permitting blood-borne proteins and cells to enter inflammatory sites where they are needed.

Anaphylactic reactivity to intestinal parasites often occurs and increased intestinal motility and secretion may purge the gastrointestinal tract of them.

The acute sneezing and coughing that is part of the acute asthmatic attack may help eliminate agents in the tracheobronchial tree.

The acute reactivity may serve as a warning to avoid contact with exciting agents.

Cell-Mediated Immune Effector Mechanisms

Delayed hypersensitivity reactions are mediated by a population of specifically sensitized T lymphocytes that bear receptors for antigens. The lymphocytes that effect delayed hypersensitiv-

Delayed Hypersensitivity

ity reactions belong to a subpopulation of the T lymphocyte class: T_D cells and/or T_K cells.

The characteristic lesion of delayed hypersensitivity reactions is a perivascular mononuclear infiltrate. T_D lymphocytes reacting with antigen in tissues release lymphokines, which attract and activate macrophages. Most of the tissue damage is caused by macrophages, which have been attracted to the site of inflammation by lymphokines. T_K (killer or cytotoxic) lymphocytes may attack target cells directly. The term *delayed* is used because injection of antigen into the skin of an individual expressing delayed hypersensitivity induces an inflammatory reaction that peaks at 24 to 48 hours, in contrast to immune complex reactions, which peak at 6 hours (Arthus reactions), and cutaneous anaphylactic reactions, which peak at 15–30

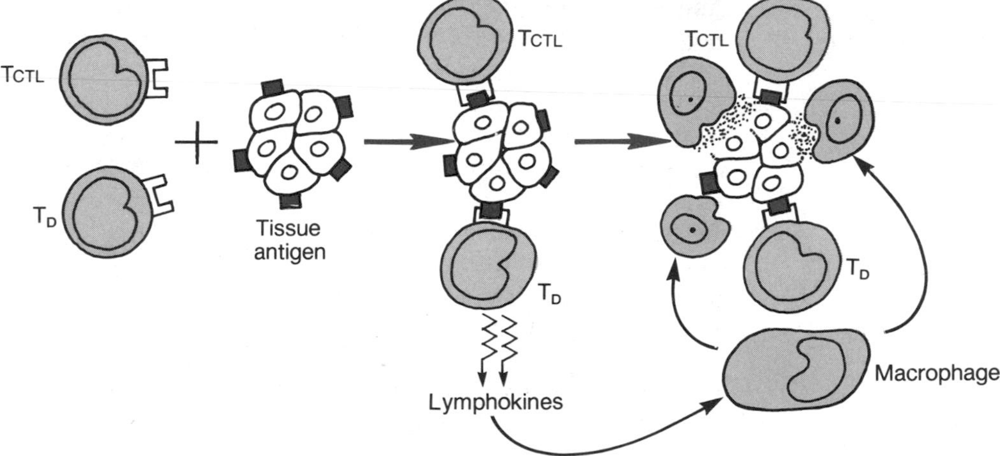

minutes. Some examples of delayed hypersensitivity reactions are tuberculin skin test, contact dermatitis (i.e., poison ivy), tissue graft rejection, virus exanthems (such as measles), and viral-associated demyelinating diseases (postinfectious encephalomyelitis, Guillain–Barré, multiple sclerosis).

Delayed skin reactions become manifest when sensitized lymphocytes react with antigen deposited into the skin. In normal skin, lymphocytes pass from venules through the dermis to lymphatics, which return these cells to the circulation. Recognition of antigen by sensitized lymphocytes (T cells) results in immobilization of lymphocytes at the site, production and release of lymphocyte mediators, and accumulation of macrophages with eventual destruction of antigen and resolution of the reaction. This results in an accumulation of cells seen at 24 to 48 hours after antigen injection. Macrophages degrade the antigen. When the antigen is destroyed, the reactive cells return via the lymphatics to the bloodstream or draining lymph nodes. In this way, specifically sensitized lymphocytes may be distributed throughout the lymphoid system following local stimulation with antigen.

The protective function of delayed hypersensitivity is directed mainly to intracellular agents, such as viruses, and to fungal and mycobacterial infections. Although delayed hypersensitivity reactions to infectious organisms may result in extensive tissue damage, the damage is a secondary effect of the immune attack on an infecting agent. It is incorrect to think, as in the past, that delayed hypersensitivity is a deleterious type of reaction. Delayed reactions are particularly important in eliminating intracellular virus infections when the viral antigens are expressed on the cell surface. It is unfortunate if the infected cell is one that performs a unique vital function, such as a neuron, because in elimination of the infected cells, irreversible tissue damage may result. The role of T_K cells in vivo remains unclear, but appears to be important in contact dermatitis, tissue graft rejection, and some autoimmune lesions.

Granulomatous Reactions

A granulomatous reaction is a characteristic type of space-occupying chronic inflammatory lesion. It may be considered a variant of delayed hypersensitivity or immune complex reaction in which the antigen is poorly catabolized and remains as a chronic irritant. Indeed, the early lesions resemble delayed hypersensitivity reactions or are associated with necrotizing vasculitis. However, instead of macrophages clearing away the antigen, there is a prolonged accumulation of macrophages and lymphocytes, which organize into granulomas. Typical granulomas consist of a ball-like mass of macrophages resembling epithelial cells (epithelioid cells) and multinucleated giant cells admixed with lymphocytes. Frequently the center of larger lesions is necrotic. Grossly this form of necrosis looks like cheese and is described as *caseous* necrosis. The major destructive mechanism is simply the occupation of organ space. The lesion may become so extensive that the normal function of the organ is impaired. Granulomas serve to isolate the infectious agent by walling off infected areas of tissue. This operates when the delayed hypersensitivity mechanism is unable to eliminate the agent. Infectious diseases in which granulomatous reactions play a major role are tuberculosis, leprosy,

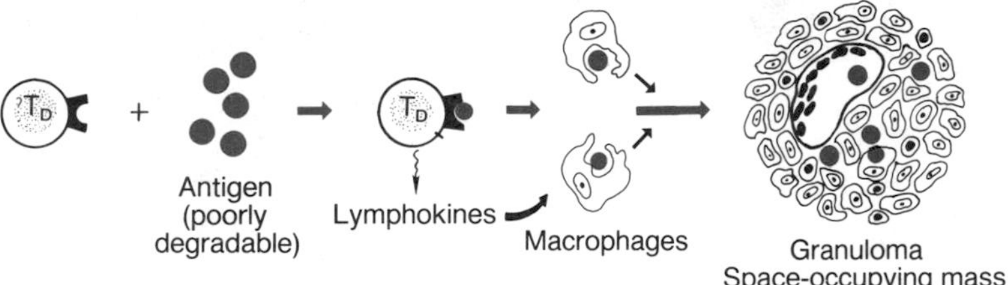

parasite and fungus infections, and syphilis. Granulomas occur in children who have a deficiency in macrophage digestive function (granulomatous disease of children). In these individuals, granulomas form where macrophages ingest material that cannot be degraded and large numbers of macrophages collect in the tissue.

Summary

Specific antibody and sensitized T effector lymphocytes provide mechanisms for directing protective defense mechanisms to foreign invaders. These directed immune effector mechanisms serve to focus nonimmune specific inflammatory accessory systems on the specific infectious agent. Six protective mechanisms are recognized: inactivation, cytotoxic, immune complex (Arthus), anaphylactic (atopic), delayed hypersensitivity, and granulomatous reactions. Each of these mechanisms has important protective functions, but may also cause tissue damage. Immunopathology is the study of how immune mechanisms cause disease.

References

(First Editions)

Bellanti JA: Immunology. Philadelphia, Saunders, 1971.

Boyd WC: Fundamentals of Immunology. New York, Interscience, 1943.

Criep LH: Clinical Immunology and Allergy. New York, Grune & Stratton, 1962.

Gell PGH, Coombs RRA: Clinical Aspects of Immunology. Oxford, Blackwell, 1963.

Humphrey JH, White RG: Immunology for Students of Medicine. Oxford, Blackwell, 1963.

Miescher PA, Muller-Eberhard HJ: Textbook of Immunopathology. New York, Grune & Stratton, 1968.

Raffel S: Immunity, Hypersensitivity, Serology. New York, Appleton–Century–Crofts, 1953.

Roitt IM: Essential Immunology. Oxford, Blackwell, 1971.

Sampter M, Alexander HL (eds): Immunological Diseases. Boston, Little, Brown, 1965.

Sell S: Immunology, Immunopathology, and Immunity. Hagerstown, Md., Harper & Row, 1972.

Concluding Remarks: Immunity and Immunopathology

Immune reactions of both humoral and cellular types play critical roles in the defense of the host against infectious agents. Antibody is generally operative against bacteria or bacterial products, whereas cellular reactivity is primarily operative against viral and mycotic organisms. The protective effect of immune reactions is called *immunity*. However, we increasingly recognize instances in which the immune reaction of the host produces tissue damage (disease). The disease state produced by the destructive effect of immune reactions is termed *allergy* or *hypersensitivity*. *Immunopathology* is the study of tissue alterations produced by various types of hypersensitivity or allergic reactions.

The terms *immunity* and *allergy* should be reserved for effects mediated through immune mechanisms. Many instances of altered reactivity as a result of a previous exposure are not reactions of allergy or immunity. These phenomena include adaptive enzyme synthesis (substrate selection of enzyme production), anaphylactoid reactions (pseudoallergic reactions resulting from liberation of pharmacologically active agents that may also be liberated by allergic reactions), reactions to drugs caused by nonallergic physiological hyperreactivity (idiosyncrasy), and other types of environmental adaptations produced by nonimmune physiological or psychological mechanisms.

The term *immunopathology* incorporates a double meaning: *immune* means "protected or exempt from"; *pathology* is the study of disease. Thus *immunopathology* literally means the study of the protection from disease, but in usage it means the study of how immune mechanisms cause diseases. *Allergy* is frequently used for a particular type of reaction (anaphylactic) and *hypersensitivity* for delayed or cellular reactivity. The term *immunity* was once restricted to the protective effects of immune reactions, but by common usage, this is no longer the case.

In the systemic study of disease, pathogenic changes are classically described according to their anatomic location. In the study of diseases due to immune mechanisms, however, more than one organ system may be involved with the same process. Because the alterations in different organ systems caused by the same process have pathologic similarities, the lesions caused by allergic reactions are best classified by the particular type of immunopathologic effector mechanism involved. These effector mechanisms also serve as protective immune mechanisms; thus, immune mechanisms represent a "double-edged sword," cutting down our enemies with one edge and causing disease with the other edge. Some examples of protective and destructive effects of immune effector mechanisms are listed in the table below.

The "Double-Edged Sword" of Immune Reactions

Immune Effector Mechanism	Protective Function: "Immunity"	Destructive Reaction: "Allergy"
Neutralization	Diphtheria, tetanus, cholera, endotoxin neutralization, blockage of virus receptors	Insulin resistance, pernicious anemia, myasthenia gravis, hyperthyroidism
Cytotoxic	Bacteriolysis, opsonization	Hemolysis, leukopenia, thrombocytopenia
Immune complex	Acute inflammation, polymorphonuclear leukocyte activation	Vasculitis, glomerulonephritis, serum sickness, rheumatoid diseases
Anaphylactic	Focal inflammation, increased vascular permeability, expulsion of intestinal parasites	Asthma, urticaria, anaphylactic shock, hay fever
Delayed hypersensitivity	Destruction of virus-infected cells, tuberculosis, syphilis, immune surveillance of cancer	Contact dermatitis, autoallergies, viral exanthems, postvaccinial encephalomyelitis
Granulomatous[a]	Leprosy, tuberculosis, helminths, fungi, isolation of organisms in granulomas	Beryllosis, sarcoidosis, tuberculosis, filariasis, schistosomiasis

[a] Granulomatous reactions, like other inflammatory lesions, may result from nonimmune stimuli as well as from an immune reaction activated by antibody or by sensitized cells. The frequent association of granulomatous reactions with delayed hypersensitivity reactions has resulted in the inclusion of granulomatous reactions as a subset of delayed hypersensitivity.

Modified from Sell S: Introduction to symposium on immunopathology: "Immune Mechanisms in Disease". Hum Pathol 9:24, 1978.

Why a "Double-Edged Sword"?

Much of what we recognize as immunopathology may result from artificial stresses put on a system that normally would not occur. The use of abnormally high doses of exogenous agents in therapy and the delivery of these agents by unnatural routes (such as intravascularly) may produce deleterious reactions such as anaphylaxis, serum sickness, transfusion reactions, drug allergies, and graft rejections that do not occur naturally. However, there are many naturally occurring hypersensitivity diseases, including autoimmune hemolytic anemias, erythroblastosis fetalis, hay fever, anaphylactic shock, polyarteritis nodosa, collagen diseases, poison ivy, and allergic granulomas. In many of these diseases infectious agents are not the primary pathogenic agent. It may thus be said that the immune response is being used for the wrong purpose, yet the very same processes that are responsible for the pathogenesis of these diseases are also essential for protective responses that are required for life.

Appendix: Cluster Designations

Revised Nomenclature (Cluster Designations) for Human Lymphocyte Markers Detected by Monoclonal Antibodies

Cluster Designation	Antibody
CD1	OKT6, anti-Leu-t, NA1/34
CD2	OKT11, anti-T11, anti-Leu-5, 9.6
CD3	OKT3, anti-T3, anti-Leu-4, UCHT-1
CD4	OKT4, anti-T4, anti-Leu-3
CD5	OKT1, anti-T1, anti-Leu-1, 10.2, T101
CD6	12.1, T411
CD7	Anti-Leu-9, 3A1, WT1, 4A
CD8	OKT5, OKT8, anti-T8, anti-Leu-2
CD9	BA-2, SJ-9A4, Du-ALL-1
CD10	J5, BA-3, anti-CALLA
CD11	Mol/OKM1, Mo5, OKM10, OKM9
CDw12	20.2
CDw13	DUHL60.4, MY7
CDw14	Mo2, MY4, MOP-15, FMC 17
CD15	FMC10, VIM-D5, 82H5, 1G10
CDw15	TG-1, FMC 13, 80H.3, DUHL 60.1, DUHL60.3
CD16	VEP13
CDw17	T5A7
CD19	Anti-B4
CD20	Anti-B1
CD21	Anti-B2
CD22	SHCL-1, HD6, HD39, 29-110
CD23	PL13, MNM6, Blast-2
CD24	BA-1
CD25	Anti-Tac

Anti-T9 and anti-Ti are not included in cluster designations.

Modified from Reinherz E, Haynes BF, Nadler LM, Bernstein ID (eds): Leukocyte Typing II (3 vols). New York, Springer-Verlag, 1986.

Glossary

ABO blood groups. Major carbohydrate antigens on red blood cells; responsible for transfusion reactions.

Absorption. Use of antibody or antigen to remove corresponding antigen or antibody from a mixture.

Accessory cells. Monocytic, epithelial, or lymphocytic cells that cooperate with T or B cells in the induction of antibody formation or T cell sensitization. Accessory cells express class II MHC markers.

Acidophilic. Having affinity for acidic dyes resulting in a red-to-pink color (used to describe tissue staining).

Acquired immunity. Protection that develops as a result of immunization.

Activation. Process of changing lymphoid cells (lymphocytes, macrophages) or proteins (complement, kinin, coagulation systems) from resting or inactive state to functionally active cells or effector molecules.

Activation factors. Proteins produced by activated cells or protein systems that serve to activate other cells.

Active immunity. Protection due to induction of an immune response by immunization or infection.

Active phase substances. Nonantibody factors that appear in increased amounts in blood soon after induction of inflammation: α_2 macroglobulin, C-reactive protein, fibrinogen, α_1 antitrypsin, etc.

Adaptive differentiation. Process whereby thymocytes acquire the ability to recognize class II major histocompatibility markers during maturation in the thymus to T helper/inducer cells.

Adaptive immunity. Specific acquired protection against infectious agents or product as a result of immunization.

Adjuvant. Material capable of enhancing an immune response.

Adoptive immunity. Transfer of state of immunity via immune cells or serum from an immune individual to a nonimmune individual.

Adoptive tolerance. Transfer of tolerance by cells from a tolerant individual to a normal individual.

Adult respiratory distress syndrome. Respiratory failure in adult humans caused by pulmonary edema secondary to increased vascular permeability.

Affinity. Strength of binding of antibody combining site (paratope) to antigenic determinant (epitope).

Agglutination. Joining together of visible antigenic particles or antigen-coated visible particles by reaction with antibody that can be seen by the naked eye.

Aggretope. Postulated product resulting from combining of part of an antigen with class II MHC components of a processing macrophage that is recognized by the MHC antigen receptor on T helper/inducer cells.

AIDS (acquired immunodeficiency syndrome). Severe immunodepression associated with human immunodeficiency virus (HIV) infection characterized by multiple opportunistic infections and death.

Allele. One or more genes at the same chromosomal locus that control alternative different forms (phenotypes) of a particular inherited characteristic.

Allelic exclusion. The phenotypic expression of only one of the two allelic genes in cells containing two different allelic genes (heterozygous cells).

Allergen. Antigens that induce or evoke atopic or anaphylactic reactions.

Allergy. Altered state of immune reactivity (usually used to refer to atopic/anaphylactic reactions).

Alloantigens. Antigens recognized by different individuals of the same species (see *allogeneic*).

Allogeneic. Used to describe genetically different phenotypes present in different individuals of the same species, such as human blood group antigens or immunoglobulin allotypes.

Allograft. A tissue graft between two genetically different individuals of the same species.

Allotypes. Genetically different antigenic determinants on proteins of individuals of the same species (see *allogeneic*).

Alternative pathway of complement activation. Activation of complement involving factor B, factor D, properdin, and C3.

Alums. Compounds of aluminum used to precipitate proteins. When used as antigens, alum-precipitated proteins form a tissue deposit that has an adjuvant effect.

Anamnesis. Immune memory or secondary immune response.

Anaphylactoid reaction. A local or systemic reaction due to physical stimuli (heat, trauma, etc.) that mimics an anaphylactic reaction.

Anaphylatoxin. Activated complement components C3a and C5a, which cause increased vascular permeability.

Anaphylaxis. Immediate hypersensitivity reaction (wheal and flare, systemic anaphylaxis) due to release of mediators from mast cells sensitized by IgE antibody.

Anergy. Inability to respond to skin test antigens, usually due to loss of delayed hypersensitivity reaction secondary to a debilitating disease.

Antibody. Protein, produced in response to immunization with an antigen, that specifically reacts with the antigen.

Antibody combining site (paratope). Area on antibody molecule that binds antigenic determinant (epitope); that part of an immunoglobulin antibody or T cell receptor that binds antigen.

Antibody-dependent cell-mediated cytotoxicity (ADCC). A form of lymphocyte-mediated target cell killing, requiring immunoglobulin antibody reacting with the target cells and binding of killer lymphocytes through Fc receptors.

Antigen. A substance that induces an immune response. A *complete* antigen both induces an immune response and reacts with the products of the response. An *incomplete* antigen (hapten) cannot induce an immune response by itself but can react with the products of an immune response. Incomplete antigens induce an immune response when complexed to a complete antigen (carrier).

Antigen binding capacity. A measurement of the ability of an antibody to bind antigen, based on the effects of dilution of the antibody.

Antigen binding site (paratope). That part of an immunoglobulin antibody or T cell receptor that binds antigen.

Antigenic determinant (epitope). That area of an antigen that reacts with antibody or T cell receptors for antigen.

Antiserum. Component of blood without cells or coagulation factors (serum) that contains antibody of known specificity.

Antitoxins. Antibodies that neutralize the effects of toxic products.

Appendix. Gastrointestinal lymphoid organ located at junction of ileum and cecum.

Arthus reaction. Dermal vascular inflammation caused by immune complexes formed when antigen is injected into skin of animal containing antibody to the antigen.

Association constant (Ka value). Mathematical measure of affinity of binding between antigen and antibody.

Atopy. "Strange" reaction; a term now used for genetic predisposition for anaphylactic reactions.

ATxBm. Designation for an adult thymectomized, irradiated mouse treated with a bone marrow transplant (B cell mouse).

Autoantibody. Antibody to self antigens.

Autoantigens. Substances that are recognized by autoantibodies.

Autochthonous. Arising in the same individual; synonym: *autologous.*

Autograft. Tissue graft from one part of the body of an individual to another part of the body of the same individual.

Autoimmunity. A state of immunity to self antigens.

Autologous. Derived from self: (1) grafted tissue and recipient are from the same individual; (2) origin of immune response and antigen are from the same individual.

Avidin–biotin technique. A system used to label antibodies or antigens by means of the strong binding affinity of avidin and biotin.

Avidity. Strength of union between antibody or a receptor and antigen or a ligand.

Bb. A protein of MW 65,000 active in the alternative complement pathway.

B cell domain. Area of lymphoid organ containing high proportion of B cells.

B cell growth and differentiation factors. Substances that enhance B cell proliferation or development into plasma cells.

B cells (B lymphocytes). Lymphocytes that are precursors of plasma cells that produce antibody (term derived from *bursa-derived cells* that arise from the bursa of Fabricius in avian species).

B lymphocytes. See *B cells.*

B2 microglobulin. A peptide of MW 12,000 that is part of the class I major histocompatibility cell surface marker.

Backcross. Breeding of a hybrid of two parental strains (F_1) with either one of the parental strains.

Bacteriolysin. An antibody or other substance that is capable of lysing bacteria.

Bacteriolysis. The process of disintegration of bacteria.

Basophil. A polymorphonuclear leukocyte with granules containing acid glycoproteins that bind basic (blue) dyes. When released, these glycoproteins mediate anaphylactic reactions.

Basophilic. Having affinity for basic dyes resulting in a blue color (used to describe tissue staining).

BCG (bacille Calmette–Guérin). An attenuated strain of *Mycobacterium bovis.*

Bence Jones protein. Monoclonal immunoglobulin light chains found in the urine of patients with multiple myeloma or other paraprotein disorders; precipitated by heating acidified urine.

Benign monoclonal gammopathy. Elevated serum levels of a single immunoglobulin species in the absence of detectable disease.

Binding site. Configuration of antibody or cell receptor that binds antigen or ligand.

Birbeck granules. Rod-shaped structures found in cytoplasm of Langerhans cells in the epidermis.

Blast cell. A large cell with dispersed chromatin and ribosome-rich cytoplasm usually in an active stage of the cell cycle prior to mitosis.

Blast transformation. Process of activating small lymphocytes to enter cell cycle and form blast cells.

Blood groups. Allogeneic antigenic differences on red blood cells, responsible for transfusion reactions.

Blocking antibody. Antibody capable of interfering with binding of another antibody (IgG blocking effects of IgE) or sensitized cells (antibody blocking cell-mediated graft rejection).

Blocking factors. Substances that inhibit induction or expression of an immune response.

Bone marrow. Soft internal tissue in bones, containing proliferating precursors of blood cells.

Booster. A dose of antigen given after primary immunization to induce a secondary response.

Bradykinin. A nine-amino-acid peptide, split from a larger serum α-globulin molecule by the enzyme kallikrein, that causes a slow, sustained contraction of smooth muscle.

Buffy coat. A thin white layer between red cells and plasma in blood that has been allowed to settle; contains white blood cells.

Burkitt's lymphoma. Tumor of B lymphocytes believed to be caused by Epstein–Barr virus.

Bursa of Fabricius. Lymphoid organ, located in the cloaca of avian species, from which B cells are derived.

Bursa equivalent. Postulated organ site of B-cell precursors in mammals (liver, GI tract, bone marrow, yolk sac).

Bursapoietin. Substance produced by epithelial cells of bursa of Fabricius that is responsible for B cell maturation.

C1–C9. Abbreviations used for components of classic complement sequence.

C3 convertase. C42, activated enzyme of complement system that converts C3 to C3a and C3b.

C1 esterase inhibitor. A serum protein that inactivates activated C1, reducing levels of formation of C2b, which has a kinin-like activity causing edema.

C-reactive protein. Serum protein of MW 105,000 that increases markedly during inflammation. It reacts with somatic C substance of *Streptococcus pneumoniae.*

C region. Constant region carboxyterminal portion of immunoglobulin H or L chains that is identical for a given class or subclass.

Capping. Movement of surface molecules on a cell towards one pole, induced by cross-linking by mitogen, antibody, or antigen.

Carrier. An immunogenic molecule that, when coupled to a nonimmunogenic incomplete antigen (hapten), renders the incomplete antigen immunogenic.

Caseous necrosis. Death of tissue resulting in a gross appearance that resembles cottage cheese (from Latin *caseus,* cheese).

CD (cluster designation). A term used to identify identical lymphoid cell markers detected by different monoclonal antibodies. For instance, *CD4* refers to phenotypes of T lymphocytes identified by monoclonal antibodies: OKT4 and Leu-3.

Cell-mediated immunity. Immune effects caused by sensitized lymphocytes or activated macrophages.

Cellular immunity. Immune state due to action of sensitized or activated lymphocytes or macrophages.

Central lymphoid organs. Lymphoid organs essential for development of lymphoid system, i.e., thymus, bone marrow, bursa of Fabricius.

CH_{50} unit. The amount of serum (dilution) required to lyse 50% of antibody-coated red blood cells in a standard assay for hemolytic complement.

Chemotactic factor. Substance that attracts inflammatory cells.

Chemotaxis. Process by which cells are attracted by chemicals or factors.

Chromium release assay. Measurement of cell death detected by release of intracellular radiolabeled chromium in vitro.

Class I major histocompatibility markers. Tissue antigens responsible for graft rejection, encoded by HLA-A, B, and C loci in humans and H2K and D loci in mice.

Class II major histocompatibility markers. Tissue markers responsible for self recognition and graft rejection, encoded by HLA-D in humans and H2I region in mice.

Clonal restriction. Limitation of an immune response to expression by a few clones of reactive cells.

Clonal selection. Theory of antibody formation stating that the individual recognizes different antigens through many individual clones of cells. A given antigen selects those clones that react with that antigen and stimulates proliferation and differentiation of the clones.

Clone. A population of cells that arises from a single precursor cell.

Coagulation system. System of 12 proteins in serum that results in formation of fibrin that blocks bleeding from injured vessels.

Cold antibodies. Antibodies that are detectable at higher titers below 37°C than above 37°C; cryoglobulins.

Cold target inhibition. Assay in which addition of unlabeled target cells blocks antibody- or cell-mediated release of radioisotope from labeled target cells.

Colony-stimulating factors. Substances that enhance the clonal growth of cells.

Competitive inhibition. Process in which one population of cells or molecules inhibits the reaction of antibody or cells with another population (e.g., cold target inhibition, radioimmunoassay).

Complement. A system of at least 13 serum proteins that are activated by enzymatic cleavages and aggregrations to produce components with biological activity.

Complement fixation. A test for antibody–antigen reactions that depends on binding (consumption) of complement by antibody–antigen complexes.

Concanavalin A. A lectin, derived from the jack bean, that reacts with carbohydrate residues (mannosides) and stimulates mitosis of T cells.

Concomitant immunity. Resistance to infection or transplantable cancer growth in an individual who already has the infection or is bearing the cancer.

Constant regions. See *C regions*.

Contact sensitivity. An epidermal cell-mediated immune reaction to chemicals placed on the skin.

Contrasuppressor cell. A subpopulation of T cells that inhibits the function of suppressor cells.

Cords of Billroth. Medullary cords of spleen.

Cortex. The outer parenchymal layer of an organ (*medulla* refers to inner part).

Cross-reactivity. Reaction of antisera or sensitized cells with different antigens, due to some shared antigenic determinants or shared structures within the determinant.

Cyclic adenosine monophosphate (cAMP). Adenosine 3′,5′-(hydrogen phosphate); key intracellular regulator; derived from adenosine triphosphate by adenylcyclase; activates protein kinase C; functions as "second messenger" during activation of cells by hormones; decreased levels in mast cells associated with *increased* responsiveness of mast cells to degranulation signals.

Cyclic guanosine monophosphate (cGMP). Guanosine cyclic 3′,5′-(hydrogen phosphate); an antagonist of cAMP, formed by conversion of guanosine triphosphate by guanylatecyclase; increased levels in mast cells associated with *increased* responsiveness to degranulation signals.

Cytolytic reaction. The effect of antibody or sensitized cells that results in lysis of a target cell.

Cytophilic antibody. Antibody that binds to the surface of effector cells through the Fc fragment (IgE to mast cells, IgM to macrophages).

Cytotoxic T lymphocytes. Specifically sensitized T cells that are capable of killing target cells (also termed *T killer cells*).

D region. Segment of gene coding diversity region in hypervariable region of immunoglobulin H chain.

Degranulation. Process of fusion of cytoplasmic granules of cells (mast cells, phagocytic cells) with cell membrane so that contents of the granules are released from the cell.

Delayed hypersensitivity. In vivo inflammatory reaction mediated by sensitized T cells (T_D cells). The classic skin reaction reaches a maximum 24–72 hours after injection of antigen.

Dendritic cells. Cells of macrophage lineage present in lymph nodes (follicular and interdigitating), spleen, other lymphoid organs, and skin (Langerhans cell), that bear class II MHC markers, have Fc receptors, and can process antigens for an immune response.

Dermatographism. Immediate wheal and flare reaction produced by scratching the skin. The reaction is caused by the release of mediators from mast cells by physical stimulation (anaphylactoid reaction).

Desensitization. Production of a temporary loss of immune reactivity in a sensitized individual following administration of antigen due to consumption of antibody or sensitized cells.

Diapedesis. Passage of cells from small vessels into adjacent tissue, due to constriction of endothelial cells.

Dick test. Lack of an inflammatory response in the skin to scarlatina toxin of streptococci in individuals with neutralizing antibody.

Differentiation factors. Substances that induce maturation of cells.

Disulfide bonds. Chemical bonds between sulfhydryl-containing amino acids that bind together polypeptide chains.

Domains. (1) Segments of polypeptide chains that are folded together and stabilized by disulfide bonds. (2) Zones of lymphoid organs that contain different proportions of lymphoid cell populations.

Double-diffusion test. Antibody–antigen precipitation reaction in agar, in which antigen and antibody are allowed to diffuse toward one another and react at equivalence in the agar.

DTH. Delayed-type hypersensitivity.

E rosette. A lymphocyte surrounded by a cluster of red blood cells. Human T lymphocytes form E rosettes with sheep red blood cells.

EA. Erythocyte coated with antibody; will be lysed if complement is added.

EAC rosette. A cluster of red cells sensitized with antibody and complement around lymphocytes that have cell surface receptors for complement (human B lymphocytes).

ECF-A. Eosinophil chemotactic factor: an acidic polypeptide of MW 500 that attracts eosinophils.

Ectoderm. Outermost of three cellular layers of embryo. Gives rise to epidermis and neuronal tissue.

Edema. Swelling of tissue, due to extravasation of fluid from intravascular space.

Endoderm. Innermost of three cellular layers of embryo. Gives rise to gastrointestinal lining and some internal organs such as liver and pancreas.

Effector cell. Cell capable of mediating a function.

Electroimmunodiffusion. A double-diffusion-in-agar technique in which antibody and antigen are pulled toward each other in an electric current.

Electrophoresis. Separation of molecules in an electrical field.

ELISA (enzyme-linked immunosorbent assay). An immunoassay system employing enzyme bound to antibody or antigen.

End cell. A terminally differentiated cell, no longer capable of dividing.

Endocytosis. Process whereby material is taken into a cell.

Endoplasmic reticulum. Membrane-like structure in cytoplasm of cells in which proteins are synthesized.

Endotoxins. Lipopolysaccharides, derived from the cell wall of gram-negative bacteria, that have pyrogenic, toxic, and stimulatory effects.

Enhancement. Prolonged survival of skin grafts or tumor grafts in individuals with humoral antibody, presumably due to blocking antibody.

Eosinophil. A polymorphonuclear leukocyte with granules that stain red (acidophilic) and contain basic proteins believed to modulate inflammatory reactions.

Epithelioid cells. Cells of macrophage lineage in granulomas that resemble epithelial cells morphologically.

Epitope. Antigenic determinant; the smallest structural area on an antigen that can be recognized by an antibody.

Epitype. A family of restricted epitopes.

Epstein–Barr virus. The virus that causes infectious mononucleosis and Burkitt's lymphoma in humans.

Equilibrium dialysis. A technique used to measure the affinity of antibody–antigen binding, based on diffusion of unbound antigen across a dialysis membrane.

Equivalence. The ratio of antibody to antigen that gives the maximum precipitation in the quantitative precipitin reaction.

Exhaustive differentiation. Process whereby cells mature and die.

Exon. Portion of a structural gene that is expressed in transcribed RNA.

Exotoxins. Diffusible toxic substances produced by microorganisms.

Exudation. Inflammation in which blood cells and fluid containing high-molecular-weight serum proteins are present in tissue.

F_1 hybrid. The first generation of a mating between two inbred strains.

f-Met peptides. Tripeptides released by bacteria that are chemotactic for inflammatory cells (formyl-Met-Leu-Phe).

Fab. The monovalent antigen-binding fragment of an IgG antibody molecule produced by digestion with papain.

$F(ab')_2$. The bivalent fragment of an IgG antibody molecule produced by digestion with pepsin.

Fc. "Crystallizable fragment": the non-antigen-binding fragment of an immunoglobulin molecule produced after digestion with papain. When first recognized using rabbit IgG this fragment formed crystals, but Fc of most species does not.

Fd fragment. Part of the heavy chain of immunoglobulin that lies on the N-terminal side of the site of papain hydrolysis.

Fc receptor. Structure on surface of some lymphocytes that binds aggregated Fc portion of immunoglobulin.

FACS. Fluorescence-activated cell sorter.

Factor B (C3 proactivator). A component of the alternative pathway of complement activation that interacts with factor D.

Factor D. A serine esterase of the alternative pathway of complement activation that, when activated, cleaves factor B when the latter is complexed to C3b to form C3bB.

Farr technique. A primary binding assay for antibody activity employing radiolabeled antigen.

Fibrinoid necrosis. Death of tissue resulting in debris that looks like fibrin microscopically, produced by enzymatic digestion of tissue by proteases released from neutrophils or deposition of fibrin in tissue.

Flocculation. Precipitation reaction of antibody and antigen in which the precipitate appears as flakes of insoluble protein, usually seen with horse antibody–toxin reactions.

Fluorescein. Yellow dye used to label antibody for fluorescence technique.

Fluorescence. Emission of light of a given wavelength by a substance activated by light of a different wavelength.

Follicles. Round-to-oval areas in lymphoid organs, containing a high proportion of B cells.

Forssman antigen. A common carbohydrate antigen on sheep cells, goat cells, human type A red cells, certain bacteria, etc. Antibody to Forssman antigen appears in patients who recover from infectious mononucleosis.

Framework regions. Sequences of amino acids other than hypervariable sequences in the variable regions of H or L immunoglobulin chains.

Freemartin. Female twin of a male calf. These twins share a common placenta and exhibit mutual tolerance to each other's tissues as adults. Female twin is sterile.

Freund's adjuvant. A water-in-oil emulsion that enhances immune responses when antigen is included. Freund's complete adjuvant includes killed mycobacteria; Freund's incomplete adjuvant does not.

Gamma globulins. Serum proteins with least mobility to positive electrode during electrophoresis. Gamma globulins contain immunoglobulins and antibodies.

Gastrointestinal associated lymphoid tissue (GALT). Lymphoid organs or tissue located along the gastrointestinal tract: tonsils, Peyer's patches, appendix, and submucosal lymphocytes.

Gel diffusion. Technique of allowing antibodies and antigen to diffuse toward each other and react in agar.

Germinal center. A lymphoid follicle with a clear center and dense margin; a site of active proliferation of B cells.

γ-Globulin. Obsolete term for immunoglobulin (e.g., *γG* vs. *IgG*).

Glomerulonephritis. Inflammation of glomeruli of kidney, often due to deposition of immune complexes.

Gm. Allotypic marker on human IgG heavy chains.

Golgi apparatus. A collection of tubular cytoplasmic structures involved in rapid secretion of proteins.

Granuloma. Tissue reaction of modified macrophages (epithelioid cells), lymphocytes, and fibroblasts to poorly degradable antigens.

Growth factors. Substances that stimulate or enhance the proliferation of cells.

Graft vs. host reactions. The systemic effects of reaction of transferred immunocompetent cells to the cells or tissues of a histoincompatible host.

H-2. The major histocompatibility complex of the mouse.

H chain (heavy chain). One pair of identical polypeptide chains of four-chain immunoglobulin molecules. The other pair of chains are the L (light) chains.

H substance. Core carbohydrate of ABO blood group system.

Hageman factor. Factor VII of the coagulation system; activated Hageman factor initiates the intrinsic coagulation system as well as generation of inflammatory peptides.

Haplotype. Phenotypic characteristics inherited through closely linked genes on one chromosome.

Hapten. An incomplete antigen. A hapten cannot induce an immune response unless complexed to a carrier. A hapten can react with immune products induced by a hapten–carrier complex.

Hassall's corpuscles. Whorls of epithelial cells in the medulla of the thymus, believed to be the source of thymic hormones.

Helper factor. Substance secreted by T helper cells or accessory cells that contributes to B cell activation.

Helper T cells. A subpopulation of T lymphocytes that cooperate with macrophages and B cells during induction of antibody formation.

Hemagglutinin. Antibody or substance that causes aggregation of red blood cells.

Hematologist. An individual who specializes in study and/or treatment of diseases of the blood and blood-forming system.

Hemolysin. An antibody or substance capable of destroying red blood cells.

Hemolysis. Process of lysis of red blood cells.

Heparin (heparinic acid). A glucoside anticoagulant present in liver and mast cells.

Heteroclitic antibody. Antibody produced to one antigen that actually has a higher affinity to another antigen.

Heterocytotropic antibody. Antibody that has greater affinity to fix to mast cells of a different species than that from which the antibody is derived; usually tested by ability to fix to skin, i.e., passive cutaneous anaphylaxis.

Heterologous. Used to describe: (1) a donor–host relationship between two different species (synonymous with *xenogeneic*); (2) a substance derived from a foreign source.

Heterophil antigen. An antigen found in different apparently unrelated organisms and/or tissues, usually carbohydrate.

High endothelial postcapillary venules. Specialized vessels in lymphoid organs where circulating cells pass into parenchyma.

Hinge region. Amino acid segment, between the first and second constant regions of the immunoglobulin heavy chain of IgG, that permits bending of the molecule.

Histamine. A bioactive amine of MW 111 present in mast cells and platelets that causes immediate effects of anaphylactic and anaphylactoid reactions.

Histiocytes. Phagocytic cells of the macrophage series that are fixed in tissues.

Histocompatibility. Relationship between tissues of different individuals; compatible organs or tissues will not evoke an immune rejection reaction.

Histocompatibility antigens. Antigens on cells responsible for tissue transplantation rejection.

HIV (human immunodeficiency virus). A term identifying the family of retroviruses that causes human acquired immunodeficiency syndrome (AIDS).

HLA (human leukocyte antigen). The major histocompatibility complex genetic region of the human.

Homocytotropic antibody. An antibody that binds better to cells of animals of the same species than to cells of animals of different species.

Homologous. Used to describe: (1) a substance derived from the same source; (2) a donor–host relationship within the same species (allogeneic).

Horror autotoxicus. A concept proposed by Paul Ehrlich in 1900 whereby individuals do not make an immune response to their own tissues.

Hot spots. Short amino acid sequences in the variable regions of H and L chains of immunoglobulin that appear together in the paratope (antigen binding site) of the folded antibody molecule. Also referred to as *hypervariable regions*.

HTLA. Human T lymphocyte antigen; obsolete term replaced by cluster designations (see Appendix).

HTLV. Human T cell leukemia virus (a subgroup of HTLV is now designated *HIV*–human immunodeficiency virus).

Humoral. Pertaining to blood or tissue fluid.

Humoral immunity. Immunity due to immunoglobulin antibody in blood or tissue.

Hybridoma. A transformed cell line formed by the fusion of two parental cell lines.

Hyperplasia. Reversible increase in the size of an organ due to an increase in the number of cells. Usually related to a physiological response to a stimulus.

Hypersensitivity. A state of increased reactivity or sensitiveness.

Hypervariable regions. See *hot spots.*

Hyposensitization. Decreased immune reactivity due to production of blocking antibody.

I region. That segment of the mouse major histocompatibility complex genome that controls immune responses and expression of Ia and Ie phenotypes; class II MHC region of the mouse.

Ia antigens. Cell surface markers controlled by the I region (a and e); class II MHC antigens of the mouse.

I-J. Subsegment region of mouse I region that codes for a postulated antigen on suppressor cells and/or suppressor factor.

Idiotope. An epitope on the V region of antibody molecules.

Idiotype. A set of unique antigenic determinants (idiotopes) on the V region of homologous or monoclonal antibodies.

Idiotype network. A series of idiotype–anti-idiotype reactions that is postulated to control production of idiotype-bearing antibody molecules or cells.

Ig. Immunoglobulin.

IgA. Secretory immunoglobulin class; dimeric.

IgD. Immunoglobulin class on surface of B cells.

IgE. Immunoglobulin class that fixes to mast cells and is responsible for anaphylactic sensitivity.

IgG. Predominant immunoglobulin class in adults.

IgM. Pentameric immunoglobulin; first class of antibody produced to most antigens.

IL. See *interleukin.*

Immediate hypersensitivity. Inflammatory reaction that occurs within minutes of exposure to antigen (see *anaphylaxis*).

Immobilization test. An assay for antibody or factor that stops the motion of motile organisms.

Immune adherence. Binding of antibody–antigen complexes or antibody-coated particles to primate erythrocytes, rabbit platelets, or white blood cells, due to activation of C3 and formation of C3b.

Immune complex reactions. Tissue inflammation mediated by antibody–antigen complexes.

Immune deviation. Substitution or exchange of one immune effector mechanism for another (e.g., IgG antibody in preference to delayed hypersensitivity in lepromatous leprosy).

Immune elimination. Rapid clearance of an antigen from the circulation due to reaction with antibody and removal of immune complexes by the reticuloendothelial system.

Immune memory. Secondary response; property of more rapid and more intense immune response after the first exposure to an antigen (anamnesis).

Immune paralysis. Inability to detect antibody to a nondegradable antigen, due to repeated consumption of the antibody.

Immune surveillance. Postulated function of the immune system to prevent tumor cells from growing.

Immunity. State of protection from injury, due to previous experience or special state of responsiveness.

Immunization. Process of inducing a state of immunity.

Immunoabsorption. Removal of an antigen by reaction with antibody, or removal of a subset of antibodies by an antigen in a solid phase system or by precipitation.

Immunoblot (Western blot). Reaction of labeled antibodies with proteins absorbed on nitrocellulose paper.

Immunodeficiency. Defect in immune system resulting in decreased resistance to infection.

Immunodiffusion. Test for antibody–antigen reaction involving diffusion in agar precipitation.

Immunodominant epitope. That epitope on an antigen that best binds or absorbs the antibody made to that antigen.

Immunoelectrophoresis. A technique involving separation of proteins in an electric field followed by a precipitation reaction in agar or gel with antibodies to the separated proteins.

Immunofluorescence. A histochemical technique employing fluorescence-labeled antibodies or antigens for localization in tissues or cell suspensions.

Immunogen. A complete antigen; an antigen that can both induce an immune response and react with the antibodies of T cells elicited.

Immunogenic. Capable of inducing an immune response.

Immunoglobulins. A family of glycoprotein molecules having similar structure, to which antibodies belong.

Immunoglobulin classes. Subfamilies of immunoglobulin based on large differences in H-chain amino acid sequence: IgA, IgD, IgE, IgG, IgM (isotypes).

Immunoglobulin subclasses. Subpopulations of an Ig class based on somewhat more subtle structural or antigenic differences in the H chains (e.g., IgG1, IgG2, IgG3, IgG4) than are class differences.

Immunoglobulin supergene family. Set of related genes coding for immunoglobulins and cell surface molecules (T cell receptors, MHC surface markers).

Immunologically competent cell. A lymphocyte that has the ability to recognize and be activated by an antigen.

Immunologist. An individual who studies immunology.

Immunology. The study of immunity.

Immunopathology. The study of how immune mechanisms cause disease.

Immunotherapy. The use of immunization or immune products to modify disease.

Incomplete antibody. Antibody that binds antigen but does not precipitate or agglutinate the antigen.

Inducer cells. A subpopulation of T lymphocytes that cooperate with macrophages and precursor T cells during the generation of active T cell subpopulations (T suppressors, T CTL).

Inflammation. The process whereby blood proteins and cells enter tissue in response to infection or injury.

Inflammatory cells. Blood and tissue cells that take part in inflammation.

Inflammatory mediator. A substance involved in the inflammatory process.

Innate immunity. Protection from injury or infection that does not require immunization.

Innocent bystander. A cell that is destroyed by an immune effector mechanism specifically directed to a different cell population.

Instructive theory of antibody formation. An obsolete theory that antigen directs immune responsive cells to produce antibody of a given specificity by imposing a conformation on the antibody formed.

Interdigitating reticulum cells. A subclass of antigen-processing macrophages found in the paracortex of lymph nodes.

Interferons. A group of low-molecular-weight protein molecules produced in virus-infected cells that inhibit infection of noninfected cells.

Interleukins. Substances produced by one mononuclear white cell population that act on other white cell populations.

Interleukin 1. A macrophage-derived substance (MW 15,000) that has multiple biologic properties, including the ability to promote short-term growth of T cells (previously called *leukocyte-activating factor*).

Interleukin 2. A substance (MW 35,000) derived from activated T helper cells that promotes growth of other activated T cells or B cells (previously called *T cell growth factor*).

Interleukin 3. Substance (MW 40,000) derived from activated T cells that stimulates proliferation of bone marrow cells.

Internal image. Epitope on an anti-idiotype antibody (Ab2) subpopulation that binds to the paratope of the antibody induced by the "foreign" antigen (Ab1).

Introns. Segments of a structural gene that are not transcribed into RNA.

InV. Allotype on κ light chains of humans.

Ir region. Genes in MHC that control immune responses (class II MHC).

Isohemagglutinins. Antibodies that react with antigens present on red blood cells of different individuals of the same species.

Isologous. Derived from the same species (see *allogeneic*).

Isotype. Antigen that defines class or subclass specificity.

J-chain. A polypeptide chain that joins individual 4-chain immunoglobulin units in polymeric immunoglobulins (IgA, IgM).

J region. That postulated portion of the mouse I region that controls suppression.

Jones–Mote reaction. A form of delayed hypersensitivity skin reaction to soluble proteins that involves a high proportion of basophils.

K and D regions. Class I MHC genomic regions of the mouse.

Kallikrein (kininogenase). Activated by cleavage of prekallikrein found in tissue fluids, kallikrein acts on kininogen to produce kinins.

Kappa (κ) chains. One of two major types of immunoglobulin light chains.

Killer cells (K cells). Lymphocytes that mediate antibody-dependent cell-mediated cytotoxicity (ADCC).

Kinin system. A humoral amplification system for inflammation, involving activation of substrate protein molecules to active polypeptides by enzymatic cleavage.

Kinins. Inflammatory peptides formed by action of kallikrein on kininogen.

Koch phenomenon. The classic delayed hypersensitivity skin reaction to tuberculin in guinea pigs following infection with mycobacteria tuberculosis.

Kupffer cells. Fixed mononuclear phagocytic cells in the sinusoids of the liver.

L chain (light chain). A polypeptide chain of MW 22,000 present in all immunoglobulin molecules in two forms, κ and λ. Each four-chain Ig molecule has either two κ or two λ light chains.

Lacteals. Small lymphatic vessels that drain intestinal villae.

Lambda (λ) chain. One of two major types of immunoglobulin light chains.

Lamina propria. Thin layer of connective tissue supporting the epithelium of the gastrointestinal tract.

Langerhans cells. Antigen-processing, class II MHC marker–positive monocytic dendritic cells in the epithelial layer of the skin.

Large granular lymphocytes. Lymphocytes in the NK/K series with large cytoplasmic lysosomes.

LATS (long acting thyroid stimulator). An anti-thyroid cell antibody that stimulates thyroid hormone production.

LE cell. Neutrophil containing phagocytosed lymphocyte nucleus because of opsonization by antinuclear antibody, found in sera of patients with systemic lupus erythematosus.

LE factor. Antinuclear antibody found in patients with systemic lupus erythematosus that allows formation of LE cells.

Lectin. A substance derived from a plant that binds to, and sometimes is mitogenic for, lymphocytes. Some lectins also bind red blood cells.

Leukocyte. White blood cell.

Leukotrienes. Metabolic products of arachidonic acid, some of which have inflammatory properties.

Levamisole. An antihelminthic drug that may potentiate immune responses or effector mechanisms.

Ligand. A molecule that binds to another molecule (receptor).

Light chain. See *L chain.*

Linkage disequilibrium. The tendency for a set of genetically determined characteristics to be inherited together in a given population.

Lipopolysaccharides. (See *endotoxins.*) Substances produced by gram-negative bacteria that may have pyrogenic, inflammatory, or mitogenic effects.

Low responder mice. Inbred mice who produce a low, usually IgM-only, antibody response to antigens that induce normal responses in other strains of mice. Low responsiveness is controlled by the class II MHC region.

L3T4. A mouse lymphocyte marker defined by a monoclonal antibody that identifies T helper cells.

Ly antigens. T-lymphocyte antigens of mice.

Lymph. Fluid in lymphatic system.

Lymph node. Organ of lymphoid system that filters lymphatics. Major site of immune responses.

Lymphatics. Vessels that collect interstitial fluid and deliver it back to the bloodstream.

Lymphocytes. Small mononuclear cells with round nuclei containing densely packed chromatin. Many different subpopulations may be identified.

Lymphoid organs. Organs of the body that contain dense populations of lymphocytes (thymus, spleen, lymph nodes, GALT, etc.).

Lymphoid system. Lymphatics and lymphoid organs.

Lymphokines. Soluble substances, produced and secreted by lymphocytes, that act on other cells.

Lymphokine-activated killer cells (LAK). A population of killer cells activated by lymphokines (IL2, interferon).

Lymphoma. Cancer of lymphoid organs.

Lymphotoxin. A lymphokine that lyses selected target cell lines.

Lysosomes. Granules that contain hydrolytic enzymes; present in many cells.

Lysozyme (muraminidase). A cationic low-molecular-weight enzyme present in tears and other secretions that digests the mucopeptides of bacterial cell walls.

Lyt1, Lyt2, Lyt3. A set of surface antigens defining subpopulations of mouse T cells. Lyt1 is associated with helper T cells, Lyt2 and Lyt3 with suppressor T cells. In practice the helper phenotype is now defined by a monoclonal antibody that detects a marker termed *L3T4*.

M protein. (1) Monoclonal immunoglobulin found in myelomas. (2) Type-specific cell surface antigens of group A β-hemolytic streptococci.

Macroglobulins. Glycoproteins of MW greater than 200,000.

Macrophage. Large bone marrow–derived phagocytic cells in the monocyte series, which function as accessory cells in induction of immune response and as effector cells in inflammatory responses.

Macrophage activation factor. A lymphokine that increases the phagocytic activity of macrophages.

Macrophage chemotactic factor. A lymphokine that attracts macrophages.

Macrophage migration test. In vitro test for cellular immunity that depends on ability of antigen to induce formation of a lymphokine that inhibits migration of macrophages on agar.

Major histocompatibility complex. The set of genes that code for histocompatibility and related markers.

Mantle. Tightly packed zone of lymphocytes that surround a germinal center.

Marginal zone. Outer layer of lymphoid follicles of spleen, containing loosely packed T and B cells and capillary networks involved in lymphocyte circulation.

Margination. Attachment of blood cells to endothelium of vessels during inflammation.

Mast cell. A polymorphonuclear cell with large cytoplasmic granules containing basophilic mediators of anaphylaxis, related to blood basophils.

Medulla. Central portion of parenchyma of an organ. *Cortex* refers to outer layer of parenchyma.

Medullary cord. Area of medulla of lymph node separating lymphatic sinusoids.

Megakaryocyte. Large multinuclear giant cells in bone marrow from which portions of membrane-bound cytoplasm break off to form blood platelets.

Memory cell. Hypothetical immune-competent cell that has ability to recognize and respond more vigorously to antigen because of previous exposure (immunization).

Mesoderm. One of the three cellular layers of developing embryo. This layer of cells gives rise to connective tissue and blood cells.

Microglia. Phagocytic cells in the central nervous system.

Migration inhibitory factor. A lymphokine that inhibits the movement of macrophages.

Minor histocompatibility antigens. Cell surface molecules not coded in the major histocompatibility complex that contribute to tissue graft rejection.

Mitochondria. Cellular organelles where metabolism takes place.

Mitogens. Substances that activate resting cells to transform into blast cells, synthesize DNA, and divide.

Monoclonal antibody. A homogeneous antibody population produced by a clone of antibody-forming cells.

Monocyte. Cells in the macrophage series found in the blood and lymph.

Monokine. Generic term for factors produced by macrophages (monocytes).

Monomer. A single polypeptide chain. Basic components of Ig molecules are four monomers: two H chains and two L chains.

Mononuclear cells. Cells in the leukocyte lineage with rounded single nuclei (i.e., lymphocytes and macrophages in contrast to polymorphonuclear cells).

Multiple myeloma. A neoplasm of plasma cells.

Myeloblast, myelocyte. Immature precursor cells in the polymorphonuclear leukocyte series.

Myeloma protein. A homogeneous immunoglobulin molecule or part of an Ig molecule produced by myeloma tumor plasma cells (see *multiple myeloma*).

Myeloperoxidase. Major enzyme in the granules of phagocytic cells that catalyzes peroxidation.

Natural antibody. Antibody present in the serum of an individual with no known previous contact with the homologous antigen with which the antibody reacts.

Natural killer cell (NK cell). Lymphocytes present in nonimmunized normal individuals that are cytotoxic for a variety of target cell lines.

Natural selection. A theory of antibody formation in which antigen selects immunocompetent cells that already have the ability to recognize and react with the antigen.

NBT test (nitroblue tetrazolium reduction test). A test to determine the activity of the hexomonophosphate shunt in phagocytic cells.

Necrosis. Death of tissue.

Neoantigens. New antigens that appear on cells during development or in tumors.

Nephelometry. An assay that measures the turbidity or cloudiness of a suspension.

Network theory. A theory that immune responses are controlled by a series (network) of anti-idiotypic reactants.

Neutralization. Process by which an antibody inactivates a toxin or activity of an infectious agent (e.g., virus neutralization).

Neutrophil. A polymorphonuclear cell whose granules stain neither strongly acidophilic nor strongly basophilic.

Nude (athymic) mice. A hairless mouse strain that congenitally lacks a thymus and T cell function.

Null cells. Lymphocytes with no defining cell surface markers (i.e., neither T nor B cell phenotype).

Nylon wool. A substance that will bind mouse T cells; used in fractionation of T and B cells.

NZB (New Zealand black) mice. An inbred strain of mice that spontaneously develop autoimmune diseases.

Oligoclonal response. Immune response restricted to a small number of individual clones resulting in limited number of immunoglobulin bands in agarose electrophoresis.

Ontogeny. The process of development of an individual from conception to maturity.

Opsonization. The process of enhancing phagocytosis (e.g., by aggregated antibody or activated complement).

Original antigenic sin. The tendency of an individual to produce antibody specific to an antigen to which he was previously exposed when challenged with a cross-reacting antigen, even though the cross-reacting antigen may not contain some of the epitopes recognized by the antibodies.

Osteoclast-activating factor. A lymphokine that promotes resorption of bone by activating osteoclasts.

Ouchterlony technique. Double diffusion in agar; antibody–antigen precipitation occurring in gel when antigen and antibody diffuse toward each other, react, and form a precipitate.

Oudin tube. Single diffusion in agar. Antigen in solution is placed over agar containing antibody in a capillary tube. Antigen diffuses into agar and forms a precipitin band at equivalence.

OZ. Allotypic markers on human λ chains.

PAP (peroxidase–antiperoxidase). An enzyme labeling technique employing complexes of antibody and peroxidase and anti-immunoglobulin to bind the complexes to antibodies that have reacted to tissue antigens.

Papain. Proteolytic enzyme from papaw plant, used to hydrolyze immunoglobulin.

Paracortex. T-lymphocyte domain between and beneath follicles in cortex of lymph node; thymus-dependent area.

Paratope. Antigen (epitope) binding site of antibody.

Pathologist. An individual who studies disease.

Passive cutaneous anaphylaxis (Prausnitz–Kustner test). In vivo passive transfer of antiserum containing skin-sensitizing antibody (IgE) into skin of nonreactive individual. Challenge of skin site with allergen results in wheal and flare reaction.

Passive transfer. Transfer of immunity from an immunized individual to a nonimmune individual by serum or cells.

Paul–Bunnell test. Agglutination of sheep red blood cells by serum of patients with infectious mononucleosis; due to reaction to Forssman antigen on sheep cells.

Pepsin. Gastric enzyme used to hydrolyze immunoglobulin.

Peyer's patch. Submucosal gastrointestinal lymphoid tissue containing follicles and diffuse lymphoid areas.

Phagocytic index. An in vivo measurement of clearance of foreign particles.

Phagocytosis. Engulfment of particles by cells.

Phagolysosome. A membrane-limited cytoplasmic vesicle formed by fusion of a phagosome and a lysosome.

Phagosome. A membrane-limited vesicle containing phagocytosed material.

Pharyngeal pouch. Embryonal organ in the neck that contributes epithelial cells to thymus, parathyroids, and other tissues.

Phenotype. Characteristic of a given cell or individual that reflects which genetically determined properties are expressed.

Phylogeny. The evolutionary history of a given species.

Phytohemagglutinin (PHA). Lectin derived from red kidney bean that agglutinates red blood cells and is mitogenic for lymphocytes.

Phytomitogens. Glycoproteins derived from plants that stimulate blast transformation of lymphocytes.

Plaque-forming cells. Cells producing antibody to antigens on red blood cells suspended in agar that result in a clear zone of cell lysis in the agar.

Plasma. Fluid component of uncoagulated blood after cells are removed.

Plasma cell. Mature cells of the B cell series that synthesize and secrete immunoglobulin. These cells have small nuclei and prominent cytoplasm filled with endoplasmic reticulum.

Plasminogen activator. Enzyme that converts plasminogen to plasmin.

Platelet. Small cytoplasmic fragments in blood, responsible for activation of coagulation.

Pokeweed mitogen (PWM). A lectin extracted from the plant *Phytolacca americana* that is mitogenic for lymphocytes and stimulates differentiation of human B cells.

Polyclonal. Derived from many clones.

Polyclonal activation. Stimulation of a number of different clones of cells (lymphocytes), resulting in a heterogenous immune response.

Polymers. Molecules made up of more than one repeating unit.

Polymorphonuclear cells. Leukocytes (white blood cells) with lobulated nuclei; these cells take part in acute inflammatory reactions. Major subpopulations are neutrophils, eosinophils, and basophils.

Postcapillary venules. Small vessels through which blood flows after leaving capillaries and before reaching veins. Often the site of migration of inflammatory cells into tissue during inflammation.

Prausnitz–Kustner test. See *passive cutaneous anaphylaxis.*

Pre-B cells. Immature cells in the B cell lineage with cytoplasmic μ chains but no surface Ig.

Precipitation. Formation of insoluble complexes from a mixture of soluble antigen and soluble antibody, producing a macromolecular hydrophobic complex that precipitates from solution.

Primary follicles. Tightly packed aggregates of small lymphocytes in cortex of lymph node and white pulp of spleen. Site of B cells that develop into germinal centers.

Primary response. First immune response to an immunogen not previously recognized; predominantly IgM antibody.

Private specificity. Epitope defined by a single allele and only expressed when the allele is active.

Privileged sites. Places in the body where the immune system cannot function.

Properdin system. A group of serum proteins (factor B, factor D, properdin, and C3) that interact to activate complement through the alternative pathway.

Prostaglandins. Aliphatic acids derived from arachidonic acid metabolism that have a variety of biological activities, including increasing vascular permeability, causing smooth muscle contraction, and decreasing the threshold for pain. Originally identified in prostatic fluids.

Protein A. Protein extracted from cell wall of *Staphylococcus aureus* that binds the Fc of most IgG molecules.

Protein kinase C. A cytoplasmic enzyme activated by Ca^{++} that is involved in activation of different cell types.

Prothymocyte. A postulated thymocyte precursor that arises in the bone marrow and circulates to the thymus.

Prozone. Suboptimal precipitation or agglutination that occurs in antibody excess.

Pseudoallergic reaction. Clinical state that mimics allergic reaction not caused by immune mechanism (anaphylactoid reaction).

Public specificity. Antigenic specificity coded by more than one allele of an alloantigenic system.

Pyrogens. Substances released from white blood cells, bacteria, or tissues that cause fever.

Qa locus. Genetic region between H2D and TL in mice that encodes the Qa antigen found on T cells.

Quelling test. The swelling of the capsules of pneumococci exposed to antibodies to pneumococci.

Radioallergosorbent test (RAST). Measurement of IgE antibody by binding serum antibody to specific insoluble antigen; the nonbound IgE is washed off, and the IgE bound is detected by binding of radiolabeled anti-IgE.

Radioimmunoassay. A competitive inhibition assay in which an unknown amount of antigen competes with radiolabeled antigen binding to antibody.

RAJI cell test. A test for immune complexes that utilizes binding to the cells of a lymphoblast (RAJI) line that has receptors for complexes.

Reagin. Originally used for the complement-fixing antisyphilis antibody detected by the Wassermann reaction with cardiolipin; now used synonymously with *skin-fixing antibody.*

Red pulp. Area of cords of Billroth and sinusoids of spleen.

Reticuloendothelial system. A composite of the phagocytic cells of the body, primarily the sinusoidal cells of the liver (Kuppfer cells), spleen, and lymph nodes.

Rheumatoid factor. Anti-immunoglobulin autoantibody (usually IgM) directed against denatured or allotypic determinants usually on IgG; present in sera of patients with rheumatoid arthritis and other connective tissue diseases.

Ribosome. A subcellular cytoplasmic organelle that serves as a site for amino acid incorporation during synthesis of proteins.

Rocket electrophoresis. A technique to measure antigens by electrophoresing antigen into an agar layer containing antibody, resulting in a rocket-like pattern of precipitation in agar.

Rosette. A central cell (usually a lymphocyte) surrounded by cells of another type (usually red blood cells); used as a way to detect cell surface receptors or antigens.

Round cells (mononuclear cells). Tissue cells with round or oval nuclei; usually lymphocytes and monocytes.

Russell body. A fully mature plasma cell with large immunoglobulin containing cytoplasmic granules made up of swollen endoplasmic reticulum.

S region. Chromosomal region of mouse MHC complex that codes for a serum β-globulin component of complement.

S value (Svedberg unit). Sedimentation coefficient obtained by ultracentrifugation of a protein.

Schick test. A skin test for neutralizing antibody to diphtheria toxin. The test is positive if the characteristic 5–6-hour inflammatory reaction to toxin does not occur after injection of toxin.

Schultz–Dale reaction. In vitro assay for anaphylactic reactivity employing contraction of smooth muscle sensitized by IgE antibody upon exposure to antigen.

Secondary follicle. See *germinal center.*

Secondary response. The more rapid and intense immune response that occurs upon rechallenge of a previously immunized individual with antigen.

Second set rejection. Rapid rejection of a tissue graft by an individual previously sensitized.

Secretory IgA. IgA dimers prominently found in external secretions.

Secretory piece (T piece). A molecule of MW 70,000 produced by epithelial cells and found in secretory immunoglobulins.

Selective theory. A theory of antibody formation in which antigen selects cells that have cell receptors for the antigen and stimulates them to proliferate and differentiate.

Sensitized cell. An immunologically reactive cell induced by exposure to specific antigen.

Serologically defined (SD) antigens. Antigens of the MHC detected by antibodies; originally class I, now both class I and II.

Serotonin (5-hydroxytryptamine). A catecholamine of MW 176 present in mast cells and platelets that contributes to anaphylactic reactions.

Serum. Fluid component of coagulated blood; serum is different from plasma in that serum does not contain fibrinogen.

Serum sickness. A systemic vasculitis, glomerulonephritis, and arthritis due to immune complex formation following injection of foreign antigen (serum).

Shwartzman Reaction. (1) Disseminated intravascular coagulation produced in an animal with blockade of the reticuloendothelial system by injection of endotoxin (systemic). (2) Local inflammatory reaction caused by thrombus formation at skin sites injected with two doses of endotoxin 24 hours apart (localized).

Side chain theory. A theory of antibody formation proposed in 1896 by Paul Ehrlich, which first postulated cell surface receptors for antigens.

Single radial diffusion. An in vitro gel diffusion test in which antigen diffuses into agar containing antibody, forming a ring of precipitation.

Skin reactive factor. A lymphokine that produces a mild inflammatory reaction when injected into the skin.

Skin-sensitizing antibody. Antibody (usually IgE) that fixes to mast cells in skin. Synonym: *reagin*.

Slow-reacting substance A. An acidic lipoprotein of MW 400, derived from arachidonic acid, which has a prolonged constrictive effect on smooth muscle.

Somatic mutation. Acquisition of genetic variability that occurs within a given individual after conception.

Spleen. Lymphoid organ that filters circulating blood; located in left side of abdominal cavity.

Split tolerance. State in which one form of immune response (e.g., antibody) to an antigen is active, while another form (delayed hypersensitivity) is not active.

Staphylococcal protein A. Protein extracted from staphylococci that binds the Fc of most immunoglobulins and is mitogenic for some lymphocytes.

Stem cell. A multipotential precursor cell that may give rise to different functionally and phenotypically differentiated cell types.

Sulzberger–Chase phenomenon. Abrogation of delayed hypersensitivity to simple chemicals by oral feeding.

Suppressor cells. A subset of cells that suppress immune responses; usually a T cell subpopulation, but other cell types may also suppress.

Suppressor factors. Substances produced by suppressor cells that down-regulate immune responses.

Switch region. Segment of amino acids at the junction of variable and constant regions of H or L Ig chains coded for by D and J genes.

Syngeneic. Used to describe the relationship between genetically identical individuals of the same species (e.g., identical twins, inbred strains of mice).

T1–T12. Designations for T cell developmental phenotypes detected by monoclonal antibodies (obsolete terms; see Appendix).

T cell domains. Zones of lymphoid organs predominantly occupied by T cells.

T lymphocyte (T cell). A thymus-derived lymphocyte.

TAC. Transferrin receptor on activated lymphocytes detected by monoclonal antibodies.

Terminal deoxynucleotidyl transferase (TdT). An enzyme found in immature lymphocytes, but not in mature lymphocytes. Also found in leukemias and lymphoma cells.

Thy (θ). Antigens present on mouse thymocytes and most mouse T cells.

Thy 1+ dendritic cells. Intraepithelial cells in mouse epidermis of T cell lineage. Human equivalent not yet identified.

Thrombocytopenia. A condition of bleeding caused by low numbers of platelets in the blood.

Thymectomy. Removal of the thymus.

Thymic hormones. Substances produced by thymic epithelium that induce differentiation of thymocytes.

Thymic nurse cells. Large epithelial cells in thymus believed to effect maturation of thymic lymphocytes.

Thymocytes. Lymphocytes in the thymus.

Thymopoietin (thymin). A thymic hormone of MW 7000.

Thymosin. A thymic hormone of MW 12,000.

Thymus. A central lymphoid organ that is the site of differentiation of T cells.

Thymus-dependent antigens. Immunogens that require T cell cooperation to induce an antibody response.

Thymus-dependent areas (TDA). Zones of lymphoid organs that do not develop in neonatally thymectomized animals; zones that contain a high proportion of T cells in lymphoid organs of normal animals.

Thymus-independent antigens. Immunogens that do not require T cell cooperation for induction of antibody formation.

Tingible bodies. Macrophages containing phagocytosed debris found in lymphoid organs, particularly in areas of the dome of the appendix and in germinal centers of lymph nodes, tonsils, and spleen.

Tissue-fixed macrophages. See *histiocytes.*

TL (thymic–leukemia antigen). A membrane antigen, found on thymocytes of TL^+ mice, that is lost during maturation of T cells but reappears in leukemia.

Tolerance. Active state of unresponsiveness to a given immunogen while immune responses to other immunogens are normal.

Tolerogen. An antigen that induces tolerance.

Tonsils. Gastrointestinal lymphoid organs located at the junction of the oral cavity and the pharynx.

Toxin. A substance that produces deleterious effects.

Toxoids. Altered forms of toxins that are immunogenic but not toxic.

Transfer factor. A dialyzable extract of immune lymphocytes that is capable of adoptively transferring to nonsensitized humans delayed hypersensitivity to a specific antigen (e.g., tuberculin).

Transudation. Passage of fluid, electrolytes, and low-molecular-weight proteins from intravascular to extravascular tissue during mild or early inflammation.

TSF. T suppressor factor.

Tuberculin hypersensitivity. Delayed hypersensitivity to tuberculin.

Tumor-specific antigen (TSA). An antigen found on cancer cells, but not on normal cells. TSAs have been demonstrated in mice by transplantation rejection *(tumor-specific transplantation rejection).* Such antigens have not been convincingly demonstrated in man.

Type I reactions. Synonymous with *anaphylactic reactions.*

Type II reactions. Synonymous with *cytotoxic reactions.*

Type III reactions. Synonymous with *immune complex reactions.*

Type IV reactions. Synonymous with *delayed hypersensitivity reactions.*

Ubiquitin. A polypeptide of MW 8451 found in many organisms that induces both T and B cell differention and is related to the lymphocyte homing receptor on high endothelial venules.

Uremia. Condition of renal failure due to chronic renal disease with increased uric acid in the blood.

V region. Variable region of N-terminal portion of immunoglobulin H and L chains.

Vaccination. Immunization for prevention of infectious diseases; originally used for administration of vaccinia virus to induce immunity to smallpox.

Valency of antibody. The number of epitopes with which one antibody can combine. The valency of most antibodies is 2. IgM may have a valency up to 10; IgA has different valencies depending on degree of polymerization.

van der Waals force. A weak force of attraction between all molecules that is active only over very short distances.

Variable region. See *V region.*

Variolation. Intentional immunization with unmodified smallpox (variola) virus.

Vasoactive intestinal polypeptide. A 28-amino-acid polypeptide present in mast cells, neutrophils, and nerves that induces vasodilation and potentiates edema produced by bradykinin and C5a des-Arg.

Vasoconstriction. Contraction of precapillary arterioles, leading to decreased blood flow.

Vasodilation. Dilation of precapillary arterioles, leading to increased blood flow through capillaries.

Viral interference. State of resistance to infection by one virus in cells already infected by another virus.

Waldeyer's ring. Lymphoid tissue of tonsils and adenoids located around junction of pharynx and oral cavity.

Wasting disease (runt disease). A chronic fatal illness associated with weight loss and lymphoid atrophy in (1) neonatally thymectomized mice, (2) late stages of a graft vs. host reaction, (3) immune deficiency diseases, including AIDS.

Weil–Felix reaction. Diagnostic test: agglutination of *Proteus* X bacteria by the sera of patients with typhus.

Western blot. Localization of antigens present in nitrocellulose paper using labeled antibodies after transfer of antigens from separation media.

Wheal and flare. A skin reaction due to histamine release initiated by trauma or cutaneous anaphylaxis, characterized by central raised edema (wheal) surrounded by a rim of erythema (flare).

White blood cells. Polymorphonuclear leukocytes, lymphocytes, and monocytes in peripheral blood.

White pulp. Areas of splenic parenchyma surrounding penicilli arterioles containing high numbers of lymphocytes.

Widal reaction. Bacterial agglutination (by antibody) reaction used in diagnosis of enteric infections by *Salmonella*.

Xenogeneic. Denotes a relationship between two members of different species.

Xenograft. A tissue or organ graft between members of two different species.

Zymosan. Preparation of cell wall of yeast that can activate the alternative pathway of complement.

Index

(For quick definition of terms, see Glossary.)